Classic — Keep

Public Health Nursing Practice

SECOND EDITION

RUTH B. FREEMAN, R.N., Ed.D.

Associate Professor of Public Health Administration
The Johns Hopkins University
School of Hygiene and Public Health

W. B. Saunders Company

Philadelphia   1957   London

Library of Congress Catalog Card Number: 57–11272

Foreword

RUTH FREEMAN's contribution to public health is widely known through her field service, her teaching and her previous writing.

This book on public health nursing will be acclaimed by students, by workers on the job, by administrators and supervisors and by educators in public health nursing. It should find a substantial audience in those schools of medicine and of nursing where the concepts of preventive medicine and public health are the motivations in education. It will provide a much-needed text for students in social work whose work with families will be closely related to that of public health nurses and also in schools of public health preparing the several specialists who now form the team for a comprehensive community health program. The multiplication of specialists in a field where the public health nurse has become established as the general family worker makes mutual understanding of each role respectively an imperative need, to whose understanding this book will contribute.

Gradually over the years there has been brought about a change in the meaning of health service which in turn has brought about a change in the meaning of nursing. Prevention of disease and promotion of health are fast becoming the keynotes in the medical world. Striking progress has been made in the design to make health services available to the people who need them. Public health facilities have been expanding in scope; voluntary health insurance has increased sharply, and an encouraging degree of unselfish inter-professional and inter-agency cooperation is being demonstrated. It is not unrealistic to believe that the next decade will bring us more nearly to the point where all the forces of clinical and preventive medicine, mental hygiene and public health and welfare will have become coordinate services considered essential to maintain healthy family life in a highly complex society.

iii

In the light of these developments the public health nurse in particular symbolizes the new concepts, for it is she who has become the coordinating link between the individual or family in need of health service and the community health facility with a service to offer. The role of the hospital nurse in the field of prevention is gradually emerging but needs clearer definition against the background of changing medical practice which itself has not as yet bridged the gap between the traditional pattern of practice and the newer concept of preventive medicine and public health.

Miss Freeman's discussion proceeds in logical sequence to explain in interesting and practical fashion the work and methods of public health nursing and she gives a comprehensive idea of the potentialities of an evolving order of nursing in the expanding medical and health care service for the nation. Her book is a timely addition to the public health literature.

MARION W. SHEAHAN

Preface

Since publication of the first edition of this work, many changes have occurred that profoundly affect the direction and emphasis of public health nursing. The burgeoning public and scientific interest in long-term illness, and particularly in mental illness, have precipitated an aggressive treatment program that seems bound to involve community agencies in extensive home care of the sick. The searching studies of nursing functions and of nursing services undertaken by the nursing associations and by governmental agencies give new dimensions to the potential force of nursing and rouse deepened concern with the process of nursing. Group experience is taking its place as one of the methods of providing nursing service, and offers vast new opportunities.

While the basic philosophy underlying public health nursing has not changed, the content of this book has been completely reorganized and extensively rewritten to bring it into alignment with these new developments. The material has been organized around the recent official statement of functions of public health nursing issued by the American Nurses' Association. A new chapter has been added on definition and process, and those aspects of the work that deal with direct care of patients and their families have been more fully considered. Counseling and group work have been given greater emphasis.

Again it is necessary to acknowledge the generous assistance of many individuals who have helped to clarify ideas, to locate materials, and to review parts of the manuscript. In particular I would like to express appreciation to Pearl McIver who provided much background material and helpful advice, to Marian Sheahan for valuable suggestions and constant encouragement, and to Janice Mickey, Vera Fry and Martha Rogers who discussed and argued about the ideas included.

Thanks are also due to Miss Marie Barile and Mrs. Grace Beveridge who helped with the preparation of the manuscript, and to Anselm Fisher who assisted in innumerable ways throughout.

RUTH FREEMAN

Washington, D.C.
August, 1957

Contents

The Pattern of
Public Health Nursing

CHAPTER I

The Emerging Pattern of Public Health Nursing

Public health nursing, like any other public service, grows out of the socio-economic and the cultural patterns of the world in which it functions. In the world of Phoebe and her associates, dominated by compelling religious values and characterized by appalling lack of provision for the multitude of the sick and poor, nursing became quite naturally an outlet for devoted religious expression. The settlement houses and visiting nursing of Rathbone's and Lillian Wald's day grew naturally out of the crowding, poverty, disease and filth that characterized the burgeoning populations of London, New York and Chicago, and the struggle to adjust to the transition from hand to machine production.

Public health nursing in the latter twentieth century must adapt itself to a different world—to automatization, to rapid cultural change, to the stresses of cold war, to family mobility and suburbanization. It must take advantage of the benefits of fabulously rapid scientific discovery in the midst of a new appreciation of the practical as well as ethical values of the old-fashioned virtues of love and family solidarity and self-determination.

The forces that are molding public health nursing today vary greatly among different countries. The chapters which follow will be concerned primarily with the process and problems of providing public health nursing in a technically advanced, economically favored situation with well-developed health and social services. In this setting, public health practice will be affected by the pressures and changes in the socio-technical-economic environment; the psycho-cultural environment; and in the medical-nursing-public health environment.

THE SOCIO-ECONOMIC ENVIRONMENT

Never has the pace of discovery and change been as rapid as it is today. Planes that can cross our largest oceans give way to ones which can travel faster than sound and have much greater range; machines that relieved the worker from the grinding physical aspects of production are being replaced by those which can remember and think, grade and assemble, carry on many steps in a process independently of the men who run them—and become obsolete with dizzying rapidity; countries and communities change in size, importance and configuration in a matter of weeks with the development of huge hydroelectric plants, the exploitation of needed natural products such as uranium, tin or oil, or the mass production of houses in a suburban development.

Large Unit Group-Controlled Production.   In the early days of the industrial revolution, production units were relatively small and the employer and his men represented an independent group. Disagreements, while often violent, were essentially personal and local.

This situation has given way to one in which ownership is in the hands of diffuse stockholders rather than individuals, and control is vested in "boards" rather than a single person; units of production embrace thousands of workers and may be international in coverage; a middle group called "management" comes between worker and owner.

Agriculture as well as industry reflects this change to large unit production. The recently coined word "agribusiness" describes a pattern in which farming is combined with freezing or other processing and packaging of foods; the high costs of efficient farm equipment are producing new distinctions between the farm owner and farm laborer; farmers' cooperatives are bringing the force of size to bear in the production and bargaining aspects of agriculture.

Such large unit organization brings with it questions of relative liability of the individual, of industry and of government for health action and responsibility. It is difficult to maintain a philosophy of personal and individual responsibility when a man's ability to earn his livelihood depends not on his own competence and industry, but upon the maintenance of a given technological pattern that requires his skill, and upon the caprice of public demand for the goods he helps produce; when his right to work may be defeated by failure in a remote situation over which neither he nor his employer has control, as when an automobile plant in Detroit must close because there is a miners' strike in Pennsylvania, or a housing construction job in Illinois must be postponed because of failure to recruit lumberjacks in Oregon. Many questions arise as to who carries responsibility. For example, to what extent should industry be expected to provide special diagnostic services such as periodic x-ray examination of the chest; should public or voluntary agencies or industry foot the bill for home care of the sick; whose is the primary responsibility for the housing of migratory workers or usual health facilities when a temporary sharp expansion of production outruns the existing facilities?

Labor and its agricultural counterpart are taking action largely through group rather than individual expression, and are playing an increasingly important and responsible part in production, and in social and political action including health action.[1]

This dependence upon group rather than individual action for furtherance of one's welfare has a significant effect on health needs and health service. An individual's capacity to work with and through groups with discrimination and satisfaction is intimately related to his emotional health.[2] It poses particular problems for the individual whose competence and personality lead him to work in isolation—perhaps far ahead of his group—and whose capacity for effective social contribution may require him to be "different."

Automatization, too, will bring problems as well as benefits. Upgrading for workers may be accompanied by anxieties growing out of decreasing manpower needs and by personal insecurity growing out of rapid obsolescence of processes or trade skills.

Organized groups may also have a profound effect upon the way in which health care is provided. The American Medical Association and the American Federation of Labor–Congress of Industrial Organizations, for example, are both energetically

1. *Social Work Yearbook, 1954.* New York, American Association of Social Workers, 1954, pp. 305–308.

2. Fromm, Erich, *The Sane Society*, Chapter 5, "Man in Capitalistic Society." New York, Rinehart & Co., 1955.

studying and acting with considerable effect on matters relating to tax-supported health services.

High Standard of Living.   On the whole, a favorable economy has produced a relatively high level of income and standard of living. This has had the effect of diminishing some health problems such as malnutrition due to underfeeding and family stress arising from unemployment. At the same time, because it produces people who want more things, there may be danger of anxiety and stress due to striving for better levels of living. It produces a society that has high demands for health care—especially for care of overt illness. Koos[3] has shown that the use of medical services goes up as income goes up. There is also a high potential for purchasing the care demanded.

Increasing Mobility of the Population.   Industrial shifts, a favorable labor market and the broadened knowledge of different localities growing out of greatly expanded opportunities for travel and communication have resulted in much shifting of population; groups of employees of a New England cotton mill may move south as the company relocates; a New York City resident stationed on the west coast for military service may decide to return there to live. Shifting is international as well as intranational, stimulated by the search for a more acceptable political climate or more favorable economic situation.

Such mobility makes many demands on health services, and necessitates fast expansion or contraction of services. New population groups may bring new types of health problems; the introduction of different cultural patterns may create tensions and strain; people must learn to adapt to new environmental conditions.

Suburbanization.   The trend toward suburbanization seems to characterize most large urban areas.[4] In this search for a better place for living and especially for child rearing, a distortion in the usual age and class distribution occurs in the community.[5] The suburban community tends to have a high degree of uniformity—people are essentially of the same age, the same income, and often with a fast-growing population of young children. Large unit production methods also result in a very rapid increase in population, that produces very real problems of expansion of

3. Koos, Earl, *The Health of Regionville.* New York, Columbia University Press, 1954.

4. Woodbury, Coleman, Suburbanization and Suburbia. *American Journal of Public Health,* 45: 1–9, January, 1955.

5. Ibid.

health services in the suburban area. At the same time the urban center may find itself burdened with a disproportionate number of low income, low tax potential, families, while suburbanites continue to use the city's expensive medical facilities.

Retirement communities are another modern phenomenon—sometimes large mass constructed units built for the express purpose of housing retired workers and their families; sometimes simply an accretion of older people attracted by a favorable climate or low living costs. Here, too, there is a skewed age distribution and a population with specialized needs for health care.

Broad and Increasingly Comprehensive Social Planning. In many countries of the world, social planning is being substituted for the vagaries of chance in protecting the individual from the major calamities of life. This may take the form of government-controlled service to individuals, guaranteeing to the individual certain basic necessities of life, or of a widespread application of the insurance principle to provide for care when it is needed. The Social Security Laws of 1935 and their subsequent amendments, with their broad provisions for old age assistance and insurance, unemployment benefits, special programs in public health and welfare, mother and baby care and care of the crippled and blind, express the concern of the government for protection of the individual from the hazards and vicissitudes from which he cannot protect himself.[6] These laws were significantly amended in 1939 and again in 1956; in each instance the amendments broadened and extended the scope of the care given. While there is no provision for health insurance or medical care in the Social Security Laws, separate legislation has been introduced in several forms, and it seems likely that some degree of protection against the economic burden of illness will eventually be included in national legislation.

The Hospital Survey and Construction Act of 1946 similarly expressed the intent of this country to assist its less privileged communities in maintaining suitable basic health facilities.[7]

While there is some concern as to ways in which such planning can be carried forward without the loss of personal and group freedom, governmental planning on a broad scale is accepted as inevitable by most people. The concept of social planning has

6. *Compilation of Social Security Laws, as amended.* Washington, D.C., Government Printing Office, 1956.

7. A Decade of Hill-Burton Hospital Funds. *American Journal of Public Health,* 46: 1576–1577, December, 1956.

broadened to international scope. The World Health Organization, an affiliated agency of the United Nations, provides a medium for mutual study, action and assistance. The International Cooperation Agency of the United States, which carries forward an extensive program of bilateral economic aid, including assistance with health problems designed to promote self-help in the country assisted, has its counterpart in many other countries. The increasing number and long-range programs of international professional organizations—the International Council of Nurses, the World Medical Association, the World Federation for Mental Health to mention only a few—give further evidence of concern with global planning.

Military Preparedness and the "Cold War."   The uneasy peace which seems likely to continue in the world for some time also has its effect on health services. Military experience affects the pattern of family life. Homemaking and family planning, as well as career planning, must be based on military obligations and demands and on what may seem an uncertain future. Young expectant mothers may be far from home and the usual sources of emotional support, or far from their husbands. On the positive side, many young men learn much of health care through the military medical program, and their dependents may enjoy and learn to expect an unprecedented amount of medical service.

To meet the uncertainties and fears which may be generated by recurring crises, by reports of the fantastically destructive new weapons, the individual needs emotional as well as physical stamina. The assurance of security and affection in childhood under such conditions may assume an importance equal to that of assuring immunization against preventable communicable diseases.

SOCIAL-CULTURAL MODIFICANTS

There is increasing recognition that patterns of culture and value systems make a vast difference in the kind of health services people need and want. The Philippine woman, for example, is apt to welcome pregnancy with a sense of satisfaction and achievement. Friends and neighbors admire and congratulate her, and the family adjusts itself easily to the new member. The American suburbanite, on the other hand, may feel quite differently about an unexpected pregnancy. It may represent another drain on a strained budget, another individual who must have a room of his own, music lessons, college, and braces on his teeth—"necessities" which in this setting good parents are expected to provide for their children. Several cultural factors may be identified as of particular importance to health care and hence to public health nursing.

The American Way of Life.   What Allen has called the "All-American Standard" represents a social environment in which differences between the haves and havenots are lessening, in which there is great mobility within the class structure and in which expectations of the population in relation to the comforts of life are high.[8] This places a premium on health and a high value on education as a prerequisite for success. It makes health care a potential "best seller." It keeps a large proportion of young people in schools for a longer time than is usual in many other countries, thus providing an unusually effective channel for health instruction. It brings the possibility of self-development and recreation to people in an unprecedented degree. At the same time, the striving and competitive nature of much of man's work life may produce anxiety, stress and the pressures of overwork. It undoubtedly increases the difficulty of adjusting to aging and retirement.

Sub Groups.   America is characterized by great heterogeneity of population and the existence of many groups which retain unique cultural patterns. Racial and social class groups, for example, have been shown by Davis to have quite different approaches to child rearing.[9] Socio-economic status may also divide communities into different groups, each with different concepts of health and health care. Koos, in describing the problem of reporting of illness, points out that persistent backache, considered by the higher socio-economic groups to be an illness, may be accepted by the less privileged as a natural and normal condition.[10] Nationality groups may retain folk medicine practices or patterns of distribution of responsibility and authority within the family that have a definite bearing on health needs or services.

Furthermore, the individual may be caught between two strong cultural forces and find himself in revolt against one to which he feels some allegiance. The high school boy may want to conform to the culture of his family group which is one of religiously dominated studiousness and relative disregard of material things,

---

8. Allen, Frederick Lewis, *The Big Change,* Chapter 15, "The All-American Standard." New York, Harper & Bros., 1952.

9. Davis, Allison, *Father of the Man.* Boston, Houghton Mifflin Co., 1947.

10. Koos, Earl, *Health of Regionville.* New York, Columbia University Press, 1954, p. 33.

while the values of his school group are quite differently weighted. Families, too, may be in revolt, striving to move upward to a group which they feel has more status, and ultimately finding that they are not at home in either the original group or the new one.

Since cultural factors will affect how a family feels about illness or preventive care and what they are willing to do about it, public health nursing must be so organized that it can adapt to this multiplicity of patterns.

Changing Family and Community Structure.   Much has been said and written about the decline of the kinship-rooted family. Mobility within family groups, centering of populations around large industrial and commercial centers, and the decreasing size of houses and households have made the two-generation single-family household much more common than the one including a variety of grandparents, aunts, uncles and servants. Increasing recognition of the rights of individuals to be themselves has made the psychologically "desirable" family an inter-dependent group of individuals rather than a single unit disciplined and molded firmly by its composite character—a pattern which some feel will actually strengthen the family's place in a democratic society.[11]

This pattern creates many difficulties as the numbers of chronically ill persons increase. It is not too much of a problem to have an aged, bedridden, sometimes mentally confused oldster if there are many family members to help with care, friendly neighbors who are concerned and helpful, and plenty of room in the home to permit other family members to carry on their usual activities. In the "efficiency" home where space is at a premium, where the mother has major responsibility for the household chores, with intermittent household help, and where the "open" plan makes it impossible to separate the activities of the sickroom and those of a social nature effectively, it may produce an intolerable family situation.

The neighborhood or small town with its stable population and face-to-face relationships and clear and generally accepted values and ways of doing things is also declining in influence. However, a new kind of determinant is arising from the grouping of people in housing projects and in suburban developments which may be expected to have much influence on patterns of living and on health problems. Certain conditions of living may be imposed, either by actual regulation or by community pressure—perhaps

11. Wilensky, H., Changing Patterns of Family Life. *Children*, 3: 163, 1956.

lawns must be kept mowed and free of dandelions, or bedclothes must not be aired from the window, or participation in civic or social activities must be undertaken to avoid being considered a "poor citizen." Planning may deliberately promote neighborly or group activities—washing machines grouped in a basement which promote conversation while the clothes "do"; play porches for rainy-day children's activities serving several families which bring parents together while the children play; community houses; and, of course, the supermarket! Even in rural areas the accessibility of towns and the availability of communication via

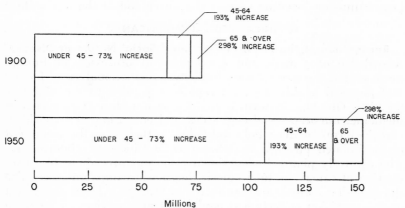

OUR   POPULATION   IS   AGING

Figure 1.   Our population is aging.

the radio and television, as well as dependence on mechanical equipment rather than individual human effort, have made isolation and self-sufficiency rare.

Shifts in Composition of the Population.   The total population of the United States is growing, and it is estimated that the 1954 population of 162,000,000 will be increased to about 190,000,000 in 1965.

The population of the United States is growing older, owing in large measure to effects of intensive health conservation measures and to limitation of immigration, as shown in Figure 1. In 1954 the proportion of the population over sixty-five years of age was over 8 percent as compared to 4.1 percent in 1900.[12]

12. *Some Facts about Our Aging Population.* Washington, D.C., Federal Security Agency, 1955, p. 1.

The illness problems and health guidance of the older age group bring problems not only to the patient, but also to those who care for him. The effect of severe chronic illness on the family of the patient has never been accurately assessed—the fears of the adolescent who sees her grandmother dying of cancer and ignorantly relates it to childbearing; the desperation of the dutiful daughter caught in the trap of seemingly unending care, the budgetary adjustments that may substitute dressings or a wheel chair for the elderly patient for needed dentistry, elective surgery, or educational preparation for some other member of the family.

There are also changes arising from changes in the birth rate which mounted from 20.4 in 1945 to 25.3 in 1954, producing larger numbers needing care at the lower end of the age scale.[13]

TECHNICAL-MEDICAL MODIFICANTS

Recognition of the Physical-Emotional-Social Nature of Disease. Knowledge of growth and developmental processes, of human needs and of the interrelationship between emotional social factors and physical health has been rapidly expanded in the past few decades. This has, in turn, brought a socio-technical approach in medicine, nursing, social case work and education that considers care in terms of the whole individual rather than the treatment of an isolated physical manifestation of illness or abnormality. The carefully planned educational programs preceding the introduction of cancer or tuberculosis diagnostic campaigns recognize the fact that control of ignorance and fear may be as important as the provision of technical equipment and services in securing early diagnosis and treatment. Hilleboe says: "The social and economic problems of elderly people, who have a variety of chronic diseases, are as demanding of considered judgment and practical solution as are the vagaries and enigmas of the diseases themselves."[14]

This has led to a deepening of approach on the part of practitioners in all fields of health care. The physician is giving more thought to environmental factors as the causative or modifying factors in care and is involving the patient and family more in decisions and methods of care; the nurse is realizing that simple ministration services may have great psychologic import and

13. *School Nursing Services.* New York, National League for Nursing, 1956, pp. 1, 21.

14. Hilleboe, Herman, M.D., Speech presented at 25th Anniversary of Columbia-Presbyterian Medical Center, New York City, October 12, 1953.

potential for care; social workers have long used the findings of psychiatry to help in social appraisal, motivation and training of practitioners; pediatricians are concerned as much with how parents feel toward their children as they are with what they feed them.

"Care of the whole patient," "consideration of the entire patient-family-community complex" and "comprehensive patient care" appear over and over in the literature of a variety of health fields.

Rapidly Expanding Care Potentials. The potential for preventing or alleviating illness has grown at an astounding rate. This may be attributed to the rapid pace of discovery, aided by public confidence and willingness to support research, and to the decreasing lag between scientific discovery and its practical application. It was several decades before the work of Semmelweis and Holmes was translated into patient care, despite its obvious applications and importance to human welfare. The Salk vaccine was made available to the public through concerted voluntary and governmental efforts within months after it was found to be potent and safe. The development of health surgery, of the use of tranquilizing drugs for mental illness, and of chemotherapy for tuberculosis has similarly spread with phenomenal speed throughout the country, aided by training programs, communications through organized professional groups, television demonstrations and a host of other distributive measures.

This vigorous pushing back of the frontiers of knowledge makes possible an aggressive and concerted attack on diseases formerly felt to be hopeless or amenable only to palliative treatment. What Scheele calls "wide-spectrum" health services—attempts not only to control communicable disease and environmental hazards, but to tackle such problems as the psychologic and physical precursors of accidents, more intensive preventive and treatment measures for mental disease and other chronic conditions—place a new dimension on public health service, and emphasize the constantly broadening area of possible control.[15]

Expanding knowledge in related fields also provides greater opportunities. In the behavioral sciences, new study techniques are making it possible to predict more accurately the effects of various conditions that surround learning or behavior.[16] The

15. Scheele, Leonard, The Wide Spectrum of Our Health Services. *Public Health Reports*, 71: 26–33, January, 1956.

16. Homans, G. C., *The Human Group*. New York, Harcourt, Brace and Co., 1950.

effects of group action open up new avenues for health services—
working with problems in groups produces a result different from
working in a one-to-one relationship since the force and strength
within the group itself may be brought to bear on the problem.[17]
Foster demonstrated that the skills of the anthropologist may provide a valuable approach to the evaluation of health programs.[18]

New tools are constantly being provided for influencing behavior toward health and for developing and safeguarding personality through health service and for predicting what people
are liable to do under given circumstances, and what they will
accept and under what conditions.

New problems, of course, continue to appear and to require new
methods—problems of air pollution, of stress and the use or alle-
viation of its effects, identification and control of industrial
hazards associated with new processes, to mention only a few.[19]
Problems tend to be attacked intensively and promptly and with
constantly growing public concern and support.

Team Approach to Care.   Growing out of the recognition of
the physical-emotional-social basis of disease and the rapid
changes and increasing complexity of treatment is the need for a
variety of professional skills in the treatment of health problems.
The traditional pattern of the physician and nurse team is giving
way to a treatment or preventive team that includes social workers, physical therapists, anthropologists, medical specialists, health
educators, nutritionists and a host of others. Most important of all
is the recognition that in today's health problems the patient,
family and community must be considered as full-fledged members of the team also. Home care for a psychiatric patient, for
instance, may be helped or hindered by the attitudes and knowledge of his family and his neighbors. "Conditioning" of the neighborhood group through community educational measures as well
as education of the family may be necessary to ensure understanding and support for the returning patient.

Full use of all the skills included in the treatment team will
affect the outcome of patient care. For example, in a school-age

17. Chase, S., *Roads to Agreement*, New York, Harper & Brothers, 1951; K.
Lewin, Dynamics of Group Action, *Ed. Leadership*, 1: 195–200, 1944.

18. Foster, George (ed.), *A Cross Cultural Anthropological Analysis of a
Technical Aid Program*. Washington, D.C., Smithsonian Institution, 1951.

19. Williams, Huntington, and Sir Allen Dailey, Public Health Practice, An
Ounce of Prevention Is Worth a Pound of Cure. *Baltimore Health News*, 33:
41–59, June-July, 1956.

child with rheumatic fever, the physician diagnoses, prescribes and supervises care. But he must recognize the contribution of the public health nurse in the school and community in helping the child to live comfortably with his condition, and in instructing and counseling the family; the nurse in the school must recognize how the teacher's attitude and intimate knowledge of the child can help keep the child properly identified with his class group and find physical changes early; parental skills must be used by professional workers to implement the over-all plan for care.

In a treatment team characterized by mutual respect and understanding of one another's functions there will be shifts in leadership. When the problem is primarily one of health counseling the physician may defer to the skill of the nurse; when it is one of evaluation and prognosis the physician will take the leadership; if deep-seated family problems are interfering with care, the social worker may assume major responsibility for some phases of the care. Often the functions of different members of the team will overlap.

Trust and understanding among the team members themselves, as well as careful planning and coordination, are essential for full and intelligent use of all of the skills needed for care.

Increasing Professionalism of Nursing. Francis Brown has advanced the notion that the measure of professional status lies in the potential impact of the particular profession on society.[20] By force of numbers, coupled with public affection and confidence in nursing, nurses may be assumed to have a very real impact on the lives of a large segment of the population. Continuing study and deepening of nursing functions, improvement of schools of nursing and increasing recognition of the nurse's role in therapy and in education have resulted in great advances in professional status and capacity.

The tradition of self-study by the profession with full use of related professions in conducting the research has been described by Roberts, and is exemplified in the Brown Report.[21, 22]

A series of researches on nursing functions is currently being

20. From address given to Graduate Nurses' Association, Washington, D.C., 1956.

21. Roberts, Mary, *American Nursing,* Chapter 15, "Fact Finding Studies of Nursing and Nursing Education." New York, Macmillan Co.

22. Brown, Esther L., *Nursing for the Future.* New York, Russell Sage Foundation, 1948.

sponsored by the American Nurses' Association.[23] Nursing Research, a periodical developed specifically to report on studies and study methods in nursing practice and service, was first published in 1951. The Public Health Service, the Veterans Administration and military services have developed new methods in analysis of service components, needs and estimation of outcomes of nursing service which have been reported and proved useful in other situations. Recent federal legislation specifically supports nursing research efforts, and during the fiscal year 1955–56 nearly $500,-000 was awarded by the Public Health Service to qualified researchers for projects in nursing.[24]

From these many and varied approaches there has come a new concept of the depth and impact-potential of nursing.

Increasing Proportion of Students in Collegiate Programs. Nursing, unlike other professions, relies primarily upon service institutions rather than academic institutions for the basic preparation of its practitioners. In 1955, students enrolled in hospital "diploma programs" constituted 86 percent of the total enrollment in schools of nursing.[25] However, although degree students for 1955 constituted only 14 percent of the total enrollment, this must be compared with the less than 6 percent enrolled in degree programs in 1946.[26] While the proportion is still low, the trend seems to be definitely and sharply upward.

Increasing Recognition of Nursing.   Less easy of documentation, but quite apparent, is the trend toward increasing recognition of nursing in health planning and action. Community support of nursing surveys, nursing membership on local and national planning and action bodies, and the important place allotted to nursing in the development of new programs such as that of home care are indications of increasing professional stature and recognition.

Public health nursing operates in a milieu characterized by rapid technical and social change, and by increasing interdependence among social, technical and professional activities. The people with whom the nurse will work are beset by many threatening experiences despite an unprecedented prosperity, an abun-

23. *Nurses Invest in Patient Care.* New York, American Nurses' Association, 1955.

24. *Nursing Research,* 5: 86, October, 1956.

25. *Facts About Nursing,* 1955–56 Edition. New York, American Nurses' Association, 1956, p. 76.

26. Ibid. p. 75.

dance of material benefits, and an increasing life span. Increasing professionalization of nursing is broadening the potential contribution of nursing to health and welfare efforts designed to protect the individual from adverse conditions that are outside his control. These conditions set the stage for a professional service that is challenging, creative and demanding.

CHAPTER II

Present Pattern of
Public Health
Nursing

Pᴜʙʟɪᴄ ʜᴇᴀʟᴛʜ nursing today reflects the adaptation of nursing competences to a changing society.

The pattern of public health nursing may be indicated by the numbers and distribution of nurses employed for public health work, by the types of public health nursing service afforded to the public and envisioned by nurses as desirable, and by the organizational structures through which public health nursing services are transmitted.

Numbers and Distribution. The number of nurses employed for public health work has shown a sharp upward trend from the first reported figures of 130 in 1901 to over 16,000 in 1931, with a somewhat less rapid increase after the latter date as shown in Figure 2. The number of nurses employed for public health work in the United States on January 1, 1955 was 27,112.[1] In addition, approximately 12,000 nurses were reported as employed in industry.[2]

The concentration of public health nursing service may be

1. *Census of Nurses Employed for Public Health Work* in the U.S., in the Territories of Alaska and Hawaii and in Puerto Rico, and the Virgin Islands on January 1, 1955. (Mimeo) Washington, D.C., U.S. Department of Health, Education, and Welfare, p. 3.

2. Number reported January 1, 1952, 11,096, from *Facts About Nursing,* 1955–56 Edition, p. 45.

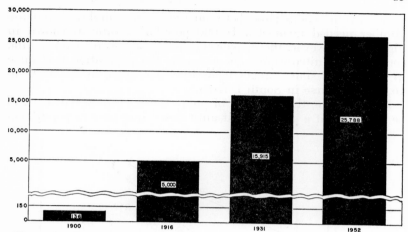

Figure 2. Total number of nurses employed in the United States. (Source: 1900 and 1916—Mary S. Gardner's Public Health Nursing; 1931—National Organization for Public Health Nursing Census; 1952—Public Health Service Census.) (From Bureau of State Services, Public Health Service, Department of Health, Education, and Welfare.)

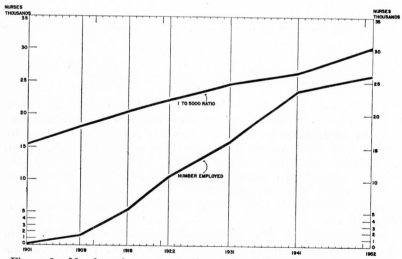

Figure 3. Number of nurses actually employed in public health compared with the number of nurses needed to reach a 1:5000 population ratio. (Source: Gardner, Mary, Public Health Nursing, 3rd Ed., p. 463; Annual Census Public Health Nursing; Division of Public Health Nursing; U.S. Public Health Service.) (From Bureau of State Services, Public Health Service, Department of Health, Education, and Welfare.)

shown by the comparison between the nurses employed and the number needed to meet a 1:5000 population ratio as shown in Figure 3. However, the distribution is by no means even. In the continental United States, for example, the population per nurse in the various states ranges from 1984 per nurse in Delaware to 16,675 per nurse in South Dakota.[3]

Furthermore, the numbers of public health nurses will need to be increased at a sharp rate if anticipated increases in population

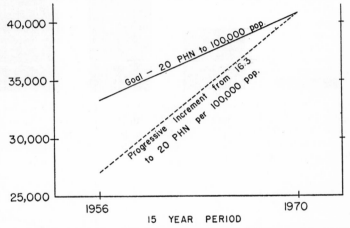

Figure 4.   Increments required between 1956 and 1970 to reach 20/100,000 ratio. (Source: National League for Nursing.)

are to be served, as shown in Figure 4. The goal of 20 public health nurses per 100,000 population is considered a minimal one.

Types of Nursing Services.   Services offered in various localities will differ greatly in pattern and scope, depending upon the facilities available, economic resources, and citizen and professional attitudes regarding services. However, some trends seem to have rather general application.

There seems to be an increasing load of noncommunicable morbidity service, and—particularly in voluntary agencies—of long-term illness service. This is clearly indicated in a recent study of 513 agencies made by the Department of Public Health Nursing of the National League for Nursing.[4] Table 1, taken from this

3. Loc. cit. p. 40.

4. *Nursing Activities of Public Health Nursing Agencies.* New York, National League for Nursing, 1955.

study, reveals that between 1943 and 1955 the percentage of home nursing visits for care of noncommunicable disease increased in the county health departments reporting from 1.4 percent to 7.9 percent; in the city health departments, from 0.7 to 5.7 percent;

Table 1. Percentage Distribution of Visits in the Home Visiting Programs of Public Health Nursing Agencies by Type of Visit and Type of Agency, 1952 and 1943*

Type of Visit	Median Percent						
	County Health Departments		City Health Departments		Nonofficial Agencies		Combination Services[a]
	1952	1943	1952	1943	1952	1943	1952
Maternity	11.2		10.2		8.1		10.8
Antepartal		6.6		2.5		4.7	
Postpartal		5.8		1.7		8.9	
Infant	14.8	15.8	19.7	11.5	10.5	17.4	13.5
Preschool	13.4	13.1	12.5	9.8	3.1	2.7	9.5
School	16.7	11.0	10.3	11.8	1.5	0.3	5.4
Adult	2.5	0.6	1.6	none	1.7	0.8	2.6
Tuberculosis	13.9	8.6	9.8	8.5	2.2	0.4	9.5
Venereal disease	b	4.0	b	1.9	b	—	b
Communicable other than TB	5.0	7.7c	4.5	11.1c	2.3	3.0c	3.9
Noncommunicable disease	7.9	1.4	5.7	0.7	68.8	48.8	36.6
Crippled children	d	1.8	d	0.1	d	0.1	d

a Not available for 1943.
b Included in communicable other than TB.
c Excludes VD data.
d Included in noncommunicable disease.

* Table prepared by Department of Public Health Nursing, National League for Nursing in *Nursing Activities of Public Health Nursing Agencies.* New York, National League for Nursing, 1955, Table 9.

and in voluntary (nonofficial) agencies, from 48 to 68.8 percent.[5] Undoubtedly much of this increase, especially in the voluntary agencies, is associated with expanding programs for home care of long-term illness. A study of the Instructive Visiting Nurse Association of Baltimore showed that long-term illness made up 19 percent of the total case load in 1954, and that another 8 percent of the load, the status of which was undetermined, consisted, in the opinion of the director, largely of long-term illness. Long-

5. Loc. cit. Table 9.

term illness accounted for a much larger proportion of visits than of cases. Although it was not possible to separate visits to long-term illness patients from those to other patients with noncommunicable illness, noncommunicable morbidity visits accounted for 60 percent of the visits in 1954.[6] The trends in relation to acute and long-term illness in this same organization are indicated in Figure 5.

The National League for Nursing report indicates that the proportion of visits in maternal and child health continues to be

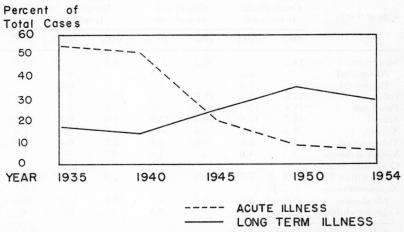

Figure 5.   Percent of long- and short-term diagnoses in case load, IVNS Baltimore, 1935–54.

high in all types of agencies. When home visits for pre- and postnatal care, to infants, and to preschool and well school children are combined, the median percent of these home visits in 1952 was 56 percent in county health departments, 53 percent in city health departments, 23 percent in voluntary agencies, and 57 percent in combination agencies. Communicable disease, including tuberculosis and venereal disease, accounted for 19 percent of home visits in county health departments, 14 percent in city health departments, 5 percent in voluntary agencies and 13 percent in combination agencies. The study also showed a re-

6. A study of the Instructive Visiting Nurse Association of Baltimore, conducted by The Johns Hopkins School of Hygiene and Public Health, June, 1955, (mimeo) p. 40.

duction in all types of agencies in communicable diseases visits other than tuberculosis, and in infant supervision in county and nonofficial agencies, but an increase in infant supervision in city health departments.[7] This might reflect greater dependence on private medical care among the clientele in the first two agencies named. In city health departments there may be a shift of responsibility from the voluntary to the official agency, or the figures may represent relatively greater needs growing out of lowered family economic capacities in the city-suburban group.

Home care programs have, of course, existed from the earliest visiting nurse days, but so-called "organized home care programs" designed to provide, for patients ill at home, *multiple* professional and supportive services ordinarily afforded only in the hospital setting came into being only during the 1940's. By 1955 there were about fifty such programs in operation, and in all instances some home nursing care is provided for those who need it.[8] The great variations and pattern of these programs are described in a recent study of eleven selected organized home care programs.[9]

The methods used in providing nursing care also influence the type of service given. There is growing interest in the use of group methods as part of the nursing program, especially in the so-called problem solving or discussion group. The National League for Nursing survey showed that 238 of the 513 agencies studied—over 40 percent—included group instruction among their activities.[10]

The distribution of time between home visiting and various types of activities to reach people in groups (clinics, group instruction, school nursing) shows sharp differences between types of agencies. In 1955, 411 agencies reported that 70.3 percent of nursing time was spent in home visiting.[11] However, this ranged from 38.8 percent in city health departments to 89.9 percent in nonofficial agencies. Clinic service took 18.4 percent of the time in city health departments and only 3.4 percent in nonofficial agencies.

7. Loc. cit. Table 9.

8. Commission on Chronic Illness, Chronic Illness in the U.S., Vol. II, *Care of the Long Term Patient*. Cambridge, Harvard University Press, 1956, pp. 63–79.

9. A Study of Selected Home Care Programs, *Public Health Monographs #447*. Washington, D.C., Government Printing Office, 1955.

10. Loc. cit. Chart 1.

11. Loc. cit. Table 3.

"Giving advice" as a means of health teaching is being replaced by "health counseling," which is a more delicate and complex skill. This will undoubtedly influence both the time per visit and the number of visits per case when health education is the major purpose of the visit.

There is also a growing tendency (a suggestion rather than a trend!) to place more emphasis and time on program evaluation and to experiment with new methods of work. Reports and records of nursing service are being markedly altered to permit easier analysis; reference to the "pilot program" appears more and more often in nursing literature, and small studies that can be done by the practitioner without special research skill are being encouraged in a growing number of agencies.

Commitment to Comprehensive Nursing. Comprehensive nursing has been defined as the provision of all necessary nursing service including bedside care, health teaching guidance and supervision of ancillary nurses such as home nurses or practical nurses.[12] The need to assure such inclusive care with the minimum of confusion is gaining more and more acceptance by public health groups. Recognition of the need for home care of the sick was expressed in the resolution passed by the American Public Health Association at its annual convention in 1942:

"Whereas the dislocation of considerable segments of the population and the dislocation of physicians, nurses and dentists emphasizes the desirability of extending nursing care to the sick in their homes, and

"Whereas the accomplishment of this objective in many areas may not be possible through coordination of all public health nursing services, including the full utilization of auxiliary services, therefore be it

"Resolved that the American Public Health Association endorse the principle that nursing care of the sick in their homes should be an integral part of a community public health nursing program."[13]

To an increasing degree such "enrichment" services as rehabilitative care and supervision, home care of patients discharged from psychiatric hospitals and counseling and supportive services to their families, and parent study groups appear in agency pro-

12. Desirable Organization of Public Health Nursing for Family Service. *Public Health Nursing*, 38: 387–389, August, 1946.

13. Resolution. *American Journal of Public Health*, 32: 1420–1421, December, 1942.

grams. Recently the medical director of a large industrial health service pointed with pride to a graph which showed that the proportion of nursing visits for "general health counseling" in relation to those for specific illness or injury was increasing.

"Depth" care, in which there is a concerted effort to work with a family intensively and with deliberative consideration of the total physical-emotional-social factors involved and in the light of individual-family-community complex, is more and more discussed in case conferences and staff meetings. Acceptance of this approach requires a different spacing of family-nurse contacts and services from the more limited service approach of the past.

Team Approach to Care. The term "team approach" has been used so freely of recent years that it has a rather hackneyed sound, but it is expressive of a concept of the broadening base of patient care. In public health nursing today, this is reflected in the increasing use of full-time or consultant personnel from other health fields in nursing services, and by greater frequency in differentiated assignment of nurses with different levels of preparation.

The Philadelphia Visiting Nurse Association, for example, includes physical therapists and a social worker as well as nurses on its staff. Clinic nurses and practical nurses are increasingly used to relieve hard-pressed public health nurses. A National League for Nursing study in 1955 revealed that 63 of 583 reporting agencies employed practical nurses on their staff and that practical nurses represented 8.2 percent of the total staff in the reporting agencies.[14] Mental health nurses, or specially prepared rehabilitation nurses, are used in some agencies for special assignments requiring preparation beyond that for generalized public health nursing.

Coordinated Inter-agency Action. The medical developments referred to in Chapter I have changed the pattern of medical care, so that most illnesses involve the services of several agencies or individuals. The man with cardiac impairment, for example, may receive nursing care in the hospital, at home and on his job, shifting from one to the other fairly frequently. This kind of situation has induced shared planning and action, not only in relation to the individual or family concerned, but also in relation to the general directions and plans for the agency as a whole. A radical change in practice in the hospital outpatient depart-

14. *Facts About Nursing,* 1955-56 Edition. New York, American Nurses' Association, 1956, p. 146.

ment, to provide for more intensive patient instruction, or a change in discharge policy involves the community nursing service. Similarly, extension of rehabilitative services in the community agency might well affect hospital discharge policy, or the hospital's outpatient service load. Development of a mutual aid service in industry which provides for more extensive health services, or the broadening of health insurance coverage to include more long-term illnesses, also affects the demands made upon community nursing services, and must be taken into account in program planning.

Coordination among nursing services within a community is secured by many devices, from routine administrative exchanges of information and referral to actual unification into a single organization with joint support. The growth of "combination agencies" in which health department and voluntary community nursing services effect some type of administrative unification has been quite rapid. From 71 agencies using 89 nurses in 1931, the number of combination agencies has increased in 1955 to 95 agencies employing 978 nurses.[15]

Several patterns of combination services have been described in a study made by the National Organization for Public Health Nursing in 1950,[16] ranging from joint direction of separately financed units, each with its own policies and responsibility-bearing bodies, to completely unified services. Unification may proceed on a contractual basis, with nursing services purchased by one agency from another, as when a city health department or industry purchases specified nursing services from a visiting nurse service rather than establish a new service or branch of service.

In other instances, coordination is achieved without combining services through a "planning umbrella" in the form of a planning council or committee embracing all agencies providing nursing care, which plans and allocates responsibility.

Increasing Public Support.   In 1912, at the inception of the town and country nursing service of the Red Cross, public health nursing was essentially an activity of voluntary associations. The

15. *Census of Nurses Employed for Public Health Work on January 1, 1955.* Washington, D.C., Public Health Service, Department of Health, Education, and Welfare, 1955.

16. National Organization for Public Health Nursing. *A Study of Combination Services in Public Health Nursing.* New York, National Organization for Public Health Nursing, 1950.

visiting nurse in urban centers was a sort of combined health and social worker, usually directing her activities toward the under-privileged segment of the population.

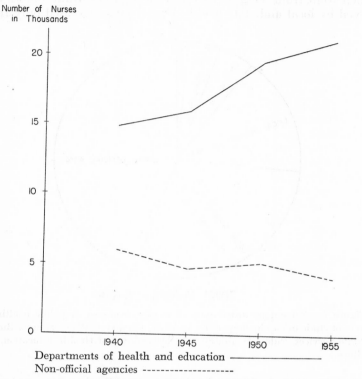

Departments of health and education ——————————
Non-official agencies --------------------

Figure 6. Nurses employed by state and local departments of health and education, and by local nonofficial agencies, 1940–1955. (Data from *Census of Nurses Employed for Public Health Work, January 1, 1955.* Public Health Service, Department of Health, Education, and Welfare. These data exclude 479 clinic nurses employed in public health agencies, and 941 employed in combination services, since both were included only in the 1955 count.)

However, as health department organization progressed, and as schools recognized their responsibility for pupil health, communities began more and more to provide basic nursing services within the official health agency and educational authority. The trend is shown in Figure 6, which indicates the changing proportion in numbers of nurses employed for local health services by health departments, school authorities, and by voluntary agencies. It must be noted, however, that much of the increase arises from increased numbers of nurses employed by Boards of Education which went from 3952 in 1940 to 7736 in 1955, while nurses employed by local and state health departments increased only from

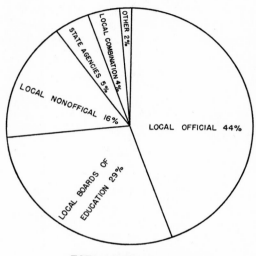

TOTAL NURSES -26,633

Figure 7. Percentage distribution of nurses employed in public health exclusive of clinic nurses by employing agencies, January 1, 1955. (Source: Bureau of State Services, Public Health Service, Department of Health, Education, and Welfare.)

10,540 in 1940 to 13,221 in 1955.[17] Distribution by employing agency is indicated in Figure 7.

The Veterans' Administration provides nursing services to its beneficiaries through its community nursing program—an extension of the home town medical care program—under contracts with local agencies. In 1956 it reported approximately 500 visiting nurse services.[18] The army health nursing service, begun in 1949 and which assists in maintaining an active preventive medi-

17. Census of Nurses Employed for Public Health Work. Washington, D.C., Public Health Service.

18. Addams, Ruth and Iva Torrens, Home Nursing Care for Veterans, *Nursing Outlook* 4: 497–499, September, 1956.

cine program for military personnel and their dependents, had grown to a staff of 86 by 1957.[19]

Modern public health nursing, then, may be characterized as functioning in a broadening sphere of influence, with a deep and comprehensive concern with the health problems of families and in a constant and complex relationship with a number of other nursing or related health and welfare services. It is increasingly governmentally sponsored and supported.

19. Personal communication, Major Elizabeth Pagels, February 14, 1957.

CHAPTER III

Public Health
Nursing: Definition
and Process

Public health nursing cannot be differentiated from other types of nursing by its functions or activities. Virtually every activity undertaken in public health work will appear in some degree in other types of nursing. It is in the emphasis and configuration of activities, and in the degree of competence that is expected in certain areas of nursing that the difference arises.

Public health nursing may be defined as a special field of nursing in which technical nursing, interpersonal and organizational skills are applied in appropriate relationship to the skills of other members of health and social professions for the conservation of community health. It includes comprehensive nursing care of individuals, families and groups and, in addition, public health measures addressed to the community as a whole, such as epidemiologic investigations, law enforcement or organization of the community for health action.

Nursing Care of Individuals and Families. Nursing care of families represents a major approach to community health conservation. A community cannot be in good health if its individual members are not healthy, and public health activities must be directed toward assuring for each individual the highest possible degree of physical, mental and social well-being. In achieving this, the efforts of the family and of private medical practice must be supplemented by community action, to do those things which the family cannot do for itself.

30

More and more, the improvement of family health depends upon individual family service rather than environmental control or mass preventive procedures, and in this type of activity the nurse is the primary purveyor of health services.

Nursing of patients is based on helping through "doing for" and "doing with." Kreuter defines it as ". . . . acting and interacting with the patient through physical and personal contact for his welfare, and intervening in his behalf between him and those stresses in the physical environment and in the social climate that impinge upon him."[1]

In distinction to nursing in other fields, the type and amount of care given to individuals and families must be related to community needs. The selection of those to be served, for example, must rest on the comparative impact on community health, rather than solely on the needs of the individual or family concerned. For example, a public health nurse could not serve a very small proportion of the population needing her care, providing excellent and comprehensive care for a few while ignoring the needs of others.

The unit of service in public health is apt to be the family rather than the individual. Because the locale of the service is often the home, families are involved in the immediate situation, and observation of family members and of the climate of family interaction is facilitated. Furthermore, health needs of individuals in a family are so interwoven and interdependent that consideration of the family as a unit is often the only feasible approach.

Ferguson, in analyzing the service load of the staff nurse in an urban health department, found that the average number of health problems per nursing visit was 4.02[2]; this is exclusive of the social, emotional and economic problems encountered in these visits. This would indicate that the presenting problem—or the primary reason for the visit—is seldom the only one in the family that requires nursing action.

The family case load in public health is also heavily weighted with well children and adults, and with minor or long-term illness. This gives unusual emphasis to the counseling and health supervisory phases of nursing.

1. Kreuter, Frances, "What is Good Nursing Care?" *Nursing Outlook*, 5:302–304, May, 1957.
2. Ferguson, Marion, *The Service Load of a Staff Nurse in One Official Agency*. New York, Bureau of Publications, Teachers College, Columbia University, 1945, p. 29.

Community-Focussed Services.   Communities, like individuals, have a state of health. Such things as defective housing, fearful and resistant attitudes toward acceptance and employment of the mentally handicapped, and over-restrictive patterns of parental control may characterize a community and represent a health problem. The existence of disease carriers, accident hazards, dangerous water or milk supplies, or inadequately housed and staffed nursing homes are other examples.

Like individuals, communities also have differing levels of competence to cope with their own health problems. In some communities, unwillingness of different cultural groups to work together for slum improvement may deprive individuals and families of the chance for better environment which can be secured only through group effort. Lack of knowledge or indifference to the health needs of school children may lead to inadequate school health service. Lack of organization may fritter away the efforts of a few crusaders for health, which, if channeled into organized effort, might have a real effect on public health.

Public health nursing involves the use of planning and community organization, of group and individual teaching, of epidemiologic procedures, of interpreting and helping enforce the laws and regulations the community has established for its own protection. The nurse's patient in this case is the community.

Whether directed toward family care or community action, the public health nurse works always in proper relationship with the many other individuals or agencies concerned. She may take leadership or serve in a supporting and participating capacity to other members of the health team, depending upon the situation and upon her own competence. She plans her own program and activities in relation to those of others, setting as her goal the improvement of community health through nursing practice.

PROCESS

Process in public health nursing may be considered in three general areas—use of technical and ministration skills, the use of self, and the use of group energy. In practice, all three are interwoven and inseparable, and incompetence in any one area seriously affects the others. It is only for purposes of analysis that any separation is justified. No attempt will be made to identify areas that are unique to public health nursing, since few, if any, parts of the process can be separated from the general nursing base.

Use of Technical and Ministration Skills. The technical and ministration skills of nursing are closely bound to the expectations of patients and the community in relation to nursing. To the public, the nurse is one who helps, and these tangible helping skills identify her.

The skills of ministration—the homely arts of comforting the patient, of bathing and positioning, of making medicine acceptable, of supporting a paralyzed arm in a colorful scarf instead of a bandage—are important not only in themselves, but also because they may have a profund effect on the patient's feelings of security, his willingness to get well, his determination to help himself. They communicate to the patient a sense of wanting to help.

In a recent article a patient describes the discomfort and fear she felt when nursing skills were inadequate. She writes: "I sensed the nurses were uncertain about the irrigating procedure . . . . . . I needed a nurse who had special training in the care of colostomies to give me specific instructions . . . . had I been properly instructed my rehabilitation time would have been cut considerably."[3]

Ministration skills must be applied selectively and with full comprehension of their relationship to and dependence upon related physical and emotional factors. For example, bathing a patient when he should be developing greater capacity for self-care may retard his recovery, however skillfully done. Similarly, withholding such care or delegating it to someone other than the nurse at a point when the patient needs the security and warmth such attention can give, or an environment conducive to talking out his problems will also have a negative effect, even though the patient or helper may be perfectly capable of providing the necessary physical care. Simple ministration skills may also contribute to or delay physical restoration. The application of a good knowledge of body mechanics may help to prevent deformity in long-term illness, or help to restore arm motion following mastectomy.

The application of therapeutic procedures is based on knowledge of the procedure and its purpose, and also upon manual skills that permit gentle and assured performance. The nurse must be sufficiently familiar with the effects of medication or other therapy to foresee difficulties. The patient with hemiplegia and his family

3. No One Knows I Have a Colostomy. *American Journal of Nursing*, 51: 703–704, December, 1951.

should know that some pain is inevitable with the physical therapy designed to restore motion to paralyzed limbs, and the nurse should be aware of and able to explain why this is so. The nurse supervising the tuberculosis patient taking medication at home should anticipate and prepare the patient for possible gastric distress.

Nursing also includes skills of observation. As in the physical care skills, the process of observation implies awareness of the interrelationhip of various factors observed. Observation of the infant, for example, will be related to many factors such as maternal history of syphilis or of extended or difficult labor, the possible presence of nitrates in the water supply, the competence of the mother and the temperament of the infant himself.

Health counseling is also an integral component of nursing. Ranging from the giving of information to supportive listening, health counseling involves a sensitive balancing of expert consultation, guidance and instruction adapted to the patient's physiologic state and to his needs as a human being. Through putting the knowledge and skills of nurse and family or group into a contributary relationship the resources of both are applied to solving health problems. For example, in rehabilitative care of the postmastectomy patient, the nurse's knowledge of anatomy, of the effects of exercise and of the physiologic and pain responses that may be anticipated with exercise is combined with the family's knowledge of the patient's resistance to pain, the rhythm of the family day, the values that the patient holds dear and that will have a high motivational force. If these are applied so that each can and does contribute, a satisfactory program for exercises can be developed. If the nurse presents her knowledge in a way that makes the family feel she doesn't appreciate their problem, it will not be accepted and hence cannot be put to effective use. If the family is avoided by the nurse and is therefore unable to analyze the patient's potential for self-help or to regard her tolerance for pain as a factor to be taken into account and made to work for rather than impede the therapy, the family knowledge cannot be put to work.

Use of Self.   The process of public health nursing includes the extension of the nurse's professional self toward the family in such a way as to influence favorably its capacity for health, and toward co-workers in such a way as to permit free and productive use of one another's competence for the health program. Peplau says: "nursing is a human relationship between an individual who is sick, or in need of health services, and a nurse especially educated to recognize and to respond to the need for help."[4] This extension of one's self is essentially the communication of aura of mutual confidence and trust, of valid personal example, and of recognition and strengthening of another's personal capacity.

Creating an Aura of Mutual Confidence and Trust. Whether working with a family to find a way to cope with the problem of tuberculosis or with a health officer to make budget adjustments, or with a teacher to talk about health inspection procedures, decisions are made and action taken much more easily if the atmosphere is favorable. A feeling of warmth, of relaxed confidence in one another, and of being valued contributes to one's capacity to think and act wisely or to use another's help.

The process of creating such an atmosphere is made up of many small actions growing out of the sincere conviction that people are important and likeable, and that ordinarily they genuinely desire to do the right thing for themselves and for others. Sometimes it is necessary to learn to express this feeling, for it must be recognized to be put to work.

Physical bearing may be a cogent method of communication. Sitting in a relaxed and unhurried manner while listening may be a tangible expression of interest. Looking at and listening carefully to participants in a planning conference (rather than doodling or gazing out the window!) emphasize the importance placed on the ideas presented. A confident, untroubled facial expression reassures the anxious in times of stress.

Physical contact, too, communicates. Shaking hands, cuddling an infant, or placing a hand on the shoulder of a troubled school child may give a sense of nearness—of being liked. The physical contact of giving care to a sick person has been mentioned before and is truly expressive of desire to help. Just "being with" or "thereness" may have importance—as when the patient first gives his own insulin, or after a psychiatric patient returns from the hospital. This factor, so important in nurse-patient relationships, is equally operative in professional contacts. No number of written referral forms or flyers distributed by the medical society to the family physician takes the place of stopping in at his office occasionally to ask about a patient; the inter-office memo cannot build the togetherness that comes from informal luncheon conversation or problem discussion.

4. Peplau, H., Interpersonal Relations in Nursing. New York, G. P. Putnam's Sons, 1952, pp. 5–6.

Words are, of course, a major channel of communication, and in establishing a good service climate the selection of words, the manner of speaking and the acceptability to the patient may have greater importance than the dictionary meaning. When the purpose is to establish a climate of relationship, verbal communication may be used to imply rather than state. For example, "Would you write out that recipe so I can give it to some of my other families?" may really say "I think you are a clever homemaker." Negatively to say "You really should try to nurse your baby" may really say "I don't think you love your baby enough." The use of noncommittal or "reflecting" words may give an assurance of interest without implying any judgment, and say in effect "its all right for you to be bitter or critical or fearful."

Through a subtle synthesis of physical expression and contact, of talking and listening, of using words with respect for their feeling tones as well as meaning, respect for personal worth and acceptance of the other as he is, are made clear. Through personal bearing and actions is conveyed the conviction that the individual has a right to his own values, attitudes, biases and hostilities. It is interesting that some nurses who find it easy to accept a patient's right to have values and judgments different from their own experience great difficulty in accepting physicians or social workers in the same nonjudgmental way.

Setting a Valid Personal Example.　　　Nursing has traditionally evoked in the minds of the public a picture of a helping person. Caplan describes this as a "wise sister" role—someone close and approachable, yet able to guide and help.[5]

The way in which the nurse practitioner acts has in itself significance in modifying the attitudes and behavior of others. The gentleness and warmth with which she handles the sick person or baby communicate themselves to others without words. The nurse's tolerance, consideration for others and compassion is "catching" because she exemplifies good attitudes. The school nurse talking of responsibility to protect others from infectious disease cannot be effective if she must interrupt her speech to cough and sniffle.

One of the best ways to teach the bases of behavior is to act consistently in relation to them. Accepting the hostility or over-demand of a hemiplegic with understanding rather than personal resentment will do more to promote family understanding than much formal instruction.

5. Caplan, Gerald, The Mental Hygiene Role of the Nurse in Maternal and Child Care. *Nursing Outlook*, 2: 14–19, January, 1954.

This valid example concept is important also in inter-professional activities. Nurses, as a rule, are rather sensitive to professional status, yet their personal example may actually negate the claims for greater professional recognition. The nurse who "fights for nursing" in the budget conference, rather than considers thoughtfully and objectively the total needs of the agency or department, is creating a picture of bias and sectionalism, while at the same time asking to be considered as a mature professional worker. Presenting and facing the facts in relation to nursing rather than blindly insisting upon maintenance of vaguely authenticated nursing "standards" demonstrate by example a true concern for professional achievement.

Recognizing and Strengthening the Personal Capacity of Others. The nurse's own attitudes and expectations will have much to contribute to the understanding and development of others. Through a sensitive kind of "feeling with" or "empathy" it is possible to gain greater insight into the motivations of others, and to learn more of how they see themselves. Empathy is described by Kandler and Hyde as "the capacity to put one's self in the other's place, both intellectually and emotionally, and to see things from the other person's point of view."[6]

This putting oneself in the other fellow's shoes makes it possible to sense the strength of certain spurs to action, or the threats inherent in what may seem a sensible and necessary course of action. The capacity of the individual to act or to cope with a problem becomes clearer. Furthermore, this understanding usually communicates itself to the family or patient and leads to a closeness of relationship which is conducive to effective service.

Reality Based Expectations. A writer in industrial management indicates that what a person does is greatly influenced by what is expected of him—as a worker, as a family member and as a citizen in a community.[7] The nurse's expectations in relation to families will be apt to influence them. If too little is expected, there may be no incentive to go forward. For example, if the nurse *expects* that the clinic patient will not report unless she makes a visit to remind him to come, the patient is likely to wait for the nurse's call before making any effort himself. If a patient is expected to want to work just as hard to restore motion to a paralyzed arm as he did on his job as a printer he is readier for the

6. Kandler, H. M. and R. W. Hyde, Changes in Empathy in Student Nurses during the Psychiatric Affiliation. *Nursing Research*, 2: 33, June, 1953.

7. Gardner, Burleigh, *Human Relations in Industry*. Chicago, Richard Irwin, 1947, pp. 168–169.

long, tedious and sometimes painful effort required than he otherwise would be. If county commissioners are expected to want to benefit their county residents in the best possible way, both commissioners and health personnel approach budget discussions in a cooperative rather than belligerent spirit.

Expectations in relation to performance must also be reconciled with the limits in the situation itself. The older parent with a long history of rigid patterns of living cannot be expected to· adapt readily to permissive handling of a young child any more than can the parent brought up in very poor and disorganized home and community be expected to adapt easily to necessary routines.

Accepting One's Personal and Professional "Role."   The process of nursing involves adapting, conveying and using expectations of others. Nursing requires helping others to develop. This is possible only if one's own needs and concepts of self do not get in the way. If the nurse sees herself as one who relieves suffering by selfless personal service to others, she may distort her function as a helper by her very zeal and devotion. The nurse who bathes the patient who could and should be bathing himself may do so because she gains a sense of fulfillment from "doing for," but the patient may in consequence lose precious time in his rehabilitation. Nursing practice requires working through and developing competence in others, being willing to forego assertion of one's own values above those of others, or the easy satisfaction which arises from letting others become overdependent. Acceptance of one's professional self also means appreciating at its true value the contribution nursing might make, and feeling comfortable about putting forward suggestions based on nursing competences. The nurse who would rather teach growth and development than develop sound and deep nursing care services for children may be rejecting her professional role.

Channeling Group Energy.   In addition to the application of technical skills and personal relationships for the achievement of nursing purposes, public health nursing includes the channeling of group energy. Much of public health nursing is done with groups—families, classes of school children or school faculties, community groups, committees and conferences. Within each of these groups there is a great amount of potential helping power, which if released and channeled may have great value.

Participating in a Team Relationship.   The emergence of the health team concept of care has been commented upon previously. The responsibilities of the public health nurse as a team member are set forth with great clarity by Coulter, who points out that team action characterizes every aspect of public health nursing practice.[8]

Someone recently said that working as a team member is "more than holding hands." It involves a process of balancing one's own goals with those of others on the team, of sharing as well as differentiating functions, of accepting as well as giving help. The additive services of the physician, the nurse, the teacher, the physical therapist and the parent provided separately to the convalescent poliomyelitis patient may result in fragmented rather than comprehensive care. The nurse must understand the objectives of the physical therapy regimen, and may share in providing treatment under the supervision of the therapist and supervise the parent in carrying out procedures. The physician must understand the nurse's concern and program for protecting the parent from strain, for developing maximum independence in the patient, and helping the teacher to avoid overprotection while at the same time making necessary adjustments in school routines. Each member of the team modifies his own contribution to conform to the whole.

The process of sharing professional responsibility involves clarifying the mutuality of respect and confidence that is basic to joint effort. The social worker must know that the public health nurse understands and respects the professional skills of social work, and that sharing certain obligations toward a family such as assistance with food budgets does not mean that either is "taking over" the work of the other. A fine balance between having each worker involved give the most comprehensive possible service while at the same time maintaining professional control by each of the several disciplines included on the team is the objective. This can be achieved only when the team is so organized that it is easy to exchange information, to develop plans and clarify mutual responsibilities and philosophy of service; when each discipline can and does interpret the functions and possible contributions of its field; when the security and confidence of each discipline can be maintained without rigidity in the lines of professional responsibility.

It is important in patient care conferences to be able to make clear to others the fundamentals of the nursing care involved, to

8. Coulter, Pearl, *The Nurse in the Public Health Program*, Chapter I, "Team Relationship." New York, G. P. Putnam's Sons, 1954.

report selectively and succinctly the critical factors that will affect the action of others on the team, to avoid professional jurisdictional disputes in favor of shared activity. The team should represent a multiple partnership rather than a hierarchy—with every member a full-fledged participant, and with the leadership shifting as one or the other members represents the greater competence in the particular area of decision or action.

Group Organization.   In addition to membership and participation in team activities for health care, administrative or planning committees, and liaison relationships, public health nursing must concern itself with the organization of groups to facilitate self-help. One such activity is described by Bond in which she compares the effectiveness of lecture and of discussion group activity in which individuals were asked to make an individual decision or commitment in a group setting. In this situation, which compared matched groups of middle-income women, a significantly larger proportion of those exposed to the discussion-decision procedure sought a physical examination and established a habit of monthly self-examination of the breast than did those in the control groups.[9] To achieve the purposes of joint decision and action, group members are so selected that the individuals in it can help one another. For example, if a prenatal study group includes multiparous as well as primiparous patients, it may be expected that the experienced mother will be able to help the new one; families of bedridden chronically ill patients meeting together, sharing their experiences and perhaps their feelings may give to each a sense of not being alone, and also some very practical ideas for care. Conversely, if the composition of the group puts together people with such antagonism or conflicts of interest that they cannot work together on the problem, the benefits will not accrue. Manipulation of the conditions under which groups meet, and guidance directed toward encouraging each member to make his best contribution to the group are also essential in this process.

In such group organization the public health nurse shares responsibility with the health educator, who may in some instances organize the groups and in others provide consultant help to the nurse in her organizational efforts.

Strengthening Group Competence.   In many instances— particularly in families—the public health nurse is working with ready-made groups. With these, as well as with groups organized

9. Bond, E., *Group Discussion Decision*. Minneapolis, Minnesota, Minnesota Department of Health, 1956.

for a specific purpose, continuing help is needed to identify and strengthen the capacity of the group to work out its own problems. It may be that there is need for factual information on which to decide what is to be done. It may be that differences in cultural background make it hard for some members to "talk up" even though they have good ideas and need recognition and support to free them of their shyness. Lack of understanding—or, in groups involving different kinds of professional workers, lack of common vocabulary—may create antagonisms and hinder action. Ways must be found through social activities or guided contributions to interpret one to the other, and to facilitate working together.

The process of identifying and strengthening group competence involves analysis based on sound knowledge of individual and group behavior, support and encouragement based on knowledge of the group members and their backgrounds, and leadership based on confidence in the group's ability to think and act wisely for itself, given the necessary facts and a favorable environment.

The process of public health nursing is a complex of doing for, of doing with, and most of all of helping others to do for themselves those things which contribute to optimum health, with each step of the process integrally related to the action taken by other professional or family members contributing to the total care of the family or community. It involves a synthesis of providing expert technical and instructional services, of using interpersonal skills to better understand, motivate and guide others in securing the best possible health care, and organizing groups to facilitate productive interchanges of skills and competence and maximum self-help. It borrows and synthesizes skills from many fields—from medicine, from social work, from education, from sociology, from psychology—adding those of nursing itself to create a service which contributes, and even more stimulates and guides others to contribute to the conservation of community health.

CHAPTER IV

Functions and
Responsibilities

THE GENERAL functions of public health nurses are described in
the official statement adopted by the American Nurses' Association in 1955, as follows:

> "Public health nurses, including school nurses and those
> in other specialties in public health nursing, work as mem-
> bers of a health team to further community health. They
> provide nursing care and treatment, health counseling, and
> organize families and community groups for health pur-
> poses. Their activities include work in the home, clinic,
> office, school, or health center. In all phases of the work
> emphasis is placed on the prevention of disease, the pro-
> motion of health, and rehabilitative measures."[1]

Within this general statement, functions are considered in two
broad areas—those concerned with nursing care of families and
groups, and those relating to agency or community planning and
management. In relation to the first area, the statement says:

> "Gives, arranges for, teaches or supervises nursing care of
> the sick and injured. Carries out nursing skills contribut-
> ing to treatment and rehabilitation. Plans for coordinated
> nursing service for individuals and families under her care.
> Appraises individual and family health needs and hazards
> —existing or potential. Provides health counseling, includ-

1. Public Health Nurses' Section, American Nurses' Association, *Functions,
Standards, and Qualifications for Public Health Nurses.* New York, American
Nurses' Association, 1955, p. 3.

42

ing emotional support, to individuals, families, and groups. Consults with and refers families to appropriate personnel within the agency, school, or other community services. Treatments and, when required, diagnostic and preventive procedures are carried out under medical direction."[2]

NURSING CARE OF THE SICK

Care of the sick is a primary responsibility in any area of nursing practice. The continuing rise in hospital admissions in the United States (from 18,483,085 in 1950 to 20,345,431 in 1954[3]) has been accompanied by a decrease in the number of days of hospitalization, due in part to more intensive treatment methods and in part to the great demand for use of the general hospital beds that were available. There has been a decided increase in the incidence of hospitalization of the acutely ill and of maternity patients, as well as of the chronically ill during the period of diagnosis and evaluation. However, early hospital discharge and absence of adequate facilities for hospital care of the chronically ill and convalescent have increased the need for prehospital and posthospital care in the home. Minor illness and childhood diseases have continued to be cared for at home and constitute a large part of the home nursing case load.

The public health nurse may (1) provide a substantial amount of direct patient care, (2) teach and supervise a practical nurse, nurse's aide or family member who will give the nursing care, (3) teach groups or individuals the methods of providing home care of the sick or (4) refer the individual or family to other sources for nursing care or instruction. The nurse's responsibility for nursing care of the sick remains constant, whether she gives such care herself or assures the provision of care by someone else.

Nursing care in public health is characterized by great variety. In hazardous industries, emergency care will play a major role; in services where bedside care is provided a great variety of treatments may be given, including intramuscular and intravenous administration of drugs, care of orthopedic appliances and supervision of exercise therapy, and other special types of care. Prehospital and posthospital care will embrace a myriad of diagnostic areas, each requiring special knowledge or skill. Accommodation must be made to many different treatment patterns even within

2. Ibid. p. 4.

3. American Nurses' Association, *Facts About Nursing*, 1955–56 Edition, p. 169.

the same diagnostic group, for the care among different hospitals or physicians will have many variations—one hospital group may recommend restricting fats in the cardiac diet, while another does not, for example. All age groups are served in public health work, with each group presenting its own particular health needs and adjustment patterns. The nurse in public health must be a generalist in nursing, with competence in many fields.

Family Health Counseling and Teaching. By health counseling is meant action that is taken to assist the individual or family to make and carry out his or its own plans for meeting individual or family health problems. Counseling is inextricably interwoven with the other aspects of nursing care. It may be provided directly as part of a nursing visit or interview, or indirectly through conferences with teachers, foremen or parents regarding the maintenance of the health of their charges. It may be provided to individuals, families or to school or community groups; it may represent a carefully conceived and extensive educational undertaking (as in a series of conferences with an expectant mother), or as an incidental adjunct to another service (as in the maintenance of exhibits or informational services in a treatment clinic). Whatever the method of administration, health counseling must be carefully and systematically planned so that it is both inclusive and individualized. Comprehensive health care must include interpretation of growth and developmental factors as well as the significance of manifestations of health or illness. Management of tension, fear, worry and other emotional impediments to health must have equal consideration with full use of preventive health facilities and satisfactory family, personal and community adjustment to illness or physical impairment. Rehabilitative measures must supplement curative and preventive care.

Medical Supportive Activities. Nursing services that conserve or increase the effectiveness of medical personnel include such activities as assisting with treatments or physical examination procedures; identifying and reporting significant conditions observed or noted in records or reports; providing inspectional services, such as examination of school children during periods of increased incidence of communicable disease, or routine inspection of exposed workers for symptoms of specific occupational disease; interpretation of home or community factors that have a bearing on the disease or its treatment; instituting appropriate referral and follow-up procedures.

As diagnostic testing procedures come into more frequent use, there is a tendency for busy physicians to depend upon the nurse for the performance of those tests that may be done without immediate medical supervision. This is especially true in rural areas where it is not easy to arrange for people to get to clinics or doctors' offices for such services. Tuberculin testing, blood pressure reading, hemoglobin determination, audiometer testing and posture analysis are often a part of the nurse's work. She may also be responsible for collecting and handling specimens, cultures and slides for laboratory examination. Venipuncture and administration of intravenous medication may be undertaken by the nurse in blood collection centers or in diagnostic and treatment clinics. There is a wide spread in the degree of responsibility assigned in this area.

Control of Environmental Health Hazards. Inspection or survey of homes, farms, schools, industrial plants or playgrounds, and periodic checks on the use and maintenance of safety equipment may be done by the nurse, or she may participate in such activities under the direction of the public health or safety engineer.

Hazards in the social or personal environment may need to be considered as well as physical factors. The tension-producing effect of poorly balanced class schedules, the hazard of the worker who refuses to stay home when he is ill and thus exposes other workers to possible infection, or an aura of insecurity in a home due to misunderstanding between parents is as much a problem as the wet and slippery floor in a factory or the exposed wiring in a farmer's barn.

In addition to the direct services she herself provides, the public health nurse promotes understanding and full utilization of other members of the health team and the community through referral and reporting. She provides for a systematic exchange of information through reports or conferences with other workers, and arranges and participates in patient care conferences.

PARTICIPATION IN PROGRAM DEVELOPMENT

The second area of general responsibility relates to the development and operation of health programs in the agency, school or community, and is described in the American Nurses' Association statement as follows:

"Plans with appropriate medical and administrative personnel within the agency or school regarding nursing participation in the health program and carries out the nursing phases. Contributes to the public relations activities of the agency. Furthers observation of health laws and regulations. Participates in planning, conducting, and evaluating inservice educational programs for public health nurses and for other workers in the agency or school. Participates in community planning and action for health and welfare and contributes to professional education in nursing, medicine, social work, education, and allied fields."[4]

Planning Responsibilities. Through membership on committees and councils, conferences with administrative officers and boards and the preparation of data relating to nursing needs and services the public health nurse participates in planning for general as well as nursing phases of health programs. Her knowledge of community conditions and the temper of the community in relation to particular programs is a vital contribution to over-all administrative understanding. Through balancing her nursing activities in relation to the over-all agency or community program she avoids duplication of effort and gives maximum support to "special emphasis" activities. For example, if the health department is stressing prevention of home accidents, the public health nurse will provide information about local conditions and the probable degree of community acceptance; she will also arrange her program so that her activities in schools, clinics and home visits give particular support to this important program area.

Managerial Responsibilities. In varying degrees, depending largely on the size of the agency, the public health nurse will take responsibility for office and clinic management. In schools and industrial plants she is usually responsible for maintenance of the health room; in rural areas, organization and management of itinerant clinics including organization of community for stimulating attendance and securing volunteer assistance, and office management are often added to her other duties.

Maintenance of individual or family case records and statistical or financial reports provides the necessary base for accounting and program planning. Progress reports of the nursing service supplement this basic data and provide an analytical interpretation that is basic to agency program planning and evaluation as well as a helpful source of information for public information.

The nurse also participates constantly in the public relations activities of her agency. She may supply data or ideas for publicity material, interpret the service through talks, radio or tele-

4. Loc. Cit., p. 6.

vision appearance or newspaper or magazine articles. Most of all, in all her contacts with the public, she exemplifies the interest and philosophy of her agency. This has particular significance, since the nurse is the representative of the health agency who is in the closest and most frequent contact with the public.

In some instances, public health nurses may take a part in the enforcement of health laws or regulations. They may participate in inspection of nursing homes or foster homes, or check on the adequacy of home isolation measures for communicable disease control. While law enforcement may be the primary purpose of the service, consultation and interpretation—the usual helping approach of nursing—are an integral part of such activities, and are usually adequate without recourse to coercion. Especially in relation to inspection of nursing homes and boarding homes, public health nursing has been shown to be very effective in improving patient care.[5]

Education and Supervision of Other Workers. The public health nurse may participate in the education and supervision of professional and auxiliary nurses, of medical or social work students and related professional workers in other fields. New staff nurses, professional and practical nurse students, nurses' aides and volunteer workers who will assist in nursing activities may be assigned to the public health nurse for training. In some areas, training and supervision of midwives may also be included as a public health nursing responsibility. In addition to students and new workers who are members of the nursing team, the nurse may participate in the field experience of students in medicine, social work, education, public health or public administration. A major contribution in these fields is interpretation of the services of the public health nurse. Observation of the nurse at work is supplemented by case discussions and sometimes by group discussion. Programs for orientation of workers in related fields may vary in duration from a single day to a period of several weeks.

These training and supervision activities necessitate careful individual planning and guidance, as well as an extensive knowledge of the objectives and programs of a variety of sponsoring institutions. The nurse must avoid giving a fragmentary experience to the individual who has a very short time under her supervision; she must likewise plan carefully for a comprehensive educational program and for continuing guidance and supervisory

5. Foote, Roberta and Lucille Tracy, We Like Working in Boarding Homes. *Nursing Outlook*, 5: 19–21, January, 1957.

assistance to those whose assignment extends over a longer period.

Participation in Research and Service Studies.   Many health and welfare research projects include nursing factors, and the nurse may make a significant contribution to the planning and conduct of such broad investigations. In epidemiologic study the nurse has long been recognized as a dependable and ingenious fact-finder, and is gaining recognition as a helpful assistant in planning for epidemiologic studies. Nursing records and studies may do much to reveal health and welfare needs of the community, and the degree to which they are being met. They may provide the stimulation necessary for a wider or more complex study of the problems so revealed. For instance, the nurse may feel that families of chronically ill patients need emotional and personal guidance to cope with the demands of the situation. She may indicate the frequency with which emotional problems occur, based on her own judgment. This may lead to a full-scale research project, using more refined and extensive procedures than the nurse herself can command.

Research in nursing itself is proceeding at an accelerated pace. Critical shortages of nursing personnel have resulted in careful investigations of the use of nursing time, and the costs of service. Analysis and evaluation of nursing practice have stimulated many independent field and statistical studies. These studies of nursing practice call for thoughtful participation of all nurses, as well as for guidance and leadership from well-prepared nurse leaders with special research competence.

Overlapping Functions among Health Professions.   The concept of public health nursing as part of a team activity designed to bring total health care to individuals, families and communities through a multidisciplinary approach and the need for a unified and integrated approach to health care makes it virtually impossible to define with exactness the scope, and limits each profession represented.

The difficulty of distinguishing between the respective responsibility of physician and nurse may be demonstrated in the care of a prenatal patient. The physician has, of course, the responsibility for diagnosis and treatment. However, when guidance in personal hygiene and emotional adjustment is considered, the division of responsibility is far from clear. Here the physician and nurse (and frequently other workers such as nutritionist, health educator or mental hygienist) share the responsibility with no very clear line of demarcation. The physician prescribes diet;

the nurse, on the other hand, may be the more expert in assisting the family to make the necessary adjustments in family eating habits. She may be better acquainted with the "fair exchanges" in foods that may be worked out to meet more completely the requirements of family tastes or pocketbook—how to substitute margarine for butter, evaporated or dried milk for whole milk, tomatoes for citrus fruit. She may discuss the effect of food preparation on vitamin content of foods, or practical ways of modifying the "no breakfast" habit. In this latter type of activity the nurse may function within the framework of medical prescription, but may also, in the absence of a medical problem, give much advice independently, since family nutrition is considered a problem of general health instruction.

Similar problems may arise in division of responsibility between nurse and medical social worker or case worker. The description of modern social work as "a professional service rendered to people for the purpose of assisting them as individuals or in groups, to attain satisfying relationships and standards in life in accordance with their particular wishes and capacities and in harmony with those of the community"[6] makes it obvious that public health nursing and social service work must be similar if not identical in some phases of their work. Social diagnosis and intensive case work are unquestionably the responsibility of the social case worker. However, in the course of her work the nurse will be faced with many problems requiring social adjustment. Helping the family with budgeting, promoting wholesome family recreation, assisting individuals to make satisfactory emotional adjustments to long-term illness or to pregnancy are common public health nursing activities. Whether such problems come within the province of the social worker or of the nurse depends upon the degree of difficulty presented, and placement of the primary responsibility for case management will be based in many instances upon a joint review of the individual situation by the nurse and social worker. The availability of prepared social workers will also inevitably influence the degree of responsibility the nurse will take.

In a similar manner, the function of the teacher places upon her the responsibility for selecting the content of the educational program, and managing the school environment so that it becomes a source of desirable learning experiences for the student. The nurse

6. *Social Work Yearbook*, 1954. New York, American Association of Social Workers, 1955, p. 506.

in the school generally assumes responsibility for individual health counseling, for consultation on health matters and provision of materials for health education. In the actual conduct of the school health program, however, the teacher will often counsel with individual students, and the nurse may become a valuable resource in planning for educational content and in participation in selected classroom activities. In industry, too, the nurse and personnel worker will frequently find areas of common concern,

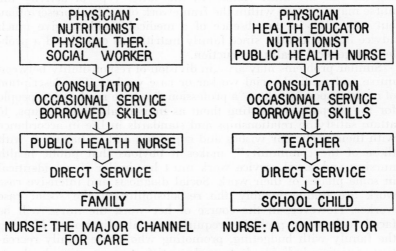

Figure 8.   Public health nursing in family health care.

as in the placement problems of a "nervous" worker or guidance of an accident-prone driver whose home problems may be influencing his job behavior. The job of the public health nurse must be flexibly interpreted and constantly adjusted to meet the demands of the particular situation. It is not always possible to separate the activities inherent in health service with sharp distinction and to assign them categorically to one or another of the members of the health team, and the nurse may be either the main purveyor of service to the family, or may be a contributing member of the team, as shown in Figure 8.

Nursing functions and responsibilities may be primarily supportive to the medical or social care plan, as when the nurse performs diagnostic tests to be interpreted by the physician, arranges for the physical set-up of a clinic, or secures information necessary for a case worker's analysis of a family's social problem. Other tasks will be essentially independent—areas in which the nurse takes the leadership in planning and action, as in the provision of nursing care, building parental skill in maintaining emotional security in infants or small children, or teaching family management of chronic disease nursing care. Other nursing activities will be directed toward securing optimal coordination of a variety of services, where the function of the nurse is essentially that of a facilitator. Examples of activities that are primarily coordinative in nature are: arranging for a conference to decide on an action program for health care of a particular family, or of a specified group, such as care of rheumatic fever victims; providing appropriate information on student health to school personnel in order that it may be used in the educational guidance of the student, or in securing needed administrative adjustments; or assisting families to make wise use of available medical resources.

JOB RESPONSIBILITIES

Within the general structure of public health nursing functions, there will be wide variations in the job responsibilities assigned in a particular situation or to a particular individual. Factors affecting job configuration include:

1. Agency purposes and program
2. Community needs and readiness for service
3. Other available health services
4. Adequacy of nursing staff
5. Specialization of service

Agency Purposes and Program.   Public health nursing may operate in agencies motivated by quite different purposes. For example, a visiting nurse service may exist primarily to serve a humanitarian purpose—to help those who need help. Direct nursing care would probably be emphasized in such a program. A health department, on the other hand, must take responsibility for protection and promotion of the public health—it may not be free to elect to minister to only a small portion of the population, or to carry expensive services that do not contribute materially to prevention of disease or general health promotion. Each agency will have its own purposes or objectives. Some agencies, both tax supported and voluntary, for example, consider research and "forward thrusting" investigations as an integral part of their work; others feel their purpose is to apply the findings of research done by others. Some agencies distinguish sharply between curative and preventive services, and may see their sphere of action only in the preventive area. In such a case the direct nursing service aspects of public health nursing would probably be minimized.

Agency objectives will be molded in some instances by legal mandates, or by restrictions placed on the use of certain funds. For example, a foundation may grant funds to be used only for providing prescribed types of care. Contractual arrangements between community nursing services and home care programs may obligate the agency to provide a large amount of simple home care, and thus lead to emphasis on the public health nurse's role in planning patient care services and in training and supervising auxiliary workers.

The range and depth of agency services will be modified also by the size and stability of the budget, and the nurse's responsibilities will be modified by this factor also. Regardless of its interest, the small agency may not be able to move into intensive rehabilitation nursing services if it cannot either secure the necessary personnel and equipment for such a program or reduce other commitments. The tax supported agency, which is obligated to supply certain services on a community-wide basis, may feel that intensive experimental services are not feasible within the financial competence of the agency, although highly desirable.

Community Needs and Readiness for Service.   What communities need and what they want from nursing services may not always represent the same thing. In an economically privileged community the demand in relation to nursing care may be for direct nursing care to the chronically ill, including custodial care. The nurse may recognize in the same community a great need for counseling in parent-child relationships, or for the reduction of stress in daily living activities. Educational services may be welcomed in some communities, and barely tolerated or even resented in another, particularly if they are offered without the more tangible nursing care of the sick. The willingness of the community to use and support particular nursing services must influence the configuration of the public health nurse's work.

Other Available Health Services.   The availability of related health services will also shift the demands made upon public health nursing. If hospital outpatient services provide an intensive family education program, and readily available hospital care for acute conditions, the public health nurse's load may be lightened. However, an almost certain concomitant in such cases is a higher level of sensitivity to family needs on the part of hospital personnel which may result in more rather than less referral of patients and families who need more intensive help than the hospital can provide. Improvement of community rehabilitation service, or extension of hospital home care programs, may also increase the amount and influence the direction of the public health nursing job.

The absence of adequate medical or social services may result in the public health nurse taking on responsibilities that would normally be handled by the physician or social worker. In remote, weather-locked areas, for example, the public health nurse may "pinch hit" as epidemiologist, physician or social worker. When there is no health educator on the staff, the public health nurse may carry community organization and public information responsibilities that she would not otherwise have.

The employment of practical nurses and aides may reduce the public health nurse's load of direct care, but increase her responsibility for supervising others. The existence of many social and health facilities in a community will lead to more responsibility for coordination and planning.

Adequacy of Nursing Staff. In the past, a ratio of one public health nurse for each 5000 of the population was rather generally accepted as the minimum safe level for the provision of administrative (nonbedside care) public health nursing service. When comprehensive nursing service, including care of the sick in their homes, is undertaken, one nurse for each 2000 to 2500 of the population was proposed.[7] More recently it is recognized that such averages are of very limited use in planning, since local variations influence needs so greatly. Several studies are now under way in an effort to find a more satisfactory measure of need, but none has been developed. When the concentration of nursing staff falls below the needs of the community to a significant degree, it becomes apparent that the work of the nurse must be adjusted to secure an achievable pattern of service. All activities will need to be weighed carefully, and some of the less productive or nonobligatory activities curtailed or omitted entirely.

The level of technical competence of the nursing staff will also influence the character of the work. Deficiencies in basic nursing education will have a definite limiting effect upon the job responsibilities the public health nurse can carry. A nation-wide survey of schools in 1949 revealed that at that time only about 25 per-

7. Haven, Emerson, and Martha Luginbuhl, *Health Units for the Nation.* New York, Commonwealth Fund, 1945.

cent of the schools met or approached standards set by the profession *in 1937*, and that half the schools were nearer the standards of 1937.[8] Increasing public and academic concern, aided by the concerted consultation and accreditation program of the National League for Nursing has resulted in much improvement. However, there are still a substantial number of schools whose programs are at a minimal if not frankly inadequate level.

Pre-service education in public health also influences the ability of the nursing staff to carry certain job responsibilities. In 1955 only 37.1 percent of the 26,110 nurses engaged in public health work for whom qualifications were reported had completed one or more years in an approved public health nursing program of study, and only 31.3 percent of those employed in a staff capacity had been so prepared.[9] Nurses who have not had the advantage of such advanced preparation will find it difficult to incorporate certain assignments into their work until they can acquire the special public health skills or knowledge for their accomplishment. Participation in epidemiologic study, intensive family guidance, group teaching and organization and guidance of citizen committees generally require preparation beyond that afforded in the diploma school of nursing.

In some instances, staff deficiencies in basic or pre-service education are compensated for by a strong and well-planned in-service education program. Such remedial education makes it possible to raise the job sights of the nurse, and to deepen or broaden her responsibilities. It is generally accepted that there is need for a continuous program of education on the job, not to make up for basic deficiencies in pre-service education, but to maintain and enrich professional competence. Job responsibilities can be most comprehensive when there is a combination of good basic and pre-service education and a continuing in-service education program for all members of the nursing staff.

Specialization of Service. In some instances, public health nursing will be carried on within a special field, with limits and perhaps with added special responsibilities entailed. The nurse working full time in school health services, for example, will have

8. *Nursing Schools at the Midcentury*, New York, National Committee for the Improvement of Nursing Services, 1950, p. 1.

9. *Census of Nurses Employed for Public Health Work* in the United States, in the Territories of Hawaii and Alaska and in Puerto Rico and the Virgin Islands on January 1st 1955, Public Health Service, 1955, Department of Health, Education, and Welfare.

added responsibilities in relation to participating in curriculum and course planning, and may include some classroom teaching among her responsibilities.

A statement of functions of the nurse in the school, propounded by the American School Health Association, uses a somewhat different approach than that of the American Nurses' Association, although both statements are essentially consistent with one another. The American School Health Association statement includes such general areas of responsibility as the provision of leadership and guidance in the development of the total school health program; participation in planning and policy making; serving as a consultant to school personnel, parents and children; and serving as a liaison worker with the community.

Specific areas of responsibility include health appraisal, emergency care, communicable disease control, growth and development, mental health and nutrition consultation, guidance and counseling, exclusion and readmission of children, working with exceptional children, home visiting and supervision of other nurses.[10] While fundamentally consistent with the American Nurses' Association, this indicates the special emphases in the responsibilities of the nurse in the school.

In new or developing programs, public health nurses may function on a specialized basis either for a limited time during the development of procedures and program or for an indefinite period when the skills required necessitate extensive additional training. Orthopedic nursing, psychiatric or mental health nursing and public health nursing in tuberculosis clinics are examples of special fields in which the job responsibilities of the nurse may be specialized in some agencies. In such cases, it is particularly important that the function of these nurse specialists be seen in relation to the needs and developments of the generalized program in public health nursing.

The job of public health nursing is many faceted. Its successful accomplishment demands maturity and understanding, deep sensitivity to the needs of people and a high level of professional skill. Even more, it requires ability of the nurse to function smoothly, confidently and cooperatively as a respected member of the public health team.

10. Recommended Policy and Practices for School Nursing, *Journal of School Health*, 26: 13–24, January, 1956.

CHAPTER V

Organization

Public health nursing is carried on under many different types of sponsorship and organization. Health departments, banks, private physicians' clinics, hospitals, visiting nurse associations, settlement houses, labor organizations, public schools, and insurance companies are only a few of the types of agency that may provide some measure of public health nursing service.

The great multiplicity of voluntary agencies offering public health nursing service reflects the strong force of public interest in and support of voluntary health work that has been a traditional factor in American life. While the trend has been toward assumption of greater responsibility by tax-supported agencies, the voluntary agency has continued to receive strong support, and its place in supplementation and in experimentation has not been questioned. Recognition of the importance of public health nursing as an adjunct to the private practice of medicine and in promotion of the health and welfare of workers has increased the number of privately or commercially sponsored services.

Organizational patterns within a given group of agencies, such as health departments, will vary greatly from one community to another, and within the different units of government. The almost complete autonomy of each state in matters of health, and the essentially local character of responsibility for administration of public health programs result in great differences in health organization in the different states and communities. Differences in source of income, community resources and needs and public attitudes create many variations in the organizational patterns of voluntary agencies providing public health nursing.

Philosophy of Governmental Responsibility. There seems to be general acceptance that the provision of basic services necessary for the protection and promotion of community health is the responsibility of the officially constituted health agency, and that services of all other health agencies should be of a supplementary or experimental character. The legal responsibility for safeguarding the health of the general public is clearly assigned to official health departments, with authority centered primarily in state departments of health. While few state constitutions make specific reference to public health, the police power of the state provides the general basis for its health authority.[1]

At the same time, it is recognized that the voluntary agency, or groups primarily organized for another purpose, may extend governmental services to reach more people, to provide services whose purposes are primarily humanitarian rather than preventive or protective in nature, and to experiment with new approaches or in new areas of services. Such voluntary activity has the added dividend of increased public interest in health services, which may affect the total health program as well as a particular agency's area of concern.

There is at present considerable disagreement as to what constitutes "basic" services, and what is encompassed in "community" health. Mustard distinguishes between public and personal health by the size and nature of the problem—if it is so large or of such a nature that it canot be handled by individual efforts, then it becomes a public health problem.[2] Perhaps in no place is the confusion more apparent than in relation to provision of medical care by health departments, where opinion may range from providing all services which families or individuals cannot secure for themselves for economic reasons, or because medical facilities are inadequate, without regard for ability to pay, to a sharp distinction between curative and preventive services which envision government-provided medical care only for those with communicable disease. In defining functions of local health departments the American Public Health Association officially states:

> "Because of the marked changes in the age distribution of the population and in the spectrum of our health problems, the theory and practice of public health has expanded

1. Mustard, Harry S., *Government in Public Health.* New York, Commonwealth Fund, 1945, p. 20.

2. Ibid.

to include not only the prevention of the onset of illness, but also prevention of the progress of disease, of associated complications and of disability and death."[3]

In 1951, practically all full-time local health departments provided medical services in varying degrees in connection with specialized programs, and 62 full-time health departments (5 percent) administered general medical services of varied scope and character, reaching over 10 percent of persons under jurisdiction of local health units at that time.[4] The Commission on Chronic Illness describes the role of the public agency with relation to medical care as "to make needed care available to persons who cannot themselves pay for it and to other special groups who are entitled by law."[5] It becomes clear that the role of the public agency cannot be sharply and clearly defined from that of the voluntary agency. In the final analysis, what Anderson called the "mandate of the people"[6] will prevail—a decision by the public regarding those services which they feel require concerted community action.

Despite the confusion in interpretation, the basic obligation of the official health agency to see that as far as possible the public gets such health services as are needed and that individuals cannot provide for themselves seems to be clear.

The voluntary agency, on the other hand, has an obligation to spend the money it collects wisely to meet human needs. It has not the same obligation to concern itself with the total health needs of the community, but may investigate or work in some small area of service in which its supporters have a particular interest. The wise expenditure of funds, however, involves assurance that the activities undertaken do not duplicate those already provided, and that they reflect a safe and useful or potentially useful approach to meeting human needs. For example, the voluntary agency might concern itself quite properly with a single disease or disease group (such as heart disease or cancer or ma-

3. The Local Health Department—Services and Responsibilities. *American Journal of Public Health*, 41: 302–307, March, 1951.

4. Terris, Milton and Nathan Kramer, *General Medical Care Programs in Local Health Departments*. New York, American Public Health Association, 1951, p. 11.

5. Commission on Chronic Illness, *Care of the Long Term Patient*. Cambridge, Harvard University Press, 1956, p. 403.

6. Anderson, Gaylord, Public Health—A Mandate from the People. *American Journal of Public Health*, 42:1367–1373, November, 1952.

ternal care), and with procedures as yet unproved in value (such as intensive family health maintenance services or special types of group work).

Acceptance of this principle implies that no voluntary health programs will be instituted or continued that in any way serve to supplant needed public action or impede the development of basic health programs in publicly supported agencies. For example, in a given community it might be easier for a voluntary agency to raise money for nursing and instructional services to prospective mothers and mothers with babies than to find tax support for such a program. It would be quite proper for the voluntary agency to institute such a service in order to demonstrate its worth during such time as tax money could not be secured or the official agency is for some other reason unable to encompass this important phase of the health program. However, it is important that the responsibility of the official agency be clearly understood. The service of the voluntary agency should not continue to the point where it usurps the place of the health department, or impedes the development of a sound maternal and child health program within the governmental organization.

This does not mean that nonofficial agencies should never undertake functions which should be, but have not as yet been, undertaken by the official agency. Coordinated initial planning, gradual transfer of responsibilities, and continuous supportive interpretation of health department functions by the nonofficial agency make it possible to meet the immediate needs of the community and at the same time to maintain the integrity and continuing development of official health services.

Even when governmental services are adequately developed, and the voluntary agency undertakes only that work that has been generally accepted as outside the sphere of official health service, all supplementary services should be integrally related to the basic health program of the community. For example, home nursing care of the chronically ill may in some localities be assumed to be a supplementary rather than basic protective health service, and be a logical function of a nongovernmental health agency. However, in developing such a program it is necessary that it be related to the existing or projected plans for diagnostic and educational services of the official health agency, and that the official agency in turn adjust its program as far as possible to take advantage of patient care services of the voluntary agency.

NURSING IN GOVERNMENTAL PUBLIC HEALTH SERVICES

In the United States the states are sovereign units of government, with the federal governmental units having only those powers delegated to it by the states, encompassing responsibilities not amenable to state control. The local health department is the basic service unit in the administration of public health and is accountable to the state agency for adequate performance of those programs which are delegated to it by state law or regulation.[7] Local school boards function in a similar manner and are subject to state laws and controls, but are administratively fairly autonomous.

National Services.　　　Public health nursing in national governmental units provides both direct service to specified individuals or groups, and leadership, consultative and technical research services to states. They provide:

1. Public health nursing care to groups that do not come under state jurisdiction or that are beneficiaries of federal health services, such as Indians living on reservations, military personnel and their dependents who live on army posts, veterans with service-connected disabilities who are receiving care at home, and employees of the federal government who need the usual occupational health services.

2. Personnel and advisory assistance for field studies, demonstrations or research projects in public health. For example, personnel may be provided for a demonstration mental health unit, for state surveys of nursing needs and facilities, or for special diagnostic or treatment investigations in specific disease areas or instructional programs in newly developing fields.

3. Data to be used by states and for nation-wide planning. The census of nurses employed for public health work compiled by the Public Health Service, facts about infant mortality compiled by the Children's Bureau, information on nursing needs and resources and on salaries of public health workers are examples of these types of data.

4. Standards, such as standards for nursing homes and for premature care, to serve as a guide for state and local agencies.

5. Public educational materials such as "Infant Care" for parents, or the Workers' Health Series for industrial workers, or guides for nursing surveys to be used by local groups.

7. The Local Health Department—Services and Responsibilities. *American Journal of Public Health*, 41: 302–307, March, 1951.

6. Field consultation services to states.

7. Assistance in the administration of grants-in-aid and of training or research funds.

Public Health nursing is a major activity in the Public Health Service and the Children's Bureau of the Department of Health, Education, and Welfare; in the Veterans' Administration and in the Army Nurse Corps; and in the Federal Goverment Employee Health Service. In several other bureaus or departments of government having some public nursing services it has a more limited role.

The Public Health Service is the principal agency of government concerned with national health. Its powers and duties were defined in the Public Health Service Act of 1944 and its subsequent amendments.

Nursing in the Public Health Service is coordinated under the direction of an assistant surgeon general who is also designated as chief nurse officer. Placed administratively in the Office of the Surgeon General, she advises on all nursing matters, coordinates nursing within the Service, and may serve as official spokesman for nursing in the Public Health Service in contacts with other groups.

Within the framework of over-all policy set at the Surgeon General's level, public health nursing activities are carried on in the various bureaus and divisions of the Public Health Service. The Division of Nursing Resources of the Bureau of Medical Services provides consultation within the bureau and to other Public Health Service bureaus, and to agencies or individuals outside the Public Health Service on nursing needs, utilization and resources, encourages and conducts surveys and confers on nursing education problems.

The Public Health Nursing Section in the Bureau of State Services provides general and continuing consultant service to the various states, working through ten regional offices of the Public Health Service. Nurse-consultants assigned to regional offices come under the administrative direction of the regional medical director, and planning for service to states is done in the regional office within the general framework of policy established by the Public Health Nursing Section at the national level. Regional office staff are in effect deputies of the Public Health Service. Professional guidance and supervision of nurse-consultants in regional offices are provided through the Public Health Nursing Section. The section also collects and compiles data on public health nursing, such as the status of public health preparation of staff, trends and patterns in employment, and carries on field research and demonstrations and pilot program studies.

The Public Health Nursing Section also coordinates the nursing work in other sections or divisions of the Bureau of State Services, and provides leadership for nurses assigned to other divisions or sections such as the Division of Special Health Services.

The National Institutes of Health is an aggregate of research institutes including a clinical research center. Public health nurses serve in several of the institutes—notably in the National Institute for Mental Health, the National Cancer Institute and the National Heart Institute. They assist with research projects, provide consultation for national planning and to the states.

The Children's Bureau was organized in 1912 and originally placed in the Department of Labor. It is now part of the Department of Health, Education, and Welfare. Its functions are summarized as follows:

1. It assembles facts needed to keep the country informed about children and matters adversely affecting the well-being of children.
2. It recommends measures that will be effective in advancing the wholesome development of children and in preventing and treating the ill effects of adverse conditions.
3. It gives technical assistance to citizens and voluntary and public agencies in improving conditions of childhood.
4. It administrates the financial aid that the federal government appropriates each year to aid the states in building the health and welfare of their children.[8]

The relatively small nursing staff provides consultation to national planning groups, compiles data regarding the special nursing problems of mothers and children and develops materials. Consultation service is provided to states through regional offices. As in the case of Public Health Service staff, nurses in the regional offices are administratively responsible to the regional medical director, but receive professional direction from the central nursing staff.

The military public health nursing services, exemplified by the *Army Health Nursing Service,* are relatively new. Their work with military personnel is a direct service similar to any local health agency service. Army health nurses are responsible to the

8. *Your Children's Bureau.* Washington, D.C., Government Printing Office, 1956.

preventive medical officer, with professional direction from the chief army health nurse in the Surgeon General's Office.[9]

The Veterans' Administration provides community nursing care for its medical beneficiaries who are on home care as part of the home-town medical care program. This care is provided through contracts with existing local voluntary agencies. The service has expanded rapidly and in 1953–54 involved a total of 932 patients.[10] Most of the patients were receiving care for long-term illness—the average number of nursing home visits per patient was 36.6.

The Employee Health Service is an occupational and preventive health service for federal employees in some governmental agencies. Similar services for civilian employees are maintained in some military posts.

State Health Departments. The *basis of authority* in state health departments rests in the power of the state to legislate for the protection of the public safety, health and morals.[11] Often its authority is implied rather than explicitly defined in the state legal code. The state is the sovereign power in most health matters; local health departments have such power as is delegated to them by the state with wide differences in the degree of delegation. State health departments are almost universally a separate division of government with over-all policy direction usually vested in a Board of Health and responsibility for administration in a state health commissioner or health officer.

The state health department is responsible for coordinating the work of all agencies dealing with public health in the state and for planning to meet the public health needs of the total population directly or through local action. The state department may have responsibility for some direct personal health services such as care of tuberculosis patients or crippled children services, and may maintain laboratory or other special services.

A major function is providing assistance to local health units.

Public health nursing responsibility in state health departments is essentially that of providing leadership and supervision to local nursing services. This function is maintained by activities such as the following:

9. *Army Regulations, No. 40-51.* Washington, D.C., August, 1955.

10. Addams, Ruth and Iva Torrens, Home Nursing Care for Veterans. *Nursing Outlook,* 4: 497–499, September, 1956.

11. The State Health Department—Services and Responsibilities. *American Journal of Public Health,* 44: 235–252, February, 1954.

1. Studying and appraising public health nursing needs and facilities within the state, and maintaining necessary data for planning, such as numbers, distribution and preparation of public health nurses, agencies employing public health nursing, and so forth.

2. Planning with other branches of the state health department and with other state health and educational agencies for (a) the promotion and development of local public health nursing programs, and (b) inclusion of nursing in specific programs, such as tuberculosis control, maternal and child hygiene, industrial hygiene or school health.

3. Assisting local health authorities in the development and improvement of local public health nursing services.

4. Assisting in the improvement of the quality of public health nursing through:

   a. Recommending desirable qualifications for personnel and interpreting requirements established by law or regulation when such are in force.

   b. Organizing continuing in-service education projects for public health nurses or encouraging and guiding other organizations to do so. This may include such activities as offering orientation programs for new public health nurses, provided either in the state health department or by state public health nursing personnel who introduces and orients the public health nurse in her own community; maintenance of library facilities; organization of conferences, institutes or workshops; development of study outlines or bulletins; providing educational consultant service to local agencies or to universities.

   c. Providing supervisory and consultant service to local public health nurses. Sometimes the state division of public health nursing has direct responsibility for supervision of nurses employed in local health departments and for certain administrative aspects of local public health nursing work. This is apt to be true when a district or local health unit plan is in effect and a member of the state staff is assigned to the district or unit as a supervisor. In other instances, state public health nursing personnel takes direct responsibility for supervision only in unorganized communities, and serves in an advisory capacity to those communities that have an organized health department.

   d. Assisting in the development of suitable training facilities in universities, colleges and schools of nursing, and participating in instruction where it is appropriate to do so. This may include assisting with the development and supervision of field training centers for public health nursing students.

e. Studying and recommending standards, techniques and procedures in public health nursing. This may be done by publication of standards for specific services or manuals of procedure, or by the official adoption of procedures or standards developed by other groups. For example, a state division of public health nursing may decide to adopt the standards for qualifications of personnel as recommended by the American Nurses' Association, or standing orders as written by the state medical society.

5. Participating in recruitment and selection of public health nursing personnel. This may include assistance in programs of recruitment for basic nursing courses, in the selection of applicants for federal stipends or other study grants; maintaining close liaison with the professional counseling and placement services of nursing associations to promote effective guidance of prospective public health nursing candidates; interviewing and recommending specific applicants; cooperating with state and local merit systems in determining methods of selection.

6. Promoting desirable personnel policies and conditions of work for public health nurses. Recommendations may be made to local employment agencies regarding such personnel problems as salary; annual and sick leave, business or study leave; tenure or insurance. When such recommended practice goes to local health departments it must, of course, be related to the personnel policies in force for other health department staff members.

In some states, especially in those that are sparsely settled, the state division of public health nursing may administer direct services to local communities either through assignment of state personnel to local health units as supervisors or administrators, or through provision of public health nursing services outside of incorporated municipalities.

State divisions may also assign additional personnel to local health departments in times of special need or for demonstration or experimentation. Occasionally, federal agencies loan personnel to states for reassignment to local health agencies.

Public health nursing in the over-all health department struc-

ture varies from state to state. In some states there is a division
of public health nursing directly responsible to the health officer
or his deputy, in others the public health nursing services come
under an intermediary bureau such as a division of local health
services or of preventive health services.

Organization of public nursing in a separate department or
unit has many advantages. Planning for the use of nursing personnel in the total health department is easier, since staffing and
allocation of nurses are related to the total agency needs, rather
than to a particular activity within the agency; it also provides
for flexibility in assigning staff that can be helpful in meeting
shifting program emphases or emergency needs.

Some states function under a *district* plan (New York and
Minnesota are examples) with a full-time state staff assigned to
each district. In such cases the district staff members are in effect
deputies of the state department of health. This plan does not
modify the essential relationships between state and local nurses
that are established for the department as a whole.

The *public health nursing divisions or sections* also differ in
organization from state to state. Variations will occur in (1) personnel assignment procedures and administrative lines associated
with assignment of staff; (2) relationships and lines of communication between state and local public health nursing personnel; (3) differentiation of function between specialized and
generalized consultant staff; and (4) use of citizen committees.

The development of the team concept of health work has neces-
sitated a new approach in *assignment of nursing personnel*. For
example, the development of a community-wide mental health
clinic service requires the *coordinated* services of psychiatrist,
social worker and nurse. Because services to children with behavior problems may require specialized nursing knowledge, it is
desirable to have a nurse or corps of nurses to work regularly on
the mental health team. In the past this problem was frequently
solved by the creation of a specialist group of nurses who were
employed by a particular division, and this plan is still used in
some instances. Recently, however, functional assignment—assignment of members of the public health nursing staff to another
administrative unit on a continuing basis—has been substituted
for a separate specialist corps. The nurse maintains her status
as a member and participates in the activities of the public health
nursing division. She looks to the director of public health nursing
for professional guidance and leadership. However, she reports

administratively to the division responsible for the *function* (maternal and child health or communicable disease control) of which division she is also a part. Daily work and long-range activities are planned with other members of working team, and the nurse looks to the bureau director for guidance in the technical and administrative phases of the work. Thus it is possible to secure a two-way coordination; public health nursing—as in maternal and child health—is related properly to the total public health nursing program, and is also integrally related to the total health service provided for mothers and children.

There will be infinite variety in arranging for such assignments of responsibility, and a clear understanding of lines of authority is necessary to permit team functioning without loss of professional nursing leadership.

Relationships and lines of communication between state and local nursing staffs have been profoundly influenced by the increasingly complete organization of local health services. As qualified local health officers become more prevalent and nursing staffs more adequate, local services become more independent. Public health nursing organizational patterns reflect this trend, and relationships of state personnel to local public health nursing services become more consultative and less supervisory and administrative as local units become stronger. However, in practice the range extends all the way from provision in the state division of public health nursing of some direct community nursing service and administrative supervision of other local services to a purely advisory or leadership relationship.

While there is seldom any interference in communication between local public health nurses and state supervisory or consultant staff, certain matters in public health nursing may pertain to administration of public health services as a whole. In that case the medical administrator should be consulted. In some instances, nurses will make their own plans and decisions in relation to the use of consultant service; in others, when such plans and decisions involve rearrangement of time or patterns of service, they should be made only with the knowledge and approval of some designated administrative officer. For example, if the state advisory nurse were consulting with a local nurse about improvement of skill in group and individual instruction, the only clearance necessary with the health officer might be in the selection of a conference time that does not conflict with other activities. However, if the consultation involves planning for an over-all operation, such as procedures to be used for follow-up after a mass chest x-ray program, the primary channel of communication will be through the health officer, since this aspect of the work cannot be considered apart from the whole program of tuberculosis control which is the medical director's responsibility.

Channels of communication may be very rigidly outlined, and all correspondence, contacts and recommendations may have to follow a prescribed routing. In some health departments, all outgoing correspondence goes over the signature of the health officer and no other staff member carries on any independent official correspondence whatever. In other instances, contacts and correspondence follow narrow professional lines, and the public health nurse may consult freely with the supervisory nurse, but seldom have a chance to discuss or help plan to meet the more general problems faced by the health officer in the administration of total service. In still other situations, there is a flexible policy that allows the nurse to communicate freely with state nursing staff and yet encourages inclusion of the local administrative officer in planning when it is appropriate. The public health nurse should find out how she can use consultant staff, what routines are used in requesting advisory visits and in implementing suggestions made by the consultant, then exercise good faith and good judgment in following the procedures in force.

Use of generalized and specialized consultant staff will also vary from state to state. In some instances, emphasis is placed upon specialized consultants, and they function freely and aggressively through field contacts to promote and improve nursing in a particular service. In other states, consultation is provided in large measure by the generalized advisory or supervisory staff, with specialized consultants planning with and functioning through the generalized supervisor. In the latter case the generalized consultant plans with the local nursing service for necessary visits by special consultants. The pattern will be modified in accordance with special needs and problems of the particular state. All consultant staff, of course, function through the director or supervisor of the local agency when there is one.

The state division or bureau of public health nursing may or may not use a *citizens' committee* or advisory committee. Some states have an advisory council to the whole health department that may consider and advise on nursing matters, or may have a subcommittee on nursing. Occasionally, a state public health nursing division has its own advisory committee, or may use a nursing subcommittee of a citizens' health committee that is organized independently of the health department as an advisory or interpretative group. In some cases, no provision is made for use of a citizen's committee at the state level, or the use of such a committee may be inconsistent with the philosophy or policy of the health department as a whole.

PUBLIC HEALTH NURSING IN LOCAL DEPARTMENTS OF HEALTH

The local health department is the basic service unit in the administration of public health. The major responsibilities are outlined in an official statement of the American Public Health Association, and include recording and analysis of health data, provision of health education and personal health services to the public, control and regulation of environmental health and sanitation facilities and coordination and planning for the health of the community.[12]

Local units of public health may be organized by a municipality, county or a combined city-county or multiple county health unit. With the widespread acceptance of the Emerson Report[13] it is likely that the less thickly settled areas of the country will commonly use the multiple county system, since only thus can they organize into population units large enough to make for effective use of public health personnel.

In very large cities, health center *districts* may be established to bring the facilities of the health department nearer to the people who use them. In this case, administration may be decentralized in varying degrees. Sometimes each health center is virtually independent administratively, with a complete health staff including physicians, nurses, technicians, clinical staff and aides. In other cities the health department as a whole does not decentralize its activities, but clinics or nursing services may be organized in districts of special need with branch offices established in this local center. For instance, a nursing office may be established in a housing unit or in a congested industrial section of the city.

The *basis of authority* for local health work lies in state public health law or regulations that define mandatory or permissive activities to be undertaken by local units of government. This may

12. The Local Health Department Services and Responsibilities. *American Journal of Public Health,* 45: 302–307, March, 1951.

13. Emerson, Haven and M. Luginbuhl, Local Health Units for the Nation. *New York Commonwealth Fund,* 1945.

be supplemented by municipal ordinances. While local health departments must conform to the standards and demands established by the state, there is a strong trend toward local support and control of health services, and in many larger cities the municipal health department is virtually autonomous. The executive officer is usually a medical health officer, and there is apt to be a board of health to advise him.

The *responsibility of the public health nursing division* in a local health unit is to:

1. Provide nursing service as needed to implement the basic services of the health department. This includes health guidance and teaching as well as the application of nursing skills. It also includes management functions associated with the administration of clinic or other group services, carrying out designated diagnostic procedures, and directing families to suitable sources for social assistance.

2. Coordinate and supervise the work of subsidiary nursing personnel employed by the health department. This may include practical nurses, nurses' aides and volunteer workers.

3. Participate in planning and administering the various programs and projects undertaken by the health department, especially in relation to present or potential use of nursing personnel. This includes planning for the nursing aspects of special campaigns, studies, field investigations, public relations efforts, as well as for continuing service programs.

4. Study and appraise public health nursing work, and make such adaptations as are necessary to meet local conditions and needs. This includes continuing careful analysis of the use of nursing time and skills; staff training in new skills or fields of information as required.

5. Provide leadership or participation in the coordination of community nursing services. Nursing service may be provided almost entirely by the health department in the small community that has practically no other nursing service available. For example, in a rural county the public health nurse may know and use the few inactive nurses, practical nurses or the few private practice or hospital nurses available, and assist in coordinating their efforts in a purely informal way. In a larger community a representative of the health department nursing staff may sit on planning boards or committees, or participate in the deliberations of a local nursing council that serves as a coordinating force.

6. Organize and use citizen groups for interpretation, promotion and guidance of the nursing service in coordination with other health department personnel concerned with community organization.

7. Participate in recruitment and training of public health nurses and related personnel as consistent with the needs and the facilities of the agency for providing such assistance. Planning and supervising field experience for nursing students and participation in the training of other public health personnel, as well as incidental services such as talks or demonstrations to selected groups, may be included in this activity.

The *organization of nursing in the over-all structure* of the local health department may be in a separate bureau or department, or it may be incorporated into another department such as administration or preventive health services. Sometimes nursing is placed in one or another of the special service divisions, such as child hygiene or communicable disease. The latter pattern presents obvious difficulties in securing a balanced public health nursing program.

Even when there is no specified division of public health nursing, a nurse-director should be responsible for general technical supervision and direction of the nursing program as a whole. In a small service, one nurse may be designated as a supervisor although she also carries direct service responsibilities as well. This director is responsible to the health officer or his designated deputy for the nursing program. In multiple country health units this administrative supervisor or director may be an employee of the state health department assigned to the local unit. She then becomes administratively responsible to the local health officer and functions under his general direction.

In multiple county units where an individual nurse in a particular county may have to work alone much of the time, a local committee may be appointed to serve in advisory capacity to her, and in some instances to take limited administrative responsibility, as in the selection of a nurse or in arranging for her annual leave. A part-time local health officer may also be employed, and the public health nurse may be responsible to him for certain aspects of her program.

Citizen's committees or advisory committees are much more frequently found in health departments than was formerly the case, and often these include a nursing committee. Such committees rarely assume more than advisory functions.

The *nursing division or component in the local health unit* is almost always organized under a director or supervisor even though the number of nurses is small. In very small independent health jurisdictions where the local health department organization is not complete, the public health nurse may work relatively independently, with general supervision and advice provided by the state public health nursing division staff. She may be administratively responsible to a part-time health officer, to a county board of supervisors, to a county board of health or to a special nursing committee. Such loose organization is, of course, fraught with danger of poor and ill-directed nursing care.

In larger services the pattern may be similar to that found in the state health departments, including generalized and specialized supervisors and consultants, as well as a director. Administrative assignment of public health nursing personnel to other divisions or service units may proceed much as described in relation to state divisions of public health nursing.

When health center districts have been organized within a local health jurisdiction, a public health nursing supervisor and staff are usually assigned to each district. The public health nursing staff works under the administrative direction of the district health officer. Nursing (technical and professional) leadership and direction will be provided by the director of the nursing bureau or division through the district supervising nurse.

Occasionally, nurses are employed for a specialized service and function entirely under the director of a bureau or division other than nursing. For example, a group of nurses may be employed by the director of the Division of Child Hygiene, and another by the Division of Preventable Disease Control, with each group of nurses working independently of the other. Such an organizational pattern is usually considered incompatible with full utilization of nursing skills and time.

Despite the bewildering variety of organizational patterns of public health nursing in local health departments, certain elements appear consistently. Some relics of the past remain in the form of uncoordinated, specialized public health nursing, or public health nursing that is not related to a soundly organized public health service. However, the trend is definitely toward the centralization of responsibility for the total nursing program under the direction of a qualified nurse director. The line of responsibility to the district, city or unit medical health officer is clear and close in most instances, without detraction from the importance of professional-technical supervision provided by the nurse director or supervisor.

PUBLIC HEALTH NURSING IN SCHOOLS

The protection of the health of children in schools is a joint responsibility of departments of health and education. The *authority* for health work in schools is derived from state and local public health and education laws and regulations.

The school accepts responsibility for providing a safe and healthful environment for learning, and for teaching healthful living as part of the total education of the student. The health department is in turn obligated to protect the health of its school-age citizens as well as the rest of the population.

Public health nursing responsibilities in schools include:
1. Providing necessary nursing care, including:
    a. Emergency care or other nursing service that is needed during the school day.
    b. Health counseling to individual students and their parents.
    c. Participation in health appraisal procedures offered by the school. This includes supervision of the teacher's daily inspection of pupils; providing inspection for special conditions as necessary; assisting with medical examinations; carrying out or supervising diagnostic procedures, such as vision tests, audiometer or other hearing tests, or tuberculosis tests; assisting in preparation for the follow-up of group-testing procedures.
2. Providing consultant service to teachers, student or parent groups or others as necessary.
3. Contribution to the instructional program as consistent with the over-all educational plan and the nurse's preparation. This may vary from serving as a "resource person" in student health projects to carrying a regular instructional program in a special field, such as home nursing. Nurses who provide regular classroom instruction must usually meet requirements for appointment as teachers.

Organization of public health nursing in schools may be under the auspices of either the health department or the department of education. In 1954 it was reported that 54 percent of the public school systems having school health services in cities of 2500 or more population were staffed with "specialized" nurses, 38 percent were served by generalized public health nurses provided through the health department, 8 percent had no nurse.[14] What-

14. Yankauer, Alfred, Public Health Nursing in the Schools. *Nursing Outlook*, 2: 197–199, April, 1954.

ever the sponsorship, the organizational pattern must take cognizance of the dual line of responsibility; public health nursing in schools is an essential part of both the community health program and of the educational program.

When public health nursing in schools is provided by the health department, it may be offered as part of a comprehensive nursing service, with a single nurse spending part of her time in the school and part in other public health nursing activities. In large cities, nurses may be assigned for school service only, either on a rotating or on a permanent basis. During the period when nurses are placed in school service on a full-time basis, they may be administratively assigned to a division other than public health nursing, such as the division of child hygiene, or the division of school health.

Whether nursing service is provided to the schools on a full- or part-time basis, it should be clear that in all matters relating to student instruction or school management the public health nursing service is the responsibility of the school authorities. This responsibility may be channeled through the school physician or school medical service, or the nurse may report directly to the superintendent of schools or school principal on certain aspects of her work. In matters relating to community health protection, such as the enforcement of regulations regarding communicable disease control, the school nursing service is the responsibility of the health department.

For instance, a school nurse would plan with the school principal or superintendent for such matters as conferences with teachers, group activities, tests or inspections, removal of hazards from the school environment. She will plan with the director or supervisor of nurses in the health department (or in some instances directly with the health officer) regarding follow-up to be provided for students with positive reactions to tuberculin tests, instruction of the family in communicable disease care and standards for testing vision or hearing.

This fundamental relationship and pattern of responsibility should not change whether the nurse is employed by the department or board of education rather than by the department of health, except that the employing body would determine conditions of employment such as salary, leave and hours of work. In practice, school nursing services may not have this direct association with both health and education departments. Cooperation and joint planning may be maintained by agreements made between boards of health and education, or between the health officer and superintendent of schools. The continuing nursing contacts between school and community nurse that produce an integrated school-community service may have to be assured by informal contacts between individual workers. However, if the basic principle of dual responsibility is accepted and opportunities for systematic joint planning and action in nursing are used to the fullest, a good functioning organizational relationship can be developed.

NURSING IN VOLUNTARY PUBLIC HEALTH AGENCIES

Voluntary health agencies may be national in scope, with or without state and local affiliated associations, or they may be regional or local in coverage. They may be primarily concerned with a specific health problem, such as tuberculosis or child health, or with a specific service, such as visiting nurse service. They may provide direct public health nursing services or be limited to consultative, standard-setting or research activities.

The *authority* for voluntary health services is usually vested in a governing board or board of directors. However, the voluntary agency must function within the legal restrictions relative to incorporation and to the establishment of a charitable agency that are part of the general welfare or public health laws of the respective states.

The general *responsibilities* of public health nursing in voluntary agencies are to:

1. Provide nursing services to implement the stated objectives of the agency. In general these objectives will be directed toward services that supplement or precede public health nursing in governmental agencies. The service may be sharply limited in scope or population served, in the types of care offered.
2. Relate nursing services of the voluntary agency to those of the official tax-supported agency. This will be done through:
   a. Periodic joint program planning;
   b. Encouragement of assumption of responsibility of governmental agencies for basic health services, and withdrawal from services that are fundamental health department responsibilities;
   c. Case management conferences.
3. Provide a channel for education of the public.
4. Provide an opportunity for expression of the community's

desire to help. Through the voluntary nursing agency, citizens have an opportunity to contribute money or services to help meet community needs not otherwise provided for.

5. Provide advisory and consultant services. This is particularly a function of national associations, such as the National Tuberculosis Association or the National Foundation for Infantile Paralysis, which provide field staff, teaching and reference materials and direct consultation upon request. At present these two national agencies provide nursing field consultation planned with and administered by the National League for Nursing.

The *organization* of nursing within the voluntary agency will, of course, vary greatly with the primary purpose of the agency, its size, scope and coverage.

In the visiting nurse association where nursing is the sole agency function, authority is usually vested in a board of directors. The nursing staff, through its director, reports to the board of directors or to an executive or nursing committee designated by the board of directors.

General medical direction is most frequently secured through the use of a medical advisory committee or through agreement to use the local medical society in such a capacity. Medical direction in relation to individual patient or family care is the responsibility of the family or clinic physician or other medical supervisor.

Within the nursing staff itself a *director* of nurses is usually the executive head of the service. General or specialized supervisors report to her; staff nurses report through the generalized supervisors.

When the voluntary agency embraces service other than nursing, as in settlement house or welfare organizations, patterns of organization are highly individualized. In such instances nurses may be assigned to work with a child health clinic, or to a welfare or relief unit. This is comparable to the functional assignment previously discussed in relation to governmental agencies. Professional direction continues to be supplied by the nurse director and supervisory staff.

ORGANIZATION OF COMBINATION AGENCIES

Sometimes two or more agencies under official or under voluntary auspices decide to join forces in order to provide more economical or more effective public health nursing.[15]

15. National Organization for Public Health Nursing, *A Study of Combination Services in Public Health Nursing.* New York, 1950.

In such situations the combination agency absorbs the general responsibilities of all of its members. Funds may come from taxes, from fees or from voluntary contributions collected independently or through the Community Chest or endowments. Authority for the various functions is the same as for the functions when carried by independent agencies.

A combination public health nursing service is by definition one that is jointly administered by both governmental and voluntary agencies with all field service rendered by a single staff of public health nurses.[16] However, many transitional programs are found and the pattern ranges all the way from two independently organized units consolidated by the employment of a single director of nurses and a small jointly used top staff, to complete amalgamation. The patterns described below are typical:

1. Administration by a single agency with the second agency buying the service which it sponsors. For example, a social welfare division may buy home nursing service for recipients of old age pensions from a visiting nurse association, or a community chest may provide funds to the local health department to pay for visiting nurse service or practical nursing care to chronically ill, to be supervised by the public health nursing staff.

2. Independent funds and control with coordinated service. For example, a visiting nurse association might raise its funds, determine scope of service, and set personnel policies for staff employed by that association with the health department maintaining similar separate budgets and policy-making procedures. However, within this framework nursing service functions under a single director, and the individual nurse, whether employed by the visiting nurse association or by the health department, would carry out the functions of both agencies, so that the service rendered to the family is given by a single worker. Coordination is maintained at the policy-making level by planning committees, councils or other policy-making bodies.

3. Completely integrated programs with pooled funds and staff and a joint directing board. In this instance, responsibility for certain aspects of the work may have to be allocated to one or the other of the component groups; for example, the health department or board of health cannot legally share its specific responsibilities with a voluntary group, nor can an incorporated voluntary group relinquish its responsibility

16. Ibid.

to account for the expenditure of its funds and to maintain adequate financial records. Some principles for the development and administration of combination services have been developed, and include essentially, recognition of the need for:

a. continuance of voluntary support;
b. inclusion of care for the sick and to make it available to all who need it, with fees adjusted to the individuals' capacity to pay;
c. a well-organized health department with a qualified medical director, and a nursing director responsible for direction of nursing service;
d. representative community planning and written agreements;
e. active use of citizen and medical advisory groups.[17]

ORGANIZATION OF INDUSTRIAL OR PROPRIETARY GROUPS

Many industrial concerns and privately sponsored health or welfare services provide public health nursing services to their employees or to their members. Some will quibble at the inclusion of nurses who work for profit-making groups as public health nurses. However, since their potential contribution to public health is great, and their functions very similar, they are included here. Instructing the pregnant wife of a steel worker contributes to the worker's peace of mind and thus reduces his susceptibility to accident with its attendant loss of work and compensation costs; talks on baby care by the department store nurse not only build good will which increases sales within the store, but also increase maternal efficiency and contribute to the infant health program in the community. Meticulous instruction in eye hygiene at the doctor's office not only increases the patient's confidence in the medical care he is receiving and discourages shopping around from one doctor to another, but it also serves a public health purpose in preventing unnecessary handicap.

Authority for such health service is provided by boards of directors of the organization either directly or through delegation to the executive or management officers of the corporation. This authority is written into the directives of the company or may be incorporated into the by-laws or regulations of an organization.

Responsibilities of public health nurses in industrial or commercial agencies include:

1. Providing nursing care as specified by company or organ-

17. *Progress Report on Combination Services in Public Health Nursing.* New York, National League for Nursing, 1955, p. 33.

ization policy. Health counseling is assumed to be an integral part of all nursing care. This may include infirmary care, emergency nursing, health instruction and counseling and home nursing care. Sometimes care of family members is provided as well and a general public health service is rendered.

2. Relating nursing care to the over-all organization objectives. For example, the nurse in industry should use nursing as a positive force in increasing production, promoting employee satisfaction, contributing to good personnel relations, as well as to provide necessary health care and instruction. The nurse in the private clinic should encourage intelligent use of clinic facilities and promote good patient-physician relationships.

3. Participating in planning and promotion of related health activities. For example, the nurse in industry will participate in safety instruction and care; the nurse in a department store will participate in the "grooming" classes that have definite health aspects; the nurse in industry or in a private clinic will participate in minimizing environmental hazards by observing and reporting conditions that may affect health. Cooperation with welfare and personnel departments in industry is especially important.

4. Interpreting and using community facilities for health and nursing care. Health department regulations may need to be interpreted to industrial workers or clinic patients; physicians' patients may be referred to a Red Cross home nursing class or to the Visiting Nurse Association for further instruction; or families of workers may be referred to hospital clinics for necessary health care.

In larger organizations, public health nursing is apt to be organized within a medical department under the direction of a medical director. In small industries, public health nursing may be organized as a unit in the personnel service, or as a separate unit directly responsible to top management, with medical direction provided by part-time physicians.

COMMUNITY ORGANIZATION FOR PUBLIC HEALTH NURSING

Community planning must be based primarily upon needs for care rather than upon agency objectives. It must consider not only those patients already under care, but also those who need care for which there is no present program.

Community planning groups must concern themselves with the needs of the well-to-do as well as those of the poor, of white and non-white, of urban, suburban and rural dwellers. They must consider whether "means tests" as a prerequisite for care are preventing those in the middle and upper income groups from getting the care they need; whether segregated services are producing a two-level pattern of care, whether the needs of those in outlying areas are given equal concern with those in the center of population. Most voluntary as well as official agencies have accepted the obligation to provide service to those who need it regardless of race, creed or color. However, there has been less agreement about the responsibility of the public agency toward the nonindigent group, and of well-organized city voluntary agencies for those people who work in the city and live outside city boundaries where visiting nurse services are not available.

Concern for community-wide needs does not negate the importance of experimental studies, or when necessary of limited service to designated types of patients. It implies, however, that such limited programs will be considered in the light of their immediate and projected impact on total community care.

The goal should be to provide comprehensive public health nursing care, including home care of the sick, for all who need it. To achieve this, each agency functioning in the community must see its place in the total structure. Frequent review and re-evaluation is necessary, since a change of program in one agency will often affect all others in the community. For example, if the health department inaugurates a cancer diagnostic service it is highly probable that the improved case finding will increase demands made upon the visiting nurse service for home care.

Such community-wide planning may be centered in the health department, or in a community health council, committee or commission or council of social agencies. Such a planning structure helps agencies and groups decide whether new services should be instituted or old ones expanded and provides the machinery for orderly allocation and rearrangement of responsibility for the various phases of nursing among the several health programs.[18] It provides a channel through which service agencies and professional organizations can synthesize their findings and actions and bring to the public a fair statement of their progress and unmet needs in health care. Community-wide planning helps to set the framework within which such cooperative action can be made effective and economical.

18. Local Leagues and Local Councils. *Nursing Outlook,* 1: 283, May, 1952.

Maximum Coordination of Existing Programs. Coordination of existing programs may be achieved through combined organizational or administrative structure, interlocking committees and planning and evaluation teams (including the community-wide planning groups referred to above) and through referral and case consultation systems.

A statement issued in 1946 by the NOPHN (now the National League for Nursing) and reaffirmed at a 1952 conference on home care of the sick suggests three possible types of organization of public health nursing services,[19] as follows:

"All public health nursing services, including care of the sick at home, administered and supported by the health department. This is the usual pattern for rural communities.

"Preventive services carried by the health department with one voluntary agency working in close coordination with the health department carrying responsibility for nursing care of the sick and for some special fields. This type of organization is the most usual one found in large areas.

"A combination nursing service jointly administered and jointly financed by official and voluntary agencies with all field service given by a single group of public health nurses. Such a combination of services is especially desirable in small cities."

Whatever the organizational pattern there should be some definite method for placing responsibility and for considering community nursing service as a whole in its relation to other nursing and health services. Provision should be made for periodic review and appraisal, and for re-planning of programs to assure maximum use of available resources.

Citizen Participation. A strong public health nursing program requires the counsel and assistance of related professional groups and of general citizens in all phases of planning and effectuating the programs. For this reason the community-wide planning groups referred to above should include representation from the consumers of nursing service as well as professional workers in the field. Voluntary agencies have depended upon such citizen guidance and support from the beginning. Health departments are more and more using citizens' advisory committees to provide a channel of communication between the department and the public, and to bring to the planning and

19. Desirable Organization for Public Health Nursing for Family Service. *Public Health Nursing*, 38: 387–89, August, 1946. Also in *Home Care of the Sick*. New York, National League for Nursing, 1953, p. 10.

operation of the community the expectations, understanding and special competences of an interested lay group.

Referral Systems. In addition to securing broad policy and directional planning and agency consideration of function in relation to total community structure, some machinery is needed to assure patients and families of continuous correlated care by the many agencies with which they will have contact. The cardiac patient, for example, may have intermittent hospital care, home care with supervision by a private physician, and convalescent home care. If nursing services are to be provided smoothly and without interruption in each phase of care, a system must be devised for referral and communication among the agencies involved. This problem is discussed more fully in Chapter XIV. Some arrangement for regular case conference for exchange of information by reports or notification systems and for agreement on who shall do what for particular types of patient is essential.

Criteria for Good Organization. Organizational patterns of public health nursing in agencies and in communities are not standardized. They must differ in accordance with many factors if they are to meet the basic requirement for any organization—that they facilitate and further the work.

However, some criteria of good organization may be identified. Good organization for community nursing care:

1. is designed to bring comprehensive, continuing nursing care to all who need it;
2. recognizes the fundamental obligation of the official health department to be concerned with the total health care of the community, and to assure basic preventive and health promotional services;
3. provides for a combined approach of all involved in care to prevent duplication or confusion in services, to hold ineffective time to a minimum, to encourage experimentation, and to make full use of voluntary as well as governmental resources;
4. recognizes the responsibility and right of the public to share in health planning and action;
5. relates public health nursing as an integral rather than a separate part of the comprehensive program for public health, and to other community services for health care;
6. provides for team assignment of public health nursing with the functional units operating public health services (such as maternal and child health service teams), and also for

identification and joint action with nursing as a whole within the agency or community;

7. provides for medical direction in all work involving medical care;

8. provides for nurse leadership for nursing phases of the work, including professional direction of nursing practice.

SUGGESTED READINGS

Part I

Addams, Ruth and Iva Torrens, Home Nursing Care for Veterans. *Nursing Outlook*, 4: 497–499, September, 1956.

A Study of Selected Home Care Programs, *Public Health Monograph*, Number 35. Washington, D.C., Government Printing Office, 1955.

American Nurses' Association, *Facts About Nursing*. New York, American Nurses' Association. Published annually.

American Public Health Association Resolution, 1953. *American Journal of Public Health*, 44: 134, January, 1954.

The Local Health Department—Services and Responsibilities. *American Journal of Public Health*, 41: 302–307, March, 1951.

The State Health Department—An Official Statement of the American Public Health Association. *American Journal of Public Health*, 44: 235–252, February, 1954.

Anderson, Gaylord W., Public Health—A Mandate from the People. *American Journal of Public Health*, 42: 1367–1373, November, 1952.

Anderson, O. W., The Effectiveness of Voluntary Health Insurance. *Hospitals*, 30: 13–24, July 1, 1956.

Bixler, G. and Roy Bixler, Professional Status of Nursing. *American Journal of Nursing*, 45: 730, September, 1945.

Brown, E. Lucille, *Nursing for the Future*. New York, Russell Sage Foundation, 1948.

Buell, Bradley and Associates, *Community Planning for Human Services*. New York, Columbia University Press, 1952.

Caplan, Gerald, The Mental Hygiene Role of the Nurse in Maternal and Child Care. *Nursing Outlook*, 2: 14–19, January, 1954.

Cleere, R. L., State Health Councils. *Public Health Reports*, 70: 1143–1144, September, 1955.

Constitution of the World Health Organization. *Public Health Reports*, 61: 1268–1279, August 30, 1946.

Coulter, Pearl, *The Nurse in the Public Health Program*. New York, G. P. Putnam's, 1954.

De Benneville, A. K., Financing Voluntary Public Health Nursing Services. *Nursing Outlook*, 2: 185–186, April, 1954.

Department of Public Health Nursing, *National League for Nursing Progress Report in Combination Services*. New York, National League for Nursing, 1955.

Derryberry, Mayhew, Today's Health Problems and Health Education. *Public Health Reports*, 69: 1224–1228, December, 1954.

Desirable Organization of Public Health Nursing for Family Service. *Public Health Nursing*, 38: 387–389, August, 1946.

Dunbar, H., *Emotions and Bodily Change*. New York, Columbia University Press, 1946.

Emerson, Haven, and Martha Luginbuhl, *Local Health Units for the Nation*. Cambridge, Harvard University Press, 1945.

Emory, Florence M., *Public Health Nursing in Canada*. New York, Macmillan Co., 1953.

Farris, W. B., Trends in Public Health: in Public Health Service Agencies. *Nursing Outlook*, 2: 356–358, July, 1954.

Fry, Vera, The Creative Approach to Nursing. *American Journal of Nursing*, 53: 301–302, March, 1953.

Financing Local Health Services. *American Journal of Public Health*, 45: 965–968, August, 1955.

Gardner, Mary S., *Public Health Nursing*, 3rd ed. New York, Macmillan Co., 1936.

Hartigan, Helen, Nursing Responsibilities in Rehabilitation. *Nursing Outlook*, 2: 649–651, December, 1954.

Hubbard, Ruth, The Nurse in the Healing Arts Team. *American Journal of Nursing*, 49: 27, January, 1949.

Joint Commission of the Association of American Medical Colleges and the American Association of Medical Social Workers, *Widening Horizons in Medical Education*. New York, Commonwealth Fund, 1948.

Kohler, A. Y., The Place of the Public Health Nurse in Private Medical Practice. *Nursing Outlook*, 1: 528–529, September, 1953.

Leavell, Hugh, New Occasions Teach New Duties. *Public Health Reports*, 68: 687–692, July, 1953.

Local Leagues and Local Councils. *Nursing Outlook*, 1: 283, May, 1953.

Mead, M., Nursing—Primitive and Civilized. *American Journal of Nursing*, 56: 1001–1004, August, 1956.

Merry, E. S. and Iris Iruen, *District Nursing*. Baltimore, Williams & Wilkins Co., 1948.

McIver, Pearl, Trends in Public Health: in Public Health Nursing. *Nursing Outlook*, 2: 352, 356, July, 1954.

Muller, J. N. and Bierman, P., Cooperation between Departments of Health and Welfare. *Public Health Reports*, 71: 833, September, 1956.

National League for Nursing, *School Nursing Services*. New York, The League, 1956.

National Organization for Public Health Nursing, *A Study of Combination Services in Public Health Nursing*. New York, National Organization for Public Health Nursing, 1950.

Nurses Invest in Patient Care. New York, American Nurses Association, 1956.

Paul, B. D., *Health, Culture and Community*. New York, Russell Sage Foundation, 1955.

The Public Health Service Today. Washington, Government Printing Office, 1955.

Roberts, Mary M., *American Nursing: History and Interpretation.* New York, Macmillan Co., 1954; Chapter 9, "The Rise of Public Health Nursing"; Chapter 20, "Changing Emphasis in Public Health Nursing"; Chapter 46, "Evolutionary Adjustments in Nursing Services."

Saunders, Lyle, *Cultural Differences and Medical Care.* New York, Russell Sage Foundation, 1954.

Saunders, Lyle, The Changing Role of Nurses. *American Journal of Nursing,* 54: 1094–1098, September, 1954.

Scheele, L. A., The Wide Spectrum of Our Health Services. *Public Health Reports,* 71: 26–33, January, 1956.

Simmons, L. W., *Social Science in Medicine.* New York, Russell Sage Foundation, 1954.

Smillie, W. G., *Public Health Administration in the United States.* New York, Macmillan Co., 1952.

Smith, Lucille, Tax Supported General Medical Care for the Needy. *American Journal of Public Health,* 42: 56–62, January, 1952.

Spicer, E., *Human Problems in Technological Change.* New York, Russell Sage Foundation, 1952.

Terris, Milton and Nathan Kramer, *General Medical Care Programs in Local Health Departments.* New York, American Public Health Association, 1951.

Wilensky, Harold L., Changing Patterns of Family Life. *Children,* 3: 163–169, September-October, 1956.

Winch, Robert F., *The Modern Family.* New York: Henry Holt, 1953.

Wishik, Samuel, M., Administrative Jurisdiction of the School Health Service. *American Journal of Public Health,* 41: 819–823, July, 1951.

Woodbury, Coleman, Suburbanization and Suburbia. *American Journal of Public Health,* 45: 1–14, January, 1955.

Wooton, Barbara, *Freedom under Planning.* Chapel Hill, University of North Carolina Press, 1945.

World Health Organization. *Nursing Outlook,* 2: 358, July, 1954.

Yankauer, A., Gross, K. G. and S. M. Romeno, An Evaluation of Prenatal Care and Its Relationship to Social Class and Social Disorganization. *American Journal of Public Health,* 43: 1001–1010, August, 1953.

Your Children's Bureau in the U.S. Department of Health, Education, and Welfare. Washington, Government Printing Office, 1956.

Services to Individuals and Families

CHAPTER VI

Objectives and
Methods in Family
Nursing Care

FAMILY HEALTH care is the concern of many agencies and professional workers—in schools, hospitals, medical care programs, and in legislative bodies that have responsibility for social and health measures. The best of prenatal nursing supervision cannot be fully effective without legislation providing for assistance that will enable the widow to care for her own child; or without the understanding and approval of the private physician for the care afforded his patients.

Health care should provide, for all in the community, the following general benefits:

1. Adequate, continuing medical supervision, preventive as well as diagnostic and therapeutic. Whether in hospitals, or at home, work or school, families should have care when it is needed, and know that licensure laws, inspectional procedures and social planning are such that medical care will be safe and adequate.

2. An environment that is conducive to health and safety. Families need safe milk and water supplies, regulations or subsidies that provide for decent housing and freedom from unnecessary exposure to illness or injury at home, work or school or on the highway.

3. Education for competent health maintenance. This should

be an integral part of the total educational program of the community, supplemented by adult education by health, educational, and welfare agencies.

4. Individual counseling or advisory services when they are needed to assist with health problems.

5. Assistance with social or economic problems as necessary to permit satisfactory health action.

In all of these, nursing will play an important part. Because she has an intimate and continuing contact with families the public health nurse has a pivotal place. She is often the channel through which vital information flows to the families who need it; she may be the medium by which scientific information is translated into family plans for action; she is often the one who first sees needs for community action to meet health problems formerly unrecognized.

The objectives and methods of public health nursing grow out of the application of comprehensive family nursing care discussed in earlier chapters to the concept of the things people have a right to expect from the total community program for health care.

Over-all Objectives of Family Nursing Care.   The first question that must be answered is "What should public health nursing *do* for families?" Within the framework of providing comprehensive nursing care, certain objectives may be identified. The objects are:

1. To discover and appraise health problems through combining public health nursing efforts with those of other professional workers, of the family and of the community.

   Ferguson, analyzing nurses' service loads found that of 2558 productive visits studied in an urban health department, 34.3 per cent involved social, emotional and economic problems, separately or in combination, and that the average number of health problems per visit was 4.02.[1] Often the reason for which nursing service was originally requested proved to be just the springboard to other, sometimes more significant, problems. Because of the commitment to a comprehensive and family-centered approach, the public health nurse is frequently a case finder. She may find need for cancer diagnostic service in a family member while visiting a woman for prenatal care, or find a need for behavioral

1. Ferguson, Marion, *The Service Load of a Staff Nurse in One Official Agency.* New York, Bureau of Publications, Teachers College, Columbia University, 1945, pp. 19–35.

guidance when the precipitating forerunner of referral was follow-up of a communicable disease.

Appraisal of the problem as a problem is also important in establishing objectives for public health nursing service. What is an overwhelming problem to one family may present no problem or a very minor one to another. For example, mothers will vary greatly in their capacity to "cope."[2] The arrival of a second baby when the mother is tense, overly concerned about the first child, and awkward and anxious in carrying out her maternal obligations may be a very real problem. For another mother who is calm, manages well with the first baby and is happy and relaxed in her attitude toward pregnancy and childbirth, the problem is a minimal one. Referral and nursing needs will differ widely even though the physical and economic situations are the same.

The nurse does not make this appraisal alone. The physician will, of course, take all responsibility for diagnosis of a medical condition, and will participate in appraising the emotional and social factors in the family that affect its meaning to the family, and may influence the methods of treatment that are indicated. The teacher or behavior clinic psychiatrist will be invaluable in assessing the degree of insecurity a school child feels, and what help he and his family needs to build greater security. Most of all the family itself will know to what extent they feel insecure or baffled by health situations which demand some action.

2. To ensure family understanding and acceptance of problems.

Often families have problems which they do not recognize or accept as such. The overstrict father may not recognize that he has a problem in a child who is "so good," but who bites his fingernails and shows other signs of tension. Or families may look upon a problem of mental illness as a disgrace rather than as an illness which needs to be accepted and treated as such.

3. To provide or secure nursing services that the family needs and cannot provide for itself.

Nursing needs are relative. Some families, for example, can give sustained care to a querulous long-term patient with safety and comfort to the patient, and without undue stress

2. Spence, J. A., *A Thousand Families in Newcastle on Tyne*. London, Oxford University Press, 1954, Chapter 18.

for the family. In other families the same situation may demand a great deal of supportive nursing service, even though the family has the physical and intellectual capacity to provide care, because attitudes of frustration and resentment interfere.

4. To develop the competence of each family and individual to think through and cope with their own health problems.

The parent who is contemplating the wisdom of having polio vaccine for a child should see the question as it relates to total health care—he or she should see why certain sources of information are better than others in health matters, why the matter should be discussed with the family physician. Home accident prevention also provides an opportunity for relation to the total problem of preventing illness, and securing early attention for accidents or any deviation from normal health. The broad approach should leave the parent informed in relation to the specific problem, but should also contribute to his or her general health competence. Similarly, the school child coming to the health room for a first-aid dressing for a cut should not only have his finger dressed, but he should also learn something about preventing such accidents, about the reasons for a sterile dressing and the ways he could give first-aid care at home.

5. To contribute to the personal and social development of individuals and families through health activities.

Health activities offer many opportunities to contribute to personal and social development. The clinic patient can learn to know and respect members of other racial or economic groups through planned grouping and communication during the waiting period; the patient with long-term disabling illness may discover a real capacity to help others if he is asked to write to new patients or to those who are discouraged or alone, or if he is taught to do special tasks for the family that they will appreciate.

6. To promote full and intelligent use of available facilities and services for medical care, health promotion and illness prevention and for related social and educational facilities.

Making facilities available does not guarantee their use—many cancer diagnostic clinics are under-attended, and recently a proved vaccine which was in short supply for one year went begging the next year because of lack of public demand. Seeking medical care only during the last trimester of pregnancy, and failing to discuss with the family physician those minor ills which may have real significance are other examples. In some cases overuse, too, may be a problem—when hospitalization coverage encourages overuse of hospital care, or thoughtlessness or lack of information results in use of private duty nurses when they are in short supply and not actually needed by the patient, or when attendance at clinic is overfrequent in relation to the health situation.

7. To bring to families an understanding of non-nursing health services, within or outside the agency in which the nurse is working, and to provide the families with the necessary information and encouragement to use resources wisely and fully.

For example, sanitation services in a rural area may include testing water for nitrates or for possible disease-causing organisms, or x-ray examination of the chest may be available at work or through the health department. The family should know the importance of using such help, what follow-up is indicated, and the relation between these and other health care activities.

In line with the discussion of process and functions in earlier chapters, it is obvious that these objectives for family service require active participation of the family, and a high level of self-determination. They also require close coordination of nurses with other professional workers, since virtually none of these activities can be carried on in isolation. The methods employed, therefore, must be suited to this "doing with" rather than "doing for" approach; they must be related to the activities of the whole health team, and they must be feasible of accomplishment in the situation.

The Family As a Unit of Service.   Public health nurses have traditionally focussed on the family as a unit of service, and there is increasing recognition of the validity of this approach by other public health disciplines. A recent article, pressing for the collection of more statistical data based on the family as a unit, stressed that many of the ills of individuals have their genesis in family maladjustments, and that health, illness or recovery of the sick almost always occurs within the context of the family.[3] The interdependence of family members, and the depth

3. Dunn, Halbert and Mort Gilbert, Public Health Begins in the Family. *Public Health Reports*, 71: 1002–1010, October, 1956.

of impact of family health upon the individual require that every public health nursing service take cognizance of this unit in diagnosis, in planning and in carrying out necessary health action.

In achieving this family approach, the nurse must recognize that there are aspects of family health that are distinct from the additive health characteristics of individual family members. Distribution of responsibility among family members or the general emotional tone of the home may have important health implications, as well as the pregnancy or illness of one of the family members.

Even when the work of the nurse is organized around individual service—as it may be in an industrial plant or clinic— and another agency assumes responsibility for other members of the family, there is need to see the individual in his relationship to his family. The accident-prone school child may be affected by a sense of isolation from his family or by family pressures on him to succeed in school; the diabetic patient in the clinic is going to have to consider his diet in the context of the eating habits of the whole family—his problem is affected by the person who does the cooking and by what foods other members of the family like or dislike. By careful planning with other health workers, or by inviting family members to come in to discuss problems in the school, industrial plant or clinic, the nurse may fulfill her obligation to be concerned about the family as a whole, even though her position is set up on an individual service basis.

Family-Nurse Contact.   The basic method of delivering public health nursing service is the family-nurse contact. This may be defined as any activity with or on behalf of a particular family or individual.[4] The nursing contact may be a home visit, clinic, or industrial or school conference, telephone conference, or group contact. It excludes services directed toward general education of the public or for general advisement or consultation with other professional workers. For example, a conference with a school-teacher to help appraise the degree of fatigue exhibited by a school child, and to work out a rest schedule to compensate for it would be a family-nurse contact. A teacher-nurse conference to consider methods of keeping school health behavior records would be a general or a nonfamily service, since it is not directed toward a specific family or individual service.

4. This is an adaptation of the term "patient-nurse-contact" developed by Ferguson in conjunction with a study of nursing needs, as the most descriptive of the nursing service unit.

Indirect services—such as relay instruction by training home nursing instructors who will in turn train family members in chronic-illness care; or instruction of the nurse in the physician's office, the nurse then teaching the patients under the physician's supervision—are also useful adjuncts to the nurse's service to families and will be considered separately.

Selecting the Type of Family-Nurse Contact.   The decision as to the type of family-nurse contact that will be made in relation to a particular family situation will be highly individualized. Many types of contact will be used by the public health nurse, and require that the nurse use considerable judgment in relation to the method selected. Basic to choosing a particular approach is some understanding of the advantages and disadvantages of each.

The *home visit* is the traditional approach of public health nursing service and remains one of the most frequently used and highly regarded methods of providing service. The advantages of the home visit over other methods are:

1. The home visit permits the nurse to see the home and family situation in action, and is apt to provide a more accurate appraisal of family relationships, facilities and competences than could otherwise be secured.
2. The home visit permits teaching in the actual situation, without need for the family to make a transition from general instruction to their own facilities or equipment. For example, the diabetic patient can be taught how to use his own equipment in carrying out insulin injections, to set aside a specific place to keep the syringe and needles, and to see that the light and furniture in his own home are such that it is a comfortable place for him to work.
3. The family members are less hesitant to raise questions than they might be in another situation, since they realize this visit time is theirs alone, and need not be shared by others.
4. The nurse has an opportunity to observe actual care given by family members and thus check on the instruction given and on the family's understanding of the basic principles involved in care.
5. The family gains confidence in this direct, personalized contact. Its members obtain support from the nurse's presence.
6. The home visit provides an opportunity to seek out new health problems. For example, a home visit to supervise the mother's ability to give a baby his bath may reveal home accident hazards, need for re-structuring homemaking tasks

to release time and energy for maternal responsibilities, or untreated health conditions in other family members.

For all of these reasons, home visits are expected to have a high productivity in relation to influencing or changing health behavior. However, there are some disadvantages to this method of providing nursing care. These are:

1. The home visit is expensive in time, and if there are a large number of families needing nursing care it may mean that not all who need care can be reached. For example, if there are 100 families needing nursing supervision during the postnatal period, there may be nursing time for home visiting for only half that number. If home visits only were used, there might be an inadequate number to each family to accomplish the purpose of the nursing service, or a large number of those who need care might not be given service. The use of a less time-consuming method for some of the group might be indicated.

2. Distractions in the home may make instruction difficult. If the mother learning about care of a new baby is diverted by having to watch toddlers or by the fact that the children or her husband will soon be home for a lunch which is still not prepared, it may be difficult for her to profit from the nursing visit.

3. The home visit does not provide an opportunity for the family to share experiences with others who have the same problem. For example, the young wife caring for a senile parent who is forgetful and messy may gain much more from talking with other young wives who face the same situation than from talking to the nurse whose knowledge is not apt to be based on similar personal experience.

The *office conference* has been used widely in institutional situations such as in school or industry, but much less in general community nursing. Properly planned, the office visit has many advantages. These are:

1. The office visit conserves nursing time, since the family rather than the nurse undertakes the travel. For example, the ambulatory patient who needs hypodermic medication which he cannot give himself might well come to the office.

2. The office visit makes possible the use of demonstration equipment that cannot be taken to the home. For example, the nurse may show the family members types of supports

or helping "gadgets" that may be made for the incapacitated home-bound patient.

3. Outside distractions are minimized.
4. In some cases, consultants or specialists on the staff may be called in to help.
5. The office conference emphasizes the individual's or family's basic responsibility for self-help.

There seems little doubt that with increasing chronic care loads this approach to care will grow in importance. However, the disadvantages must also be considered. They are:

1. The office conference does not permit first-hand appraisal of the home and family situation, and may lead to a false impression of the home problems.
2. Getting to the nursing office may represent a real hardship to the patient or family, either physically or financially.
3. Some patients may feel less at ease, less ready to talk out problems than in their own home. This is variable, however, since some patients will feel more, rather than less, at ease away from home. For example, it may be easier to talk about adolescent reactions to the presence of an ailing grandmother when away from the grandmother's presence.
4. Arranging nursing activities around the hours patients can get to the office may make scheduling of other work difficult, particularly in the one-nurse service.

Group conference methods are increasing in importance in the public health nursing program, as more information is obtained as to the potentials implicit in this method. Group work has the following advantages:

1. It provides an opportunity for members of the group to share experiences and to help one another. The potential of self-help may be higher than that of help by an expert.
2. It may stimulate leadership among members of the group. Families come to realize their competences when they see them in the light of helping others.
3. It provides an opportunity for consideration of practical and tested solutions to the problems discussed. The way in which a young mother schedules her day to accommodate to the needs of a new baby, presented by one who actually worked it out, usually has greater impact than would the same information provided by a professional worker.
4. It may provide an opportunity to air grievances or talk out bitter or blaming feelings. A group of teen-agers who are re-

stricted in activities and vocational choice by rheumatic fever may find this an opportunity to strike out at the unfairness of being so handicapped, or to blame others, with a resultant release of tension.

The disadvantages of group methods must also be considered:

1. Individual problems may get lost in the group discussion, either because the individual is too shy to bring them out, or because the problem is not common to others in the group, and therefore of no interest to them.

2. The outcomes of group work may be too generalized to be very helpful, particularly if the problems of the group differ greatly. For example, it is not much help to discuss the problems of the emotional impact of menopause with a group of women if the age distribution is broad so that some are interested and others not. There would be a tendency to concentrate on the general factors involved rather than upon the specific feelings, attitudes and physical symptoms the group has experienced or fears because the climacteric is in the present or in the immediate future. Similarly, if a child behavior discussion group includes parents with children of widely different age groups the time available to cover the problem of any one age group may limit the discussion to highly generalized content.

3. Those who need the service most may not take advantage of opportunities for group work. In general, those already highly motivated tend to respond most often to group opportunities.

The factor of cost has not been listed either as an advantage or disadvantage, because it may be less or more than that of comparable service rendered on an individual basis. Preparation time, individual follow-up services required, and the time needed to establish the commonality of problems and to emphasize the underlying principles as applied to a larger number of variables than would be found in a single family contact may increase time costs to a point above that of individual care. In other instances, when the group is homogeneous and the problems require instruction in greater proportion than counseling or problem solving, group methods may be considerably less expensive.

The *telephone contact* is also assuming increasing significance as a service unit. The telephone contact has obvious advantages:

1. It is inexpensive in time and usually in cost, both for the service and for the family.

2. It permits more frequent contact at the most desirable time, despite pressures of other work, because of the small amount of time required.
3. It relieves the family of "hostess" burdens which might be a problem in home visits.
4. It is more personalized than a written communication.
5. It provides a valuable screening device for deciding which of several situations requires a home visit. For example, calling school absentees will reveal that a good number represent no particular problem. Other calls would indicate that a nursing visit is needed.

The disadvantages are:

1. It does not afford the nurse a full opportunity to judge the situation—she cannot see either the home conditions or the small nonverbal indications in the patient that might indicate stress or failure to understand.
2. Some who most need frequent contact with the nurse will not have access to a telephone.

The *written communication*—the note sent home by the school child, the teaching materials sent with a covering personal note—also has a place in the total pattern of family-nurse contacts. This is, of course, the least individualized (though not necessarily either impersonal or cold) of the methods presented. The advantages of this method are:

1. Low cost.
2. For the competent, independent family, the advantage of placing responsibility for action on the family rather than upon the nurse. For example, the responsible parent without unusual economic problems might well prefer to make her own plans and follow-up when she knows that her child's vision screening tests indicated the need for further study and medical referral.

The disadvantages are:

1. It gives no opportunity to gauge the total family situation accurately.
2. It provides no opportunity to uncover or help with problems other than the one immediately under consideration.
3. It may not reach the persons for whom it is intended.

INDIRECT METHODS

When there are many people to be reached, and the amount of nursing time available is limited, indirect methods may be used.

Among these are training of instructors in home nursing, who may in turn teach family members or school groups; providing health teaching materials to other professional workers, such as social workers, personnel workers in industry, or community group leaders; providing advisement and materials to nurses in other situations (the nurse in clinic or physician's office, nurses in industry, or private practice nurses, especially those working with cases which have a high preventive or teaching potential) that will enable them in include services to families that might otherwise have been given by the public health nurse.

Criteria for Selection of the Type of Family-Nurse Contact. When deciding which of the several methods of approach might be used in a particular family, several factors will need to be considered, and the relative value of the method under consideration studied. In general, the effort is not to select the cheapest type of contact (otherwise we should use nothing but notes and telephone contacts), or the best (the best may be far beyond our nursing potential). The goal is to select the approach that will produce the greatest amount for the time and money expended—to find the most effective service approach. The following criteria may be helpful:

1. The approach selected should be the one which is least costly and still likely to meet the demands of the situation. For example, if a request has come for prenatal care of a primigravida, it would be obvious that a pretty full knowledge of the total home environment as well as of the mother herself would be necessary as a basis for nursing service, and that an opportunity to consider the particular home facilities for baby care would be highly desirable. Obviously, an office conference, group work, or telephone or written communication would not offer suitable opportunities for appraisal of the home situation as a whole. Only a home visit is likely to meet the needs of this situation. In another instance, however, when the family is known to the nursing service, has had one baby and indicated previously their welcoming attitude toward a larger family, a telephone screening to family and doctor followed by group work would probably be equally valuable and less costly.

2. The method should be one which provides the maximum opportunity for development and self-direction of the family. If, for example, it is assumed that approximately the same results in terms of patient care must be realized through the

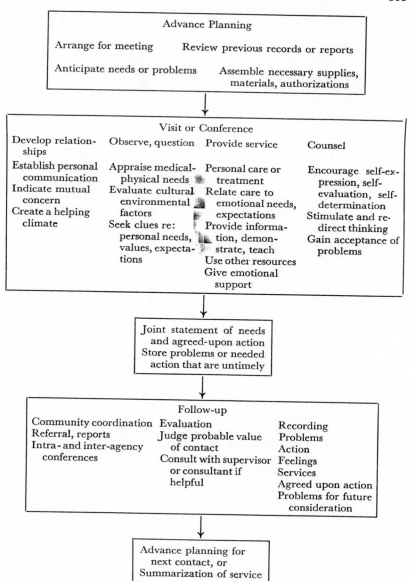

Figure 9.   Flow chart—family-nurse contact.

use of home visits or group instruction and discussion, the latter method might be selected because it would be assumed to provide more opportunity for patients and family to help themselves and one another, and hence contribute to their independence of action in health matters.

3. The method must be feasible in relation to the amounts of nursing time available and the total community needs. For example, in the face of great incidence of a communicable disease, the nurse may feel that the most desirable and effective approach would be home visits. However, this may be impossible owing to lack of nursing time and to travel problems, and a "second best" approach be required. This approach might be to get family members together in small groups for demonstration and discussion, or to rely upon telephone contacts for screening, visiting only those who seem to have particular difficulty.

4. The method must be consistent with community habits and expectations. The community may resist group activities, and its members either fail to come or fail to respond in a way which makes the group work worth while. Or it may be felt that since the former nurse visited individuals at home and if the new nurse doesn't do this it is because the latter is disinterested or lazy. Again, it may be necessary to choose the second best way temporarily, using the approach which is acceptable to the community until it learns to accept or use a better one.

Whatever the method elected for meeting the basic objectives of public health nursing services to families and individuals, the family-nurse contact will involve certain planning and action steps as indicated in the flow chart (Fig. 9). If the contact is brief or superficial, the steps will be less inclusive, but however brief there will always be need for advance planning, for family-nurse concerted thinking and action, and for evaluation and follow-up and for re-planning.

Each of these phases of the family-nurse contact will be discussed in the chapters which follow.

CHAPTER VII

Developing a Plan
for Care: Establishing
Needs and Goals

THE DEVELOPMENT of a plan for public health nursing care is the responsibility of the nurse, which she shares with many others —the physician, the teacher, the social worker, the personnel worker, and nurses working in schools, in hospitals or in industry. Most of all, the family is involved in the planning process. In planning five major phases may be identified:

1. Appraising the nursing need, including the modifying forces in the physical and cultural environment, and in the personality patterns of the individual and of the family.
2. Developing mutually acceptable goals and agreed-upon action statements.
3. Estimating and mobilizing family and community resources for care.
4. Developing a program of action.
5. Establishing measures for estimating accomplishment.

The several phases of planning are not necessarily carried out in this order. As nurse and family work together problems may be re-evaluated, or new problems may appear which modify the importance of existing ones. The process is a continuing one in which appraisal, goal setting, mobilization, action and measurement are followed by re-planning and new action.

THE NURSING APPRAISAL

If family nursing care is to be provided effectively, it is necessary to have both an accurate appraisal of the family's health needs and a comprehensive statement of these needs that may serve as a base for action. In short contacts the nurse's appraisal may be an almost intuitive sizing up of the situation, and produce a quickly achieved judgment. For example, an industrial worker with a good accident record may come to the health room with a cut finger. In the absence of a history of frequent accident and any evidence of unusual distress at this time, his needs are readily apparent. An emergency dressing, a check on whether or not the accident might have been prevented, instruction regarding prevention of future injury, and instruction in the prevention of infection can be provided without any very complex planning. There is no need to collect a great deal of information about the man and his family and his relations with his co-workers, to develop a mutual understanding of the situation and the necessary treatment.

In longer contacts, or when the situation is not clearly defined, the nurse's share in analysis of needs may be a central one, or it may be ancillary. The primary responsibility for appraisal may rest with other professional workers, individually or in a team. For example, the woman suffering from severe physical manifestations and emotional stress associated with the menopause may need the expert diagnosis of a psychiatrist, social worker, internist and nurse, with the psychiatrist taking the lead in determining the nature of the over-all problem and the nursing care that will be needed. The nurse's function may be limited to contributing her own observations to the diagnostic team, recognizing that the place of nursing care is supplementary, and that appraisal of the situation in relation to nursing needs is beyond her individual competence. In other instances the nurse may gather information from the physician, social worker, teacher or others and, with the help of the family, weld these many judgments into a statement of the nursing needs of the family.

The process of analysis of needs is discussed here in some detail, recognizing that the nurse will not need to engage in every step of the process with every family, and that at many points the nurse's judgment will represent the pooled judgments of several people, rather than her own independent appraisal.

Determinants of Family Health Needs

In general, health needs arise from four sources—from the health situation itself, from the environment, from the social-cultural milieu, and from the patterns of behavior that are characteristic of the patient and his family.

Needs Inherent in the Health Situation. In some situations the needs of the family will be determined in large part by the nature of the disease or health condition that the patient presents. For example, rheumatic fever imposes certain demands in relation to health care. The patient must have adequate rest, protection from infection, prophylactic medication and careful medical supervision and nursing observation. The post-tonsillectomy patient needs a diet that will avoid mechanical injury to the throat, rest, and instructions regarding cleansing of the mouth and throat. The cardiac patient needs instruction regarding the specific medications he is receiving, and instruction and counseling that will help him organize his patterns of living so as to avoid unusual physical or emotional strain.

A knowledge of these needs is part of the technical competence of the nurse; her recognition of them should be prompt, and her information should be comprehensive and up-to-date. Medical care changes rapidly, and shortened hospitalization combined with more accurate diagnosis has caused much change in the kind of illness treated at home. Information about chronic illness and its care, for instance, has brought greatly expanded concepts of comprehensive care requiring much greater knowledge of a variety of drugs and rehabilitation procedures. The nurse needs a constantly expanding store of information to be able to identify health needs arising from particular diseases.

The physiologic status of the individual may also produce specific health needs even in the absence of disease. Pregnancy and parturition impose certain demands for care—calcium intake must be adequate, protective foods must receive greater emphasis, postural adjustments needed late in pregnancy require instruction regarding body mechanics and the effect of restrictive clothing. Anticipatory guidance in relation to emotional changes that are likely to occur, and emotional support from the family and sometimes from the nurse or other professional worker are also needed.[1]

Fatigue is another physiologic state that may create special needs. Need for rest, need for instruction in developing habits of

1. Caplan, G., Psychological Aspects of Maternity Care. *American Journal of Public Health*, 47: 25–31, January, 1957.

relaxation, and in leisure time pursuits, changes in habits of work, and special accident precautions are examples. In periods when fatigue is apt to be high—as during the Christmas rush in a department store, or during the late afternoon hours in an industry using machinery that demands careful attention—special care to avoid accident is necessary, such as arranging for rest periods, or education to alert employees to the particular problems of these high-risk times.

The nutritional state of an individual may also create health needs. The over- or underweight individual may present a variety of physical and emotional needs, since abnormal weight may reflect unmet social or psychologic needs as well as poor habits of food selection or physical disorder. Dietary deficiencies may require information in preparation and serving of foods, or in canning or home gardening, to assure ample intake of protective foods. Nutritional requirements have been the subject of much scientific investigation, and the nurse should be alert to changes in recommended standards.[2]

Communicable disease also creates special needs. Protection of others must take its place with care of the affected individual so that neither is neglected.[3] Nonexposed individuals may need to be protected by isolating the sick person, or by excluding him from school or from certain types of work. Immunization may be needed to modify the effects of exposure. Care of bodily discharges, handling of equipment, arrangement of the sickroom and restriction of activity of the patient may be needed to protect others. At the same time the patient's need for care—for comfort-giving procedures and for the prevention of complications—must be considered. In some cases the patient or his family may feel some fear, or a social stigma in relation to the disease, and this may pose a need for emotional support.

Chronic illness also presents special needs. The burden of care for a greatly incapacitated patient may build unconscious or frank resentment that interferes seriously with family relationships. Emotional stress may also interfere with the patient's adaptation to the disease and its limitations—as when the patient feels that he is a burden on others, or that he is tolerated rather than loved,

2. Maynard, L. A., Dietary Standards in the United States. *Public Health Reports,* 67: 784–786, August, 1952.

3. Anderson, G. W., and M. Arnstein, *Communicable Disease Control,* 3rd edition. New York, The Macmillan Co., 1953, Chapter 7, "Role of the Public Health Nurse."

or that he has failed in his obligation to support his family. Frequently economic problems are important; costs of medical care, of dressings or medications may be overwhelming if the income is limited, and may require finding financial assistance through community sources. Always there is need for guidance in rehabilitation. Help in devising gadgets that will increase self-sufficiency, instruction in crutch walking or other physical adaptations to self-help, and motivation of family and patient toward maximum self-help, and interpretation of the rationale of rehabilitation are also needed.

Age is also a determinant of health needs. Each age group has its major hazards to life and health, as well as commonly encountered minor problems. The newborn infant, especially the premature, is particularly susceptible to infection, and therefore needs the protection of special care and handling, and later immunization for those diseases for which it is recommended. The school-age child is particularly susceptible to accidents; the adolescent, to emotional stress; the young adult, to the strains of job adaptation and to the physical and emotional demands associated with parenthood. The late adolescent and the young adult pose special needs in relation to venereal disease control. The person in middle years has needs growing out of the increasing incidence of long-term illness in this age period. He needs instruction in recognizing symptoms of cancer, of diabetes, of heart disease. There is need for instruction in use of diagnostic facilities, for self-examination of the breast; for developing a way of life that minimizes stress and sets the stage for enjoyment of later years. The senescent may need custodial care, as well as medical and nursing supervision for long-term illness or disability, and protection from accidental injury as accidents again assume great importance in this age group. The needs mentioned here are, of course, merely suggestive. The public health nurse needs to be familiar with the incidence of disease in different age groups, and the special risks to health that occur in the various groups.

Needs Arising from the Environment. Certain needs arise from the environment in which the individual or family functions. An industrial plant, a farm or a slum area each carries its own threats to health. Weather extremes, heavy street traffic and the presence of animal or insect vectors of disease are other examples of environmental determinants of health needs.

The working environment often creates health needs. The industrial worker may need mechanical and educational safeguards

against accident, protection from dangerous dusts or fumes, or procedures to combat the effects of working under extremes of temperature or noise. The office worker or executive may need help
in coping with stress and frustration arising from peak loads of
work, or with assuring a proper lunch in the crowded corner
drugstore during a hurried lunch hour. The housewife may need
to learn how to recognize and control accident hazards in the
home—the unguarded electric outlet or worn electric cord, the
gas jet that is within reach of the toddler. She may need to learn
proper habits of lifting heavy objects (and children!), and of
scheduling work to allow for rest periods, or of storing equipment
and supplies for safe and easy use.

Housing itself may be a problem. Unsafe or poorly lighted hall-
ways, poor sewage disposal, lack of screens or rat-proofing are
common in poorly housed groups. Lack of proper play space for
children, and crowding and inadequate provision for storage that
results in unusual energy costs in getting out and putting away
equipment may be found even in high-rental areas.

The school environment may also create health needs. Grouping of children increases the exposure to undiagnosed communicable disease, and particularly to upper respiratory infection;
handwashing facilities are often inadequate; getting to and from
school increases the hazard of accident. For the kindergartner or
for the child who is new in school the stress associated with wean-
ing from home and from the usual parental supports presents
problems.

The community, too, may create special needs. The rural environment may substitute individual control for community management in the protection of milk and water supplies and sewage
disposal, creating a need for education in sanitation. Fire and
accident hazards are increased by the fact that the farmer is in
many cases his own electrician, mechanic, power operator and
builder. Tetanus, heat prostration and injuries from animals are
other special hazards of the rural environment. In addition, reliance on the "doctors' book" growing out of the difficulty of
getting medical and hospital care may lead to unusual amounts
of self-treatment.

City environments have their own hazards. Poor out-of-door
play areas may increase accident hazards to children. Mothers
are more apt to be employed outside the home than are those in
small towns or rural areas; this creates problems in the working
mother arising from the conflict inherent in her dual responsibility

to job and family, and also problems of physical care and emotional guidance that arise from unsupervised activities of children after school hours. In low-income groups in particular, children may be left in the care of frankly incompetent mother substitutes while the mother is at work.

Suburban living, too, presents particular problems of sanitation, of crowded schools, or unusually high numbers of women needing maternity care. The relatively high degree of conformity expected of residents in a suburban area may also create problems of adaptation to this type of restriction.

Needs Arising from the Social-Cultural Setting. Social and cultural forces have a profound effect upon family life and health, and may in themselves create health problems of some magnitude. For example, the progressive deterioration of a worn-out neighborhood is associated with juvenile delinquency and crime as well as with the hazards of inadequate housing. With such a social pattern, exposure to venereal disease tends to be high, and family neglect may be common, with consequent need for more intensive supervision of children. There may be a social premium placed on being "tough" that leads to foolhardiness and accident, or to disregard of preventive health services.

Cultural groups at special risk include those whose way of life is not adapted to present-day demands, such as Indians living on reservations, or small groups living in isolation in remote mountain communities. The Indian, living apart from the rest of the community, faced with discouragingly infertile land and seeing the gradual loss of original skills, may drift into a dependent way of life and to the maintenance of old tribal customs. These customs and attitudes may be detrimental to health, such as patterns of care in childbirth that provide little protection for mother or baby, or the use of a medicine man or herbalist in preference to a physician. This may lead to high maternal and infant mortality rates, and to the spread of communicable diseases. The unfavorable economic status of Negroes in many communities may present special problems in relation to the prevention and care of illnesses associated with poverty, especially tuberculosis and nutritional conditions.

Migratory employment creates a population with a way of life different from the nonmigrant, with many hazards to health. The migratory worker and his family often live in sub-standard houses, with inadequate provision for cooking, storing and serving food. Mothers frequently work in the fields, leaving children inadequately supervised, or bring the children with them where their activities must be greatly limited.

Cultural patterns also have important health implications.[4] The family transplanted to the United States from Mexico, or from the Mediterranean area, may have food patterns that are based on different ingredients from those readily found in the new environment. The foods to which its members are accustomed may be expensive, and sometimes are bought at the expense of other necessary protective foods. The working girl, accustomed to working with others in the industrial setting, may find it hard to change her way of living when she becomes a wife and mother. She may find it hard to work alone instead of in a group, and without the pattern of required hours and ways of work. It may be very difficult not to have the tangible reward of the weekly salary, and the independence of having money of her own.

Cultural factors associated with economic class may weigh heavily in determining attitudes toward authority, values in relation to unsocial behavior such as sexual promiscuity, or in concepts of what constitutes illness. The hard-pressed group living in a marginal neighborhood may have developed mutual help patterns that contribute materially to health care. Families living in housing developments evolve a sub-culture group within the housing development itself, with characteristic patterns of health and social behavior. These patterns may affect general attitudes, such as interracial feelings or feelings of neighborliness.[5] Middle-income apartment dwellers or persons living alone may need to develop mutual help systems as an adjunct to health care. For instance, old people living alone may need to work out a "buddy" system of mutual visiting on a regular basis, so that Mr. A. calls on Mr. B. on Mondays, and the procedure is reversed on Tuesday, and so on. In this way if either should become ill there is someone available to seek help. Left alone, the individual might not be able to call for help, and might be neglected for some time. Attitudes toward conformity, regularity and orderliness in daily living habits, and responsibility toward commitments made may also be related to group values or cultures. The Alaskan native, for example, may show great responsibility toward most of his obligations, but find it difficult to do things at a prescribed

4. See, for example, Saunders, Lyle, *Cultural Difference and Medical Care.* New York, Russell Sage Foundation, 1954.

5. Wilner, Daniel, Rosabelle Walkeley and Stuart Cook, *Human Relations in Interracial Housing.* Minneapolis, University of Minnesota Press, 1955.

time during the day, since the cultural pattern grows out of a life dependent upon fishing and hunting, neither of which is done on schedule.[6]

Needs Arising from the Personal Characteristics of the Individual or Family. In addition to needs arising from the health situation itself and from the physical, social and cultural environment, there will be health problems that have their genesis in the personality patterns of the individual or of the family. If Johnny Jones is reported as having scarlet fever, and if observation reveals that his father works irregularly and that the neighborhood in which he lives is a poor one and the house run down and poorly equipped, certain needs may be anticipated. Assistance in securing medical care and nursing, instruction in the ways by which this disease is spread and how the spread can be controlled, information concerning the course of the disease and the symptoms that should be observed, and planning for home care within the limits of available equipment and money will all be required. However, because he is Johnny Jones there will be other needs that are unique to the situation. Perhaps Johnny is imaginative and fearful about illness; he may have developed habits of resistance to authority of any kind, and as a consequence find it hard to accept any restriction of his activity; he may have built up a strongly antagonistic attitude toward his mother, and look to his father for guidance and authority; he may be anxious about his school work and so find the period of convalescence particularly trying. These latter needs are personal and familial rather than categorical.

Personal factors that may produce health needs, or require modifications of health care, include:

1. Physical equipment and competence
2. Intellectual competence
3. Established patterns of health behavior and attitudes toward health care
4. Degree of personal and emotional security achieved
5. Previous experience and acquired information in relation to health care.

Physical equipment and competence will vary widely even within a given age or social group. The handicapped, the frail, the easily fatigued have special needs in relation to daily regimen and occupational and recreational adjustment. Physical status has

6. Buchan, L., and J. Allen, *Hearth in the Snow*. New York, Wilfred Funk, 1953.

importance to the individual in relation to his particular goals. For example, the young man with average health and stamina may also have an exceptional desire for occupational success. For his purposes, average physical stamina may prove inadequate, and he may need help in adjusting his ambitions and his program to meet his need to maintain the integrity of his physical well-being. A little slower pace of achievement may make it possible to move toward both physical health and occupational success.

Sometimes the individual with good physical equipment has failed to develop physical competence. The preschool child who has not had sufficient freedom for physical activity may be retarded in the establishment of good muscular coordination; the housewife may develop habits of work that interfere with proper use of her physical capacity. Previous illness or physical impairment may also create problems—a history of rickets or of severe streptococcal infection may modify the needs of the prenatal patient; a history of allergy might change the spacing of physical appraisal for the industrial worker.

Intellectual competence—the ability to think in abstract terms, to make generalizations and to foresee future consequences of present actions—is also a factor in determination of health needs. Intellectual competence must not be confused with academic achievement. The individual with very little formal education may have a highly developed ability to recognize generalizations, and to look and plan ahead. Needs for health instruction will vary greatly in accordance with this ability, since those with high intellectual competence will be able to apply the general principles taught in one situation to many subsequent similar situations. Those less well equipped will need constant repetition and reteaching to achieve the same level of understanding and competence in health action.

Established patterns of health behavior may also produce health needs. Habits of rushing to work or to school without breakfast, of snatching a hurried and inadequate lunch, or of bravely ignoring pain until it becomes insupportable create obvious problems. The habits of "not looking for trouble," and of shopping around for health care, going from clinic to clinic, or from doctor to doctor, are further examples.

Patterns of reacting to difficulty may also create or accentuate health needs, since individuals will react to health problems in ways that are similar to their reaction to other life situations.

Some people face difficult adjustments as a challenging problem, looking at the facts and the probable developments realistically and proceeding with comparative serenity and dispatch to the action that seems most suitable. Others find facing any difficulty a highly disrupting experience, and may react by withdrawal, indecision, fear, worry, procrastination, or resentment. In the latter case the program for nursing care must be modified, to keep to a minimum the delay and anxiety that might ensue.

The degree to which an individual has achieved security and maturity will also affect his health needs. The individual needs to feel secure in relation to himself, his family, and his world.[7] He needs to feel effective, and important to and welcomed by others. Without this sense of contributing and belonging, compensatory behavior patterns may develop and interfere seriously with the achievement of good health care.

Fear may cause the woman with a lump in her breast to refuse diagnostic care; overdependence on the opinion of others may cause the schoolboy to refuse instruction in preparation for parenthood as "sissified"; feelings of inferiority or insecurity may cause the young prenatal patient to deride and refuse medical supervision during pregnancy. Attention-getting mechanisms may also be detrimental to health; careless driving on the highway, overindulgence in alcohol, and horseplay in the industrial shop are examples of immature behavior that may have health repercussions.

Previous experience and acquired health information will also influence health needs. The popularization of health information and extended health instructional programs in schools, community agencies and in industry, as well as health aspects of modern advertising campaigns, have resulted in wide dissemination of health information and sometimes of misinformation. Depending on what has already been learned, the family may need more or less teaching content, or to recognize the fallacy of some health information acquired from an unreliable source. Sometimes it is necessary to combat overconfidence based on inadequate or unsound information, as when the neighborhood midwife who has practiced for years without benefit of formal training feels that her experience has left her competent to deal with any emergency.

Previous experience with health care that was not satisfactory may create new problems. The child whose only experience with

7. Witmer, Helen and Ruth Kotinsky (Editors), *Personality in the Making.* New York, Harper & Bros., 1952, Introduction.

the physician was when he went for immunization may have difficulty accepting his physical examination; the young mother whose first pelvic examination was observed by a group of interns who discussed her condition without cognizance of her as a person may insist on private medical care even though it is not desirable from a financial point of view; the old man who had to relinquish all of his little personal belongings when he went to the hospital may not want to return to the hospital even when he urgently needs the diagnostic and treatment facilities that cannot be provided in any other way.

On the other hand, previous experiences may in some cases encourage overdependence on community facilities, and avoidance of personal or family responsibility. The family may prefer to let the hospital take responsibility for the child with a physical impairment, even though home care is indicated, because it has been found easier in the past to let someone else carry the burden of care.

The nurse in public health must be constantly alert to these many determinants of health needs if she is to be sensitive to the total health requirements of the families she serves. Her proficiency in locating and appraising health needs will be dependent upon her competence to relate these determinants to the specific families and individuals under her care.

METHODS OF ANALYZING HEALTH NEEDS

In addition to knowing the sources and general nature of health needs, the public health nurse must develop techniques and methods of analysis. Some of the steps involved in analysis of family needs are of a long-range character—activities that re-enforce the nurse's general preparation and understanding and provide a richer background of professional knowledge and skill from which to draw in specific instances. Other phases of the process of analysis will be definitely related to the study of a particular family and its needs. For convenience, the procedures involved in analysis of health needs have been grouped in chronological sequence in relation to the nurse's visit, as pre-visit, intra-visit, and post-visit activities.

Pre-visit Activities Contributing to Analysis of Health Needs. Prior to the nursing visit the nurse may take several steps in the process of analyzing health needs. She may:

1. Review current medical and health practice as it relates to the cases being carried.

2. Study community and cultural factors affecting the families served.

3. Review the family or individual health record.

4. Secure information from other agencies or individuals.

Constant review of current professional health practice is imperative for the nurse in public health. Unlike the hospital nurse who is in constant contact with acutely ill patients, and with new and experimental drugs, treatment and equipment, the public health nurse may have only a small proportion of her case load made up of morbidity patients. Because public health care is apt to concentrate on prehospital and posthospital periods, the public health nurse may have little opportunity to participate in the intensive aspects of treatment that determine the needs in the early and convalescent or chronic periods of the disease. Furthermore, while the service of the hospital nurse tends to be restricted to a particular group of diseases, that of the public health nurse has a wide range; the public health nurse is expected to assist with such diverse problems as providing nursing care for cerebral palsy, recognizing symptoms of encephalitis or tetanus, and interpreting a physician's order that a baby be placed on volitional feeding. In addition, since the public health nurse often works in isolated situations she may not have easy access to the case conferences and seminars on medical care and treatment that are available in medical centers. Unless thoughtful, continuing review of professional practice is undertaken either through reading or observations, the public health nurse may become estranged from the clinical aspects of medical and nursing care.

In addition to the maintenance of general clinical expertness, it is often desirable to review current practice in relation to a specific health condition just prior to the nursing visit. If the situation is one that the nurse encounters frequently this may entail nothing more than a brief mental review of the salient points in care. When the situation is one in which the nurse feels less familiar, a more detailed check may be necessary. If she is planning to visit a family where there is tuberculosis she may want to review the current literature regarding the use of antibiotics, since there are bound to be questions about this raised by the family. Thus fortified, she is able to recognize the needs for instruction, and to provide the necessary information with confidence.

Regulations of importance in the particular situation may also need to be reviewed. Regulations regarding isolation or exclusion from school or work, forms and reports that must be submitted in industrial accident and the probable compensation status, and conditions pertaining to fees to be collected are examples of the specific kind of information that may need to be secured in advance of the visit.

The nurse needs to have necessary reference materials readily available, including recent textbooks on nursing practice and on communicable disease control. In addition to this, manuals or policy statements of her own or related agencies may supply necessary information. Clipping or pamphlet files may be developed to provide quick sources of reference of specific diseases or health conditions. There may be some information that the nurse will want to have briefed and carried with her to the home or clinic. A chart of the incubation periods, control measures and health department regulations regarding communicable diseases, for example, may be very useful.

Community and social-cultural factors can be studied in day-by-day observation. The public health nurse may notice that in some neighborhoods men tend to seek their recreation in groups, gathered at a local restaurant or in the park, while the women stay at home, or meet in each other's homes in groups of two or three. In some communities, neighborliness will be highly developed, while in others people pride themselves on not knowing anything about those who live next door. Habits in relation to the use of community health facilities are also readily observed. In some groups the use of the clinic is widespread, and any deviation from normal is quickly reported. In others, care may be sought only as a last resort.

Reports of neighborhood or city-wide surveys may be available from health or social agencies, and these may provide valuable information about housing, health problems or resources. Sometimes pertinent information about the community has been gathered and compiled for use in the nursing office, or the nurse may herself gather the information from a variety of sources into a notebook or folder on the community and its resources.

If the population contains predominant nationality groups, reading about the backgrounds, customs and sociologic problems of the group will be helpful. The public library will have valuable suggestions. Studies of cities or of small communities may be helpful to the nurse going into a situation to which she is unaccustomed.[8] The nurse working in industry, or in a community where

8. Examples of such works are Mumford, Lewis, *Culture of Cities*. New York, Harcourt Brace, 1938, and Seeley, John, R. Sims and E. Loosely, *Crestwood Heights*. Toronto, Basic Books, 1956.

one industry predominates, will find it useful to observe the plant. This type of first-hand information yields valuable clues to health needs, not only in the actual processes employed, but in the intangibles of the work environment.

When the agency already has a health record for the family to be visited, this should be reviewed prior to the visit. This will provide information on the individual's or family's health status, such as history of previous illnesses, general health condition, history of past pregnancies. The family status in relation to immunizations or other preventive care may also be found in this way. Equally important, there will be indications as to the results of previous health care. The degree to which medical advice was secured when indicated, and evidence of little change despite consultation services or of increasing independence on the part of the family are examples of the sort of indices of need that may be found on the previous record. For example, if the record showed frequent requests for nursing service when there was no real illness, or that the family had failed to learn simple procedures like temperature determination, would indicate that little responsibility had been assumed by the family.

Social and environmental factors may also be identified through record review. Economic status, housing conditions, family relationships, educational or work achievements may be found on the record, and will help to prepare the nurse for an effective visit.

When indicated, the nurse may secure information from other agencies or individuals who are concerned with the health care of the family. If the physician has visited the family in relation to this particular illness he should be called prior to the visit to secure orders for care, or any special directions he may have. If the family is under the continuing care of a social case work agency, the agency will have information of value in the analysis of needs. If the record indicates that there is a complex problem, a conference with one of the other workers involved may be indicated. The nurse may stop in to see the physician or social worker, or may arrange a conference with the hospital nurse who has cared for the patient.

Analysis during the Family-Nurse Contact. Throughout the nursing visit, activities must be planned that will make the analysis of health needs more definitive. Through observation, questioning and guiding conversation the nurse will add to her information about the family, its attitudes toward health care, and the degree of perception of health needs it has achieved, and will try to assess present health practice and knowledge.

During the visit, activities designed to secure more accurate definition of needs will in most instances be interspersed with service to the family. For example, much information may be secured during the time when the nurse is giving bedside care, or while she is explaining to the family the advice they were given by the physician.

History taking may provide an excellent springboard for analysis of health needs. Properly carried out, writing the case history can provide a discussion of health status and needs, with nurse and patient joining in the analysis. While the direction of the interview for history taking may be determined by the record form, the nurse's skill in locating and defining needs will make a great deal of difference in the final result. Supplementary questions or comments, the nurse's general attitude, or the tone of voice in which a question is asked may produce much additional information. For example, a routine question "Any children? How old?" if asked pleasantly will secure a willing answer and the information essential for completing the record form. An extra comment, such as "Oh, so John's your baby," or "You had to wait a long time for John to come along, didn't you?" may yield much more significant information—perhaps a fervent "I hope so," or "Yes, he's certainly spoiled by all of us," or "Well, we didn't really plan to have John, but now that he's here we're glad." History taking should serve as a diagnostic conference.

Simple observation of the family will yield much information relating to health needs. Observation of the individual for signs of illness or impairment, or for evidence of change in condition is an integral part of nursing. In public health work, attention must also be directed toward very early and less frank evidences of illness. Observation involves selectivity as well as sensitivity. The nurse needs to know what to look for in relation to the special needs of the particular age or nationality group, or in situations with special environmental hazards. Observation will be clearly tied to the determinants of needs discussed earlier. The listless attitude of a factory worker who says she "feels all right" may suggest the need for a more thorough periodic appraisal; the over-bright nonchalance of a clinic patient may reveal his basic fear; a mother's tension as she handles a small infant betrays uncertainty and insecurity that may indicate need for reassurance and teaching.

Attitudes toward care, as well as previous experience, may be revealed in the degree to which the family has prepared for the nursing visit. The family that has put the patient to bed, taken and recorded his temperature, and assembled supplies for his care has reached a different level of competence and hence has different needs than does the family that has waited for the nurse's arrival to decide what to do. The type of questions asked, and the kind of requests for assistance made by the family also indicate the degree of responsibility that its members are prepared to assume.

Evidences of recreational or cultural interests, or of religious interests may also be observed. Standards of housekeeping and of child care may also be obvious without special searching.

To reach maximum effectiveness, observation must be planned and properly directed. Arranging a visit at the time when the father or children are at home, or when the mother is apt to be bathing the baby may allow the nurse to see activities or relationships that would not be apparent at other times.

As has been emphasized previously, the relatedness of what is observed is extremely important. A meticulously clean home may reflect family pride in the home, or it may reflect a disregard of the social and recreational needs of the younger members of the family, and overconcern about impressing the neighbors; a woman's lack of concern about prenatal care may betoken a healthy acceptance of a normal pregnancy or a deep-seated fear or unwillingness to face the reality of the condition; overly enthusiastic acceptance of health information or advice may indicate a real interest, or it may simply be an expression of politeness and a desire to please that will lead to no change at all in health practice.

Guided conversation may be used to secure a definition of health needs. This implies leading the conversation into productive channels through questions and comments, listening, and encouraging free expression on the part of the family or individual through evidencing interest, acceptance and sympathy. Careful direction is necessary to build up the individual's confidence in his ability to define and express his health needs, and at the same time give him the assurance of the support and sustained interest of the nurse. One nurse, for instance, had been so impressed with the need to be a good listener and to reflect the patient's thinking that she felt she could not give any straightforward advice or specific direction to the family. She silently waited for the family to define their problems and indicate what they planned to do. Her patients were confused and unhappy in their relationships with her because they needed the directing questions and supporting statements from her that would help them to think through their problems. Conversation directed toward defining health needs is a two-way process, with the family members talking out their problems, desires and plans, and the nurse listening, questioning, and supplementing with information as necessary. The result should be a free discussion leading to a clear statement of family health needs.

Questions may be used to appraise present information or practice, to check information already given, or to redirect thinking. Questions such as "What did the doctor tell you about your condition?" or "Do you have any trouble following the diet the doctor gave you?" will lead to answers that define the patient's knowledge and practice. Careful wording of questions will make them an expression of interest and concern rather than a checking-up process. "Do you find it hard to get the children to take a good breakfast before they start for school?" sounds quite different from "Do you give your children a good breakfast?"

Questions may also be helpful to check the exact meaning of statements made. For example, if a man reports that he "can't sleep at night," questions such as "What time did you go to bed last night, and what time did you get to sleep?" or "Did you sleep well any night this past week?" or "Do you get any rest or sleep during the day?" may amplify the original answer.

Questions may also be used to broaden the base of the individual's thinking about his problem. For example, the mother who reports that her seven-year-old boy is a joy because he's "so good" may be asked how he gets along with boys his own age, whether he takes an interest in outdoor activities, or whether he seems to demand more parental attention than his siblings.

It is important that questions be so phrased that they elicit replies that are functional rather than verbal. "Do you know how communicable disease is spread?" is in general less productive in determining what the family knows than "What will you have to do to keep the other children from catching this?" "Do you think you could plan your housework so you could get a little rest in the afternoon?" is more apt to obtain an informative answer than "Do you know about the need to get some rest in the afternoon?"

Sometimes analysis of problems may be combined with providing information. For example, the mother of a child who has poliomyelitis may need help with home care during the convalescent period. The nurse may estimate the mother's present knowledge and needs for instruction by discussing with her a booklet describing home care. As nurse and mother review the material together, the mother's comments and questions will provide the basis for estimation of needs.

Listening and "reflecting" are discussed fully in Chapter X, but must be mentioned here because of their value in analysis of needs. Given a favorable climate, and the assurance of professional support, most people can do much to clarify and to think through their own problems. Through a relaxed and unhurried manner, and withholding her own analysis of needs and problems, the nurse can convey to the patient her willingness to let him think through what is troubling him, or what he needs to know or have to take care of his health problems. Rather than directing the conversation, the use of noncommital phrases or statements, reflecting what the patient himself has said, encourages the patient to go on in his appraisal. This approach is especially important in eliciting information about attitudes or problems of an emotional nature, where only the patient can gauge their importance to him. For example, a patient may say "I won't go back to the clinic. The doctors are inhuman and the whole set-up is badly run." The nurse may "reflect" this, saying "You don't think you'll go back," offering neither resistance, approval or disapproval. With the responsibility thus left with him, the patient may say "Well, I don't say I'll never go back," or "I don't see why I should be pushed around just because I'm not paying for care." The patient's capacity to move from a negative or hostile attitude toward greater objectivity, as well as the final status of the need his statements reveal, is highly significant in evaluating his capacity for self-direction, and in identifying his attitudes toward health care.

Listening and reflecting are not incompatible with directing conversation—each takes a place in the over-all two-way relationship between patient and nurse. The nurse needs both skill and sensitivity to recognize at which points in the patient-nurse contact to use one or the other approach.

Post-visit Analysis of Needs. The nurse may find it necessary to supplement the information relative to needs that she was able to secure before and during the nursing visit. A conference with Johnny's teacher or with the school recreational director may be necessary to determine the degree to which a physical impairment is interfering with normal activity; contact with the personnel division may help to decide whether Mr. Jones' nervousness is affecting or being affected by his work; the social worker who knew a family at some previous time might be able to throw some light on Mrs. Smith's unwillingness to accept her pregnancy. Sometimes a conference with a consultant or specialist may be needed if the nurse is to interpret what she has seen or found. Talking with the psychiatrist-consultant may help to appraise the significance of a patient's aggressive behavior; the nutritionist might review the food habits and dietary intake of a family whose diet includes many foods that are unfamiliar to the nurse, or when the disease imposes certain demands for special dietary adaptation; the public health engineer can help to determine whether a farm family needs aid in relation to protection of its water supply.

Reading records of other agencies may help to supplement the nurse's information. The hospital record of delivery and of the immediate postnatal period may provide important clues to the mother's attitude or physical condition; the cumulative school health record may help to relate observed behavior of the school age child to his total condition.

In analyzing the health needs of the family, the nurse uses her own basic professional information, records and reports that yield information about the patient, the family and the community, and observation and discussion with the patient or family to elicit facts, conditioning factors and attitudes that together indicate the needs of the patient for public health nursing care.

Organizing the Statement of Needs

Once the several sources of information regarding health needs have been investigated the results should be synthesized and a statement of needs incorporated into the nursing or health record. This may be a detailed statement of the problems and needs, incorporated into the permanent record, or the detailed statement may be used only in a working record similar to the one shown in Figure 10, and the notation on the permanent record may be a brief diagnostic one.

The statement of needs to be incorporated into the health record should be concise, clear-cut, and as far as possible related to family rather than purely individual needs. For example, if Johnny Jones needs to be vaccinated before entering school, the problem from the individual point of view is to secure the appropriate treatment. From the family standpoint, there may need to

Family 1. *Smith*, Charles (26) 2. Evelyn (24) 3. Mary (2) 4. Mrs. Sara Smith (61)
1820 Holmes Street   Ground floor

Problems	Accepted by N F M.D.			Modificants	Plan	Outcome
1. Prenatal care Fearful Poor breakfast (other meals adequate)	X	X	X	Difficult first labor Mrs. S., Sr. feels "too much fuss" Income adequate —has private M.D. Hospital physi- cian Husband sup- portive	Mothers' class— St. Albans, beg. Dec. 4 Conferences Mrs. S., Sr., get her to help Get Mrs. S., Sr., to Senior Citi- zens' Club at her church H. V. at 6th month	Attended all 6 sessions Instr. reports interested, beneficial
2. Child manage- ment Anxious mother	X			Child vigorous, active	Refer to Spock's book; Mr. S. to read, too Office confer- ences after mother's de- livery	
Play space in- adequate— Plays in kitchen		X		Mother gets irri- table if child "under foot" Worries about housework "Can't stand a messy house"	Suggest to Mr. S. gate for break- fast nook to make safe day- time play area Play in park on sunny days	
3. Cancer diag. check up Mrs. S., Sr.	X	X		Expressed worry re: this, though no symptoms	Refer to H.Dept. Multi Diag. Clinic Dec. 19, with approval from family doctor January 14, Re- appt.	Missed ap- pointment Attended— findings, negative
Overweight— Mrs. S., Sr.	X		X		Conf. with doctor Counseling re: diet	Doctor sug- gested low- calorie diet
etc.						

Figure 10.   Suggested form for family care planning sheet.

be an interpretation of the whole problem of preventive care, the relation of Johnny's vaccination to the needs of other family members, and the facilities available for the necessary care for the whole family. Needs for instruction and guidance should be included as well as needs for medical care and nursing service.

Information on health needs should be used as a basis for planning and service. For this reason it should be so placed that it is readily accessible. When indicated, priorities in service may also be noted.

Information entered on nonmedical records, such as the cumulative school record or the industrial personnel record, should be carefully selected. For example, reports of physical condition may be included in the general guidance folder to be used by teachers, counselors or special supervisors in the school. When the health findings are not extensive or of such a nature that they should be held confidential this may be adequate. For students whose problems are complex, a special medical record will be needed. In this case the medical record would be considered a confidential record, and only such information as was pertinent to the educational program would be placed in the general record.

DEVELOPING MUTUALLY ACCEPTABLE GOALS

In a recent report of a task force of the American Public Health Association the following statement appears:

"In a democratic society an individual will always retain primary responsibility for his own health and that of his family."[9]

In planning for public health nursing care, it is essential that the focal place of the family be recognized, and that the goals of the service be developed and accepted by the family as well as by the nurse and other professional workers who may be involved.

Unless the family members understand and accept the purposes of and need for the action planned, and want action to be taken when it is necessary, their ability to participate intelligently in their own health care will be limited. They may, to be sure, acquiesce in care, motivated by a respect for authority or a desire to please, without really accepting the need as valid. This response produces at best a limited outcome, since the service so accepted is without any personal significance. The immedi-

9. Report of the American Public Health Association Task Force. *American Journal of Public Health*, 47: 218–234, February, 1957.

ate situation may be met, but there is little stimulus for lasting change in behavior in health matters.

Timing is an important factor in determining the impact of a particular problem on the family. The mother who is worried about a child who is recovering from poliomyelitis may not be ready to discuss her own need for elective surgery. Once the child's acute illness and early convalescence is over, she may be ready to accept her own need for care as valid and worthy of action. The concept of need and willingness to do something about it are not always based on logical considerations. For instance, a woman may feel that it is more important to finish her fall cleaning than to go to the clinic to investigate the lump in her breast; or the student with acute abdominal distress may feel that he cannot afford to go to the hospital until he has taken a final examination. Setting goals for public health nursing care must take account of both family and professional staff concepts of need.

Securing Understanding and Acceptance of Needs. The degree to which comprehension and acceptance of health needs exists will vary greatly from one family to another, and at different periods within the same family. The nurse, too, will find that her ability to understand and accept needs will vary with her experience and preparation, and in some instances with the degree to which she possesses ancillary knowledge such as information about the community or about the physical and emotional demands of certain types of employment. The nurse is apt to have a broader concept of needs from the technical viewpoint, while the family may have deeper insight into the emotional needs of its members.

Health needs that seem obvious to the nurse may not always be understood or accepted by the family. For instance, the working mother who is faced with the problem of an adolescent daughter who is complaining of frequent ills for which no physical cause can be found may see her problem as one of forcing the child to accept responsibility, to be a "good girl." The mother may be too overwhelmed with her own work to recognize her daughter's need for assurance that life can be fun, and that she is loved and appreciated, although these needs are very obvious to the nurse.

Failure to understand health needs may be based upon inadequate or inaccurate information, or upon an inability to relate and apply known facts to the present situation. For example, a woman may refuse surgical care for cancer of the breast "because it is hopeless anyway," or a father may refuse to secure dental care for a small child because "she has only baby teeth."

In some cases the family may see only part of the problem, because of a lack of sufficiently comprehensive information. A mother may say, speaking of a child with a cardiac impairment, "I do want to learn how to give care to Mary. I've told the family they can't expect anything from me; all I'm going to do is take care of my sick baby." The mother is fully aware of the physical needs of the child. The nurse, however, may recognize that this "care of my sick baby" may lead to overprotectiveness that will interfere with Mary's emotional adjustment to her illness. The mother has not seen the child's need for independence, or the needs of the rest of the family who must share in the problem and who must also make many adjustments in the protracted period of Mary's convalescence. It is possible that the mother is welcoming this opportunity to be home nurse as an escape from the humdrum activities of housework, and might need guidance in securing better job adjustment for herself. The mother and other family members need more information and counseling to come to the realization that Mary's illness requires planning and participation by the entire family, and that her personality as well as her heart must be protected from damage due to the disease.

Sometimes the family or individual has the necessary information for health care but fails to relate it to the situation. For example, a foreman who was very particular about accident prevention in his plant saw no incongruity in having the cellar stairs of his home littered with cleaning equipment and old paint cans. His knowledge of accident prevention was applied admirably on the job, but he failed to apply it in his own home. A young woman of good family who had classic symptoms of early syphilis, and who knew what they were, failed to seek an examination because she "knew things like that couldn't happen" to her or to her husband, because they were "nice people." Perhaps the best example is that of nurses themselves; studies of their own health practices often reveal that the knowledge they dispense to other people is not applied in their own lives.

Even when the individual knows about his own health needs, he may fail to accept them or to face the need for health action. This may be due to

1. Unwillingness to face reality
2. Unwillingness to oppose family or social pressures

3. Adherence to patterned behavior
4. Failure to relate needed action to family or individual goals.

Fear may cause a man to fail to secure an eye examination when he has symptoms of glaucoma. He may recognize the symptoms, realize that something is wrong, yet fail to admit there is really a problem. As long as he does not have the examination and does not definitely know the diagnosis, he feels that he does not have to face the possibility of a long and complicated treatment or of blindness.

Sometimes family or social pressures are such that the patient finds it easier not to flout them in taking necessary health action. It may be easier to coddle mother through her heart attacks than to run the risk of being considered an ungrateful child for following the doctor's advice to treat them as the attention-getting device they really are. It may be easier to keep the toddler in "cute" clothes and white shoes, thus earning the admiration of the neighbors, than to accept his need for active play and for clothes that permit freedom of movement. Social pressures may cause a family to disregard the need for home-centered recreation in favor of a spotless house, or ignore the need for privacy in family housing in order to have less space at a "good address."

Habit may be a powerful factor in delaying or preventing acceptance of health needs. The "sandwich and coffee lunch" pattern, the "wash dishes after every meal" habit, or the habit of storing kitchen equipment behind closed doors and in inaccessible closets in order to keep a neat kitchen may cause the individual or family to fail to accept the need for new ways that will lead to decrease of fatigue. The mother who was taught as a child to respect her parents may find it hard to accept a child's need to express his rebellion; the habit of putting off things until the last moment may make it impossible for the young man to see his need for a medical examination *before* he is ill.

Sometimes individuals fail to relate health needs to their own desires and goals. For example, one young man who was told he needed surgical care for hernia said he didn't have time because of his studies—he wanted to be a foreign correspondent and was taking evening classes in journalism. He failed to recognize the relationship between his work ambitions and an unusually good health status, or to think that the rigors of travel and of daily living to which newsmen on foreign assignment are often subjected demand unusual physical stamina. The father who is anxious for his children to succeed may fail to see the importance of emotional security as a basis for a successful career in almost every field, as well as for the happiness of the individual. Once the father has seen this relationship, he may be readier to see the need to adjust the family pattern of living to reduce tension, and to place less pressure upon the children to attain high school-grades at any cost.

Stimulating Recognition and Acceptance of Needs.   The public health nurse may help the family to understand and accept its health needs by:

1. Broadening the base of the family's information
2. Helping the family to see the implications of the situation by means of questions and clarifying statements
3. Relating health needs to the goals of the individual or family
4. Encouraging wholesome emotional attitudes toward the problem.

When information is inadequate the nurse may extend the family's information by the use of health informational materials, or by serving as a source of expert information herself, or by referring the family or individual to another adviser or to a study group. For example, in discussing the care of tuberculosis it may become apparent that the family is not willing to accept the need for examination of contacts. Through the use of a booklet which clarifies the nature of spread of the disease, and the facts that the perfectly healthy appearing person may have been infected and treatment of incipient disease is hopeful and not too restricting, the family may understand the factual base on which the procedure of contact examination is recommended, and may accept the need. The nurse may provide information about the routines or the costs at the hospital, or the confidential nature of health department records. If questions arise that seem more suitable for referral to the physician, it may be suggested that the family members write down their questions before their next visit to the doctor in the clinic or in his office. The new patient may be referred to a group discussion program, where there is an opportunity for the patients to talk about their problems with other patients, and with a physician, nurse or health educator.

Sometimes the family has the necessary information, but has failed to bring it to bear on the problem, or to think through the implications of the needs. In such cases, the nurse may assist the family to see its needs in a broader way through the use of questions and suggestions. In a family where there is a child who needs surgical correction of an orthopedic defect, the family may fail to accept the need for immediate action, even though it does have the facts. By discussing the fact that Johnny is "smart for his age" it may be possible to lead to a discussion of the family's hopes for him, and this in turn may cause some reconsideration of the obligation to look at and act upon this immediate situation. The family may also be helped to see that Johnny's ability to understand other things would probably lead one to suppose he would understand and accept this need for care. The mother who "is giving up everything for her children" may know the facts about the children's need for independence yet fail to act on it. Through informal discussion and encouraging the mother to talk about herself and her relationships with the children, she may be helped to readjust her way of doing things to provide them with greater freedom and also to begin preparing herself for the period when the children will have grown up.

The nurse can do much to stress the relationship between health needs and family or individual goals, both through informal discussion of the demands of certain types of work or what goes into "providing for" a family. The working mother who never has time to spend with her growing children may feel that she is providing for them in a rather lavish way. Through discussion and talking about her plans for them and her desire to give them "the best" she may realize that the best cannot always be equated with the most in terms of material things. The relation between proper dietary and rest habits and the vitality and verve that make a girl attractive, between accident prevention and continuity of income, between the admiration of children for a mother who "does things" and relinquishing of overprotectiveness in favor of community activities can also be made clear in many ways.

Encouraging a positive emotional attitude toward health problems will also promote acceptance of them, and hence lead to action toward desirable health practice. This can often be achieved best through indirect methods. The nurse's unemotional, matter-of-fact approach to venereal disease, cancer or poliomyelitis may be much more reassuring than any amount of saying "This is just another disease." Emphasis upon the curability of the disease, and the good fortune of the individual who has discovered it early, rather than upon the dangers of delayed action; upon what the handicapped person can learn to do, rather than upon his limitations; and upon the positive aspects of the situation, rather than upon the negative ones may also serve to direct the patient's thinking and action toward productive ends.

Calm acceptance of antisocial attitudes by the nurse will also leave the way open for more constructive consideration of needs, once the hostility has been released. The mother who says she doesn't want her baby, and the man with an infectious disease who says "Somebody gave it to me, why should I worry about anyone else?" need to feel that the nurse understands and accepts them. It is then possible for the patient to talk out these feelings without restraint. Following such a release of feelings, most patients are willing to look again at their needs, and in many instances adopt a very much revised attitude toward them.

Until health needs are accepted and understood, family action toward better health care is apt to be inadequate or poorly directed. If planning proceeds on the basis of the *nurse's* concept of needs, while the family remains in doubt as to their validity or importance, the family may resist any plan, or may appear to agree to the plan for action but actually fail to follow through.

The nurse, too, may fail to understand or to fully accept family health needs. This may be due to:

1. Improper collection of facts
2. Lack of training or skill in interpretation
3. Inadequate appreciation of social factors
4. Use of a patterned approach in working with families.

Public health nurses all too often work under the pressure of heavy case loads and multiple demands on their time. When time is limited, there is always danger that there will be errors and omissions in the collection or interpretation of information relative to health needs. Failure to talk to the schoolteacher about the child who seems listless and bored at home may cause the nurse to feel that this is a continuous attitude, when actually his school behavior is exactly opposite to that at home. Careless scanning rather than careful study of an infant's clinic record may result in failure to see indications of a mother's anxiety about her child's health, and this in turn may cause her to evaluate the significance of the mother's recital of symptoms of illness incorrectly. Inadequate coordination with other health or welfare agencies interested in a family may lead the nurse to an inaccurate estimate of the health conditions of the family.

Even with carefully and completely gathered information, the nurse may fail to interpret the family's needs correctly because of lack of training or experience. For example, an inexperienced nurse may give too much weight to a recital of abuse or mistreatment by husband or children by a tired wife. A more experienced nurse might observe many informal remarks or actions that show a very real basic acceptance and affection among family members, and recognize this attitude as a temporary expression of a need to rebel. Inadequate professional knowledge, such as too little knowledge of the effects of a particular drug, or of the emotional concomitants of certain disease conditions, may make it difficult for the nurse to understand the family's needs fully. Lack of counseling skill may cause the nurse to miss tangible evidences of need that the more skilled counselor sees in minor changes of expression, or in an appearance of tension or bluntness. Often the young nurse will "overdiagnose"—seeing needs that do not require nursing care, since the family is already handling them adequately.

The nurse may fail to give sufficient weight to family attitudes and relationships that affect the family's concept of the relative importance of certain health needs. For example, in some households the new mother holds court after her delivery, while neighbors flock in to admire the new baby and congratulate the parents. The family would lose face if there were not a beautiful sheet for the bed, and refreshment for the visitors. The importance of undisturbed rest for the baby or of saving money for equipment for baby care may be of less concern to the family than are social obligations. The nurse must accept the validity of such claims for social acceptance and prestige, and take them into account when planning, even when they are in conflict with what she feels to be logical or desirable.

Sometimes there is a tendency to consider situations in a patterned manner. For example, one nurse planned for a family on the basis that its members were of limited mental capacity. Both mother and father had left school very early, one child was in an institution for the feeble-minded and three of the other four children were retarded in school. However, one child, despite great environmental handicaps, had maintained reasonably good grades in school and had never been held back. His very real ability needed to be fostered, and his needs for encouragement and support brought home to the family. Because the nurse saw the family as a *kind* of a family she had failed to look closely enough to see Jim and his special problem. Similar errors may occur if the nurse has developed habits of thinking that produce a stereotyped response to particular problems—assuming that all unmarried mothers are maladjusted; that intelligent people face problems realistically; or that all adolescents are in rebellion against the elder generation. The nurse may fail to see the needs as they really are because they do not fit into her preconceived idea of what they *should* be.

Understanding and acceptance of health needs may be a developing rather than an "all-or-none" matter. Sometimes the family's concept of its health needs and problems is quite limited in the early phases of care and later becomes quite comprehensive. For example, in the early period of caring for a patient with long-term illness the family may recognize the need for guidance in respect to the physical care of the patient and actually resist any help with emotional or social aspects of care. Later the family's concept may broaden to include emotional support of the patient, family adjustments to make the care of the patient less burdensome and less disruptive of family living, or participation in community action toward securing better care for chronic illness through legislation or increase of hospital facilities as needs with which the family want help.

Planning may have to be partial at first, expanding as the family's awareness and appreciation of needs becomes broader and deeper. The nurse must be aware of the degree to which the family understands and accepts its health problems; she must seek the reasons for nonacceptance and provide the necessary support and counseling that will promote a full realization and appreciation of its needs by the family. It is only on this sound base that effective health action can be built.

CHAPTER VIII

Developing a Plan
for Care: Organizing to
Meet Family Health Needs

ONCE THE HEALTH needs of the family have been analyzed, the next step is to estimate the resources that are available to deal with the problems presented. Such resources may be found in the family itself, or in various individuals or agencies in the community. In appraising and organizing resources for health care, maximum independence and responsibility should rest with the family. For example, in arranging for attendance at a preschool clinic in a rural community, transportation may be a problem because the family does not have a car and there is no public transportation available. The nurse may immediately take the initiative and offer the assistance of a volunteer driver who will come from a nearby town. If, however, the family is given an opportunity to work out a solution, a better plan might result. Perhaps a neighbor would be willing to arrange his weekly visit to town on the clinic day, and the mother and child could go with him, or they might ride in on the market truck of another neighbor. The family will gain a sense of pride in its ability to meet its own problem. Furthermore, since neighborly assistance is usually easily repaid, there is the added satisfaction of remaining independent—a factor that may be of great importance to the morale of the family.

RESOURCES OF THE FAMILY

Resources of the family may be financial, physical or personal; they range from the very concrete resources such as a separate bed for the family member who is chronically ill or clothes for the new baby, to such intangibles as the sensitivity of family members to the needs of one another, or the capacity to adjust and take constructive action in the face of adversity.

Economic Resources. The adequacy of the family's economic resources in relation to needed health care will depend upon the type of illness, the availability of community facilities for care, and insurance coverage as well as upon the total income and general financial obligations. The family that would ordinarily be medically independent may become medically indigent when faced with a disease of long duration, or with a high degree of disability. Sometimes even when the family is able to secure medical service, difficulty may be found in providing the drugs, dressings, glasses, orthopedic appliances or other facilities for care. Transportation costs may also present an additional strain on a limited budget.

The ability of the family to pay "going rates" for available medical and nursing services is one of the obvious measures of medical-economic resources. Ability to pay may be based upon the use of several types of care—private physician and private practice nurse, private physician and visiting nurse, pay clinic and public health nurse, free clinic with ancillary charges paid by the family, free clinic with drugs and supplies provided to the family without charge.

In considering the family's ability to pay for care, consideration must be given to the total costs involved—medical or hospital charges, transportation, home care for children if the mother is to be away, drugs, supplies and appliances.

Health insurance of various kinds may help to defray costs of illness. Hospital and medical care insurance has gained great popularity. By the end of 1954, there were over 101,000,000 people protected against hospital expense in the United States; approximately 8,500,000 were protected against costs of surgery, and 47,000,000 had regular medical expense coverage.[1]

Workman's compensation provides medical disability benefits for injury occurring in industrial employment for the great majority of workers. Provisions differ greatly from state to state,

1. *Facts About Nursing*, 1955–56 Edition. New York, American Nurses' Association, 1956, p. 83.

and among different industries.[2] Frequently, mutual aid programs are available to supplement such compensation benefits. Industrial health services may be available to workers, providing such services as physical therapy, special treatments, or certain types of home care.

Family credit may be a resource when the inability to pay for medical care seems temporary. Friends or relatives may lend money to meet short-time needs. The family doctor may prefer to accept deferred payment for his services, so the family can remain under his supervision. However, the nurse will need to help the family to face the financial demands of illness realistically, and to avoid relying too much on family credit because of overoptimism about future ability to pay. If the problem of meeting the costs of illness is complex, the medical social worker or family case worker will be needed to help the family with planning.

Resources for health maintenance are also important. An income adequate to provide the essentials of food, clothing and shelter at an acceptable minimum level is basic to health care. Sometimes an economic situation distorts the pattern of family life in such a way as to create a health hazard—as when the working mother must leave her child without proper adult supervision while she works, or when children must work to help support the family. Family income may be too restricted to allow for such services as periodic health examinations, dental care, or for the purchase of glasses.

Physical Resources for Health Care.   Provision of adequate equipment and materials for healthful living practice and for home care of the sick is important in assuring good health care. Usually it is possible to provide much that is necessary by reorganization and adaptation of available materials.

Physical equipment for healthful living practice includes facilities for maintaining personal cleanliness, particularly those needed for hand-washing; sleeping arrangements that permit freedom from disturbance; protection from disease carriers such as mosquitos and rodents through the provision of adequate screening and rat-proofing; adequate facilities for food preparation; food, water and milk supplies that are or can be made safe; and sanitary facilities for disposal of bodily wastes.

Even when these facilities are minimal, they may be made

2. Brown, Mary L., *Occupational Health Nursing*. New York, Springer, 1956, Chapter 15, "Workman's Compensation."

adequate by careful and resourceful planning.[3] Hand-washing facilities, for example, might be a pitcher and basin. Properly placed in the rural home they permit and encourage good hand-washing practice. A similar arrangement might work equally well in a tenement where a single sink must serve both for hand-washing and for food preparation and dish-washing. Folding cots may be used if there is not room for an additional bed; cloth screening will exclude insects until such time as metal or plastic screening can be obtained; a play space walled off by kitchen chairs will protect the city child from accident, while his country cousin may play in designated outdoor areas to avoid the fields where large farm equipment is in use. In other words, the facilities for healthful living may be potential rather than in actual use. In appraising resources, first consideration should be given to what could be done with the facilities that are at hand or are readily available.

Personal Resources.   Personal-social resources of the family are perhaps the most important of its contributions to health care. These include:

1. Family personnel available to provide health care
2. Intra-family relationships
3. Previously acquired knowledge or skill in health matters
4. Practical family management skills
5. Individual and family problem-solving ability.

The availability of personnel to provide care is an important factor in planning. If the mother works during the day and is not available to help and supervise children during illness and the convalescent period some substitute must be found. In the care of chronic illness with considerable disability, where care involves handling of heavy or helpless individuals, the physical capacity of the family members must be considered. An individual may be able to give difficult nursing care over a short period, but be physically unable to do so if the illness is prolonged, or if it involves much care at night as well as during the day.

The adequacy of personnel resources for home care of the sick should also be related to the maintenance of physical and emotional health of the home nurse. A high school student, for example, may be physically able to give daily care to her bedridden grandmother, but if she were to be made wholly responsible for such care it might seriously interfere with social activities within her own age group and so lead to emotional strain and conflict.

3. American National Red Cross, *Red Cross Home Nursing*. Philadelphia, Blakiston Co., 1951.

Intra-family relationships are an important factor in health care. The sensitivity of family members to each other's needs and reactions is invaluable in appraising the degree of difficulty of a health problem. It brings early recognition of any deviation from normal, and quick appreciation of emotional impediments to full use of medical or nursing facilities. Family interdependence may also be highly developed and provide a valuable resource for care. Recognition of such interdependence creates a willingness to share problems and to work together for good health. For example, big brother could consciously set an example for little brother in the matter of brushing teeth or washing hands; big sister could plan to do her homework and watch little sister while mother shops, thus permitting more economical shopping than is possible through telephoned orders; sister might agree to make-up at her dressing table rather than at the bathroom mirror to cut down on the family rush and permit a more leisurely breakfast for the whole family.

Family affection is another important personal resource. It can be called upon to build confidence and self-control of the family member who must face a difficult diagnosis. Having mother present during the clinic examination may make Junior confident and unafraid even when faced with an immunization "shot." Family affection is a prime motivating force in obtaining total family support in such activities as keeping father on a low-calorie diet, or keeping brother Joe from becoming spoiled and overdependent because he has a cardiac impairment.

Family relationships are one of the strongest forces in molding behavior. They can be used to effectuate or improve family health care, as well as for many other desirable social ends.

The problem-solving ability of the family is another valuable health resource. Habits of independent thinking on the part of families, and ability to seek answers to their own problems is of great importance in health maintenance and care.

The family that is accustomed to (or can learn) problem solving will find ways to meet such problems as organizing the home to meet the needs of a member of the family who is chronically ill. Members of the family will recognize the need for the sick person to be near others, to participate in family activities, yet have sufficient isolation to assure adequate rest, and will find some way of manipulating the environment to meet these needs. One family rearranged the kitchen so a couch could be placed there, and the sick person spend part of the day helping with simple kitchen chores that could be done in bed. Another set up the dining room as a sickroom, and turned an end of the kitchen into a dining spot. Such habits of defining problems and working out answers may be applied to many health situations. For example, in construction of equipment for a handicapped person, making a schedule for the home nurse that will prevent unnecessary fatigue; or trying new methods of food preparation when selection of foods is limited or when different tastes must be considered.

Within the family this thinking-out process may be essentially an individual matter. Mother or father may figure out the answer, and get the rest of the family to follow the program thus developed. In other families the whole family group works as a unit, discussing the difficulties and possible courses of action, making decisions and dividing responsibilities. When the latter is the case, the basis for independent, thoughtful family health action is secure.

Many individuals and families who have not developed the habit of thinking through their own problems are perfectly capable of doing so. The public health nurse can do much to provide the stimulus and the opportunity for problem-solving activity in relation to the family health.

Extent of Family Health Knowledge.   Family health knowledge and skill provides the basis for new learning. Every family has some amount of knowledge and skill relating to health care. Health information through the radio, newspapers, public schools, community education programs and classes reaches families in varying degrees, but no family is completely unaffected.

In organizing family resources for health care, it is important to know: (1) what facts and skills the family has acquired in relation to its health needs, (2) what selectivity has been developed in using sources of health information, (3) what the family has learned to do about its health problems, and (4) what attitude and competence has been developed in the use of community health facilities.

It is exceedingly important to assess the status of the family's present health competence before offering suggestions or participating in the development of new plans. The remark of the little boy who was introduced to the new public health nurse and said with disgust "I know—a quart of milk a day!" indicates how repeated instruction in matters already familiar to the individual or family may create resistance and resentment, and lead to lack of confidence in the nurse. The mother who knows how to bathe her baby skillfully (though perhaps with a technique somewhat different than that of the nurse) will probably not benefit greatly from detailed re-teaching. However, careful appraisal of what she knows already may provide the basis for discussion of material that is new, of the infant's need for activity, for affection and for security. Furthermore, this recognition of the competence of the family or individual strengthens nurse-family relationships, and provides a sound basis for cooperative planning and action.

It is also important to know what degree of selectivity the family has developed in using sources of health information. Health facts based on advertisements urging the abolishment of "B.O." or stressing the advantages of "staying on the alkaline side" may be wholly acceptable to one family, while another has learned to question such sources and to check information against that issued by the health department or other recognized educational agency.

In appraising knowledge and skill in health matters it is essential not only to discover what the individual or family knows, but also what is done about health. One young university student who got "A" on all of the hygiene examinations and who found no difficulty in outlining the essentials of a good diet had an excellent knowledge of the basic protective foods, and the sources of energy, vitamins and protein, and of the bodily effects of a poor diet. Her breakfast, however, continued to be a "coke" and a doughnut. A mother may know that children who have colds should be taught to protect others from infection, or that milk should be pasteurized, but not apply that knowledge when the situation actually arises.

Skill in the practical aspects of home management is not only a resource upon which the family may call to meet its own needs, but it serves also as a source of information for the public health nurse. The mother of nine will know how difficult it is to buy clothes for one and not for the others, and will know ways in which benefits may be fairly divided. The wife of the man on the "graveyard shift" knows practical ways of adjusting family habits so that father's sleep is not disrupted and the children are not deprived of play and study in the home. The family that must live in a low-cost housing unit has often learned how to set up values within the limits of the facilities afforded—whether less space may be preferable to a larger apartment that is close to a neighborhood bar, or whether central heating is more important than proximity to schools and playgrounds.

The resources of the family provide the framework upon which plans for family health care must be built. The nursing service and other community agencies supplement but do not replace these resources. In every contact with the family the nurse should do everything possible to strengthen and develop the family's capacity to recognize and deal effectively and independently with its own health problems.

RESOURCES OF THE NURSE

The nurse, too, has resources that may be used to meet family health needs. These include technical nursing skills, health information, vicarious experience in meeting family health problems, and teaching and guidance skills.

Technical Skill. This is the most obvious of the nurse's resources for contributing to the health care of the family. She is able to provide direct nursing care or treatments when a high degree of judgment and skill is required, to collect specimens for diagnostic study, or to perform diagnostic tests for interpretation by the physician—all of which are recognized by the family and the doctor alike as a major responsibility. Her ability to observe symptoms of disorder and to relate them intelligently to the total situation is equally important.

The degree to which nursing skills can be made available to the family will depend upon the time available and upon agency policy. If the case load is low, and the agency committed to a program of direct nursing service, the amount of technical nursing care available may be adequate to meet all needs. In other instances, even though the nurse is equipped to provide professional nursing care, the time available may make it impossible to give complete service. In estimating technical nursing resources it is necessary to know not only what skills the nurse actually possesses, but also the extent to which these skills can be applied to meet family needs.

Sometimes the nurse will stretch her own resources by teaching others to give care under her supervision. In some communities she may find professional nurses who are willing to give volunteer assistance, or family members who may be taught to give care.

The Nurse As a Source of Health Information. Many families served by the public health nurse need health information, but are not accustomed to reading. The small child needs to know something about microorganisms to appreciate the necessity for hand-washing; the industrial worker may need facts about the relationship between nutrition and fatigue, or between fatigue and accident rates; the home nurse caring for a child who has measles needs to know the symptoms of complications for which she should be alert; the family caring for a bedridden aunt needs to know what causes bedsores and how they may be avoided.

Much information of this nature will be transmitted by word of mouth, and adapted to meet the needs of the immediate situation. The family looks to the nurse to supply such help, and it is an accepted part of nursing service. When a greater degree of independence is possible, the nurse may help the family to secure authoritative pamphlets, refer the family to the public library for books on health care, suggest helpful moving pictures, or arrange for consultation with special workers of other agencies.

Vicarious Experiences. Because of her intimate knowledge of many families, the public health nurse has a store of vicarious experience in the practical problems of securing good health care. She knows what Mr. Jones did when he had to be away from work for six months owing to a nervous breakdown; she knows how Mrs. Salvatore organized her housework, using her six children as helpers and managing to keep a clean house and still find time to join in family recreation; she knows how Johnny and Evelyn and Sarah reacted to their first school health examination and what their parents did to help. Such practical information is particularly helpful to families facing similar problems.

Teaching and Counseling Skills. The public health nurse can present needed health information to families in such a way that it enables them to understand their own needs and to comprehend the principles on which action should be based. She may use various types of audio-visual aids to clarify health concepts or to demonstrate skills in health care. She can use the influence of groups to promote thinking and action of its individual members in mother's classes or in group discussions for parents. By listening, reflecting, questioning, supplementing, she can help individuals to think out their problems.

These teaching and counseling skills are essential in assisting families to consider all aspects of a problem before deciding upon a course of action, to base health action on knowledge of the available facts, and to consider remote as well as immediate outcomes of a particular behavior pattern. For example, the mother is meeting a recognized need when Johnny screams and she holds or bribes him to keep him quiet. She is stopping the irritating noise, and probably satisfying the neighbors. The possible costs in relation to Johnny's future stability and ability to live successfully with others might pass unnoticed if the nurse did not raise questions about the course of action that will be followed when Johnny's demands become impossible to meet, or provide the mother with simple material describing a child's need to blow off steam as a reaction to frustration. Such direction and supplementation of knowledge leads the mother to think further about the problem, and perhaps to work out a more satisfactory solution.

As with families, the nurse will find that some of her resources for health care are potential rather than fully developed. She may not, for example, have developed skill in working with groups, or may lack sufficient information in relation to certain disease situations, or may still find it difficult to work with resistive individuals. She should be aware of the deficiencies as well as the positive components in her contribution to total family health care, and develop the competences and skills she needs to help.

COMMUNITY RESOURCES FOR HEALTH CARE

Community resources for health care will vary greatly in their complexity and organization. While most communities provide basic resources for medical and nursing care, for social case work and other welfare services and for recreation, the pattern of resources will be very different. Medical care in community "A" may mean visits to the office of the general practitioner, or home calls by the family doctor. In community "B" it may mean the use of public clinics and hospitals for the great majority of the population, with care by the private physician assuming less importance. Recreation facilities in one community may mean settlement-house activities and organized playgrounds; to another community they may mean hay rides, picnics and fishing parties arranged by the group itself.

Community resources will include agencies and individuals who provide care for health, welfare and protective needs. Community health resources include public, voluntary and commercial agencies and individuals who provide health service, health protection or health instruction.

Health Services.   Health services may be rendered to the family by physicians, hospitals and related institutions such as nursing homes, infirmaries or clinics, by private practice nurses, community agencies such as visiting nurse associations or welfare agencies, or health departments. In most communities the private physician in general practice is the focal point in family health services. Specialists in medical practice may be readily available in some areas, but the distribution is uneven, and in some specialty fields such as psychiatry there are distinct general shortages.[4]

Sometimes specialist services are provided on an itinerant or consultant basis through state departments of health. Divisions of tuberculosis control, industrial hygiene, or maternal and child health or crippled children's commissions may provide staff or clinic facilities to meet local needs. The public health nurse through interpretation and promotional activities can do much to encourage full use of such state-sponsored services.

In addition to general hospital beds, facilities for care of tuberculosis and other communicable disease, mental disease and chronic illness will be available in varying degrees. With the increasing use of home care facilities, tuberculosis hospitals are less crowded, but facilities for care of the mentally ill and for patients with long-term illness may be less available. Nursing homes, often operated on a profit basis, vary greatly in the quality of care provided and in cost. Recently there has been emphasis upon the provision of hospital services for rehabilitation, including appraisal of work potential and occupational training as well as medical care, but such facilities have not yet been widely developed.

Facilities for professional nursing care are almost universally limited. The public health nurse will want to investigate the resources of the local nurse's registry if there is one, and find out whether practical as well as professional nurses may be obtained from that source. She will want to know the rates for private practice nursing, and the availability of nurses for home care. Nursing resources of stores or industries, visiting nurse associations, doctors' offices or private clinics should be considered. Often the nurse in the physician's office is doing an excellent counseling and teaching job, and she may be a valuable resource in extending public health teaching and guidance.

The public health nurse will find it valuable to know not only the actively practicing nurse group, but also inactive nurses who may be called upon in emergencies to assist with special projects or to take leadership in their own neighborhood groups. Local Red Cross chapters may maintain rosters of nurses who have indicated a willingness to serve on a volunteer basis in Red Cross instructional or service programs and in approved community activities.

4. Dickinson, F. G., *Distribution of Physicians by Medical Service Areas.* Chicago, American Medical Association, 1953.

Practical nurses and midwives also play an important part in the provision of nursing care. It is important to know how many practical nurses are available, what type of training or experience they have had, and the provisions for licensing and supervision that have been established in the state.[5]

Clinic services of various types may be available in the community. These may be sponsored by hospitals, local or state departments of health, charitable organizations, industrial or commercial firms.

Health Protective Services.   Health protection is generally the responsibility of governmental agencies. Departments of health, sanitation, labor, and food and milk control may participate in these services. Through such activities as enforcement of health department regulations, inspection of buildings and swimming pools, they contribute to the control of environmental hazards to health. Through control of prostitution, epidemiologic study, enforcement of isolation and quarantine measures, they help to control communicable disease.

It is important to know the adequacy as well as the existence of such agencies. For example, it is well to know the degree to which regulations regarding pasteurization of milk, compulsory vaccination of school children, required physical inspection, or examination of school children or food handlers is enforced.

A graph or description of the city or county governmental structure will provide information about the various divisions and services and their respective responsibilities. Regulations of the department of health and of the department of education may be secured from the appropriate department.

It is important to know to what degree the local health department meets the criteria for full health service; whether there is a full-time medical officer of health, and an adequate number of public health nurses, engineers and sanitarians for the population served. In some communities, health department facilities will be frankly inadequate. In others, the basic services will be covered; in a few, there will be a fully developed basic program and in addition such services as bedside care of the sick, dental services or extensive mental health or child guidance programs.

"Adequate" is difficult to define owing to differences in communities, but, in general, health departments should carry the

5. In 1955, only two states and the District of Columbia had no provision for licensing of practical nurses. However, licensing provisions vary greatly from state to state.

basic services listed in Chapter V and should be under the direction of a full-time health officer. Suggested concentrations indicated in the Emerson report are sometimes used as a base line, although they are admittedly low.[6]

Health Instruction. Health instruction may be available in the community from the public schools, in adult education classes organized by the public schools, community centers, cooperative societies, labor organizations or other groups. Local branches of national health organizations such as the National Tuberculosis Association, the American Cancer Society, local mental hygiene associations or the American Red Cross may also provide health instruction or health education materials.

Health instruction is an integral part of all health service agencies, since education of the patient and family is assumed to be a necessary part of health care. In many cases, health service agencies will offer group as well as individual instruction. Some hospitals offer lectures and courses to their patients, with instruction provided by the medical and nursing staff. Clinics may have well-organized classes for special patients such as those with rheumatic heart disease or diabetes. Hospitals, health departments or visiting nurse services may have classes for expectant mothers and fathers, or regularly scheduled lectures for the general public. Industrial health services may provide courses in personal hygiene, first aid, obesity control, or home care of the sick, or offer special opportunities such as film showings on self-examination of the breast.

Many rural agencies also have extensive health education programs. The work of the county agents and home demonstration agents of the Department of Agriculture has been outstanding. 4-H Clubs and the Future Farmers of America place health activities as one of their major activities. The Grange or farmer cooperatives also offer many opportunities for health education.

The Parent-Teacher Association has been very active in health action and in spreading health information, both as a great national organization and in its local school units. Future nurses' clubs may also offer education facilities.

Commercial sources may have well-developed and useful health informational materials, or may offer special courses or lectures. Some insurance companies produce pamphlets, moving pictures or slides on health care; utility companies frequently offer courses

6. Emerson, H. and M. Luginbuhl, *Local Health Units for the Nation.* New York, Commonwealth Fund, 1945, p. 2.

in nutrition and food preparation; department stores may sponsor parents' classes or "personal development" lectures that have a strong health component.

Commercial sources of health information should be reviewed with great care to be sure the content is scientifically accurate, and the promotional or advertising element not such that it overbalances or distorts the material. Some public health agencies and educational systems have specific policies on the conditions under which commercial materials may be used.

Welfare agencies also contribute to health care. These include public and private welfare agencies, hospital social service departments, mutual aid associations of various types and fraternal societies. They may provide intensive case work, financial assistance or friendly services that supplement the medical care of the patient. It is important to differentiate between the objectives and services of these agencies, and to refer families selectively.

The welfare agency that provides intensive family case work, under the direction of a qualified social worker, fills a very different need than does the relief agency designed to allot financial assistance in accordance with established regulations. The *Social Work Yearbook* describes the work of various types of welfare agencies, and is a helpful background for study of local welfare resources.[7]

Recreational resources may be an important adjunct in family health care, offering opportunity to develop good family relationships or to contribute to therapy. Public schools may have afterschool activities; settlement houses, day centers for the aged, parks, swimming pools, nurseries, public theaters or concerts may provide activities that contribute to health maintenance or to the treatment of illness. Commercial recreational facilities such as theaters, swimming pools, skating rinks or tennis courts may also prove to be valuable resources.

Informal resources—the helpful neighbor, the priest with a knack for and interest in working with teen-agers, the grocer who appreciates an opportunity to do small anonymous helping things —are particularly significant in many communities and should be discovered and cultivated.

ORGANIZATION AND USE OF HEALTH RESOURCES

If the nurse is to use these many different resources for health care effectively, the information concerning them must be care-

7. *Social Work Yearbook, 1954.* New York, Russell Sage Foundation, 1955.

fully assembled and organized for ready use. The public health nurse must plan to (1) locate available health resources, (2) define the scope and limitations of service, (3) construct and maintain a readily available record or reference file of resources and (4) develop suitable referral procedures.

Locating Health Resources. Information on organized resources and service agencies may be available in the nursing office in the form of a resource file, or, in some communities, may be listed in a published directory of health and welfare agencies. Informational sources on community agencies may be secured from the public library, or from libraries of local or state health or welfare departments. A Community Chest or Community Health Council may have materials on resources.

A list of hospitals approved by the American College of Surgeons is published annually by the American Medical Association, and information about local hospitals may be obtained from the local medical society or hospital association. Lists of physicians, including specialty status, may also be secured from the medical society.

In some states, lists of qualified public health nurses or of licensed professional nurses are published by State Boards of Nurse Licensure, State Nurses' Associations, or State Division of Public Health Nursing of the State Health Department. State Departments of Welfare may publish information on health and welfare agencies within the state.

Information about resources for special care may be secured from appropriate divisions of the state or local health department. Crippled children's services, mental hygiene facilities and diagnostic services for chronic disease are typical of such special services. When there are consultant nurses in these special fields they will be most helpful, and the public health nurse may request a visit through her supervisor or advisory nurse. National associations may also in some instances have information about resources for care.

Individuals who are potential health resources are usually located by the nurse in the course of her daily work. The professional nurse who has retired from active practice, the general medical practitioner who has a special interest in epilepsy, the teacher whose unusual interest in guidance gives her a position of leadership with students, the restaurateur who would take pride in offering "specials" of high nutritional value and low cost, and the foreman who has taken all the courses he could find in first aid are found by the nurse as she talks with patients or co-workers or visits homes, schools or industrial plants. Resources of the family are generally found in the course of direct contact with and service to the family. Occasionally, this will be enriched by consultation with other professional workers, by reading family health records or by reviewing reports from other agencies.

Scope and Limits of Service. If patients are to be properly referred and most effectively served, it is necessary to know what restrictions exist in the service offered; for example, whether there are geographic boundaries or residence requirements, whether there are restrictions in the age group or type of illness received for care, whether certain economic requirements have been set or a means test is enforced. The routines of treatment and frequency of visits a physician prefers, whether he wants his patients to come to him when they cannot pay for care, whether he prefers to give preventive care to small babies or have them cared for in the community clinic, all influence the way in which the nurse uses this service.

The public health nurse will want to visit the most frequently used agencies, the schools and the private physicians in her district to introduce herself and her agency and to secure additional information that will enable her to work effectively with other health and welfare agencies. In general, such visits are most productive when they can be centered about discussion of a particular case that is the joint concern of both parties involved. However, if no such occasion arises, the nurse should visit all of the major agencies shortly after reporting for work in a new community. When such an introductory visit is planned, the nurse should be prepared to request the specific information she will need. For example, she may wish to ask a private physician his office hours, what reports he would like to have on nursing visits, whether he approves the instructional material provided for maternity patients; from a clinic she may want to know the eligibility requirements, whom and when to call regarding referral of new clients, what inter-agency report forms are in use.

Recording and Filing Information. Information on resources should be carefully compiled and recorded. Information about resources of the family should be a part of the family or individual health record. Some of these resources will have significance primarily in relation to the immediate health situation, for example, the availability of adequate equipment for isolation of a child who has a communicable disease, or previous experience with a particular disease such as measles. Such information might well be woven into the first nursing notes as a guide to planning and action in this special situation. Other information about resources will have importance in long-range planning for health care. Family attitudes toward child care, the degree of civic responsibility felt by the family in protection of the health of others, general physical status or physical infirmity are important data. This type of information should be so placed on the record that it is available to the nurse when she is reviewing the record for planning family nursing care.

Limits and scope of nursing resources may be indicated in nursing manuals or directives. Regulations concerning service to the chronically ill or to those not under the care of a physician, or timing and frequency of visits to patients with specified communicable disease are examples of such definitive statements. Sometimes this information is already organized in a nursing manual.

Community resource information may be kept in a card index, in a large notebook kept in the nursing office, or in a small notebook that the nurse carries with her. The nurse who plans her daily work in the nursing office may find an office card file adequate. A suggested form is shown in Figure 11. Such a file is quickly consulted and easily revised, and may be used by nurses working in the same office. When several nurses use a file, some plan should be devised for assigning responsibility for keeping the file current. Each nurse might take responsibility for those agencies that are located in her district, or one nurse or a committee of nurses may review and revise the file periodically.

If the nurse works in a rural area and gets to the nursing office less frequently, or if the resources used cover several communities and are used relatively infrequently, a notebook that can be carried with other nursing equipment may prove more satisfactory. It is important to have such information so organized that it can be easily consulted and revised.

Whatever the form in which the information is kept, the following information will be needed for each individual or agency resource:

1. Identifying information—name, address, telephone number.
2. Type of service rendered by the agency or individual. For the private physician, specialty training or special interest might be noted.

3. Contact procedure—whom to call (medical social worker, health officer, head nurse, intake worker, etc.), hours to call for information, interagency forms to use for reporting.
4. Eligibility requirements—residence, age, citizenship, economic status.

Clinics
Diabetes

Mt. Olive Hospital
3rd and Charles Sts.   Ti. 2–8000
Nurse in charge: Mrs. Evelyn Walker
Hours: M W F 2–4.   Children S 9–11
Eligible: Census tracts 100–105
Charge: To $1.50 per visit if able
Comments: Good instructional program.
        Special interagency form for
        report.
        Request visit within 2 days after
        hospital.

Physicians

Smith,   Ellis
1402 Grove Place   Ac 2–4044
Specialty—General practice, much obstetrics
        Special interest in sterility
Office hours: 2–4 except Wednesday

Comments: Approves standing orders and
        general teaching outline for
        MCH, including relaxation
        exercises.
        Prefers telephone rather than
        written reports.

Figure 11.   Community resource file cards.

5. Referral procedures—forms, admission hours or days, admission procedures, information patient should have on application for care, hours clinic is open.
6. Inter-agency reporting procedure—type and frequency of reports requested, forms for reporting, patient conference procedures.

Information on the various agencies should be recorded in a uniform manner, with the items of information written in the same order. Space may be left on the card or page for comments to record particularized information that is not indicated on the above list. For example, a clinic may be less crowded on one day than on another; a particular physician may feel very strongly the need for reassurance techniques in handling prenatal patients; or an industrial plant may have a nurse or social worker who likes to visit sick employees at home, and would appreciate being informed of friendly services that might be helpful to the patient.

Referral Procedures. Good referral procedures promote optimum use of community resources. It is important to:

1. Get the right person to the right agency. Have all the facts before making a referral.
2. Introduce the client to the agency by sending appropriate information on the referral form, making a preliminary telephone call or personal call if indicated.
3. Introduce the agency to the client. Tell him what to expect, what to bring with him, explain the routines of the agency such as visiting hours or admission procedures in hospital.
4. Make directions explicit and accurate. Give exact times and places.
5. Personalize the referral wherever possible. Telling Mrs. Jones to report to Miss Smith, the nurse in the prenatal clinic, or to Miss Cross, the social worker, promotes easy initial contacts between family and agency. Making some comment on the interest of Dr. Smith in infant care, or how many mothers have benefited from his counsel, gives the family greater confidence in its use of this particular agency.

As nursing assumes a less isolated role in the provision of family health care, the organization and use of resources becomes increasingly important. The public health nurse is in a particularly strong position to promote optimum use of personal and community resources for family health care, and through proper use of such resources to strengthen and direct her own professional service to families.

Developing a Program of Action. Once there is understanding and acceptance of problems or needs, a specific schedule of activities for health care may be planned. Usually the nurse and family member sit down and informally map out what will be done, using information they have gathered from the physician and other health workers who may have participated in the diagnostic process or in previous health care. Sometimes other professional workers or family members may be brought in, and the planning done in conference. For example, in planning for care for a tuberculosis patient, family, nurse and physician, or family, nurse and medical social worker may confer about the care of the patient and the social and economic adjustments that will have to be made. Sometimes the plan will be fairly comprehensive, covering most aspects of the total care. At other times, either because future developments may change the situation or because the family is not ready for long-range planning, the action program may be only partial. For example, if a young mother is obviously distressed and unhappy about her pregnancy, planning in the early home or clinic visits may include only a discussion of clothing and posture adjustments that will make the pregnancy less obvious, and maintenance of a protective diet that will combat unnecessary fatigue or discomfort. As the patient's acceptance and understanding of her condition becomes more complete, plans may be made for instruction of parents in infant care, for increasing knowledge of the process of delivery, and for home adjustments.

Since health care is fundamentally the responsibility of the family itself, planning must also rest with its members. The nurse's role is to guide and supplement rather than direct. The nurse who is assisting the family to make health plans will take the following steps: (1) secure a statement of the family's plan for care; (2) supplement and help modify this plan as necessary; (3) help the family to arrange things to be done in an orderly, timed sequence; and (4) arrange for progress checks.

Eliciting the Family's Plan. Most people have a general idea of the way in which they will meet health problems. Sometimes this idea is well defined and aggressively defended; at other times it is characterized as "Well, I thought I might——." Rarely will a person say "I just don't know," or "I can't figure out what to do," or "I supposed you would tell me that." The way in which a family plans will vary with the amount of experience its members have had with community health facilities, the maturity of the members in meeting other types of problems, and with the extent of emotional trauma present as a result of the health situation. For example, an individual who needs hospitalization for tuberculosis may fail to have an adequate plan for action because he doesn't know the community and its resources or because he has always tended to postpone making unpleasant decisions, or because he is still too shocked by the diagnosis and its implications to react logically to the demands of the situation. In some instances, he may in fact have no plan of action, and want one handed to him by the nurse, doctor or social worker.

In the preliminary period of planning, it is the nurse's function to draw out whatever plan the family has already made, or the feelings about the kind of plan that would be acceptable, to use as a basis for further consideration.

In determining what plans the family has made, it is important not to phrase inquiries in such a way that the family feels forced to make an immediate definite decision, whether or not it is ready to do so. The family that is asked "What are you going to do about hospital care for Mr. Smith?" may feel that an immediate and definite reply is expected. If the family's first plan is not a sound one, changing it involves rejection of an expressed opinion, and that is not always easy. An exploratory question such as "Have you thought where you might go to the hospital?" or "Did Miss Smith talk with you in the clinic about what hospital you might go to?" leads to discussion rather than an immediate answer, and gives the patient and family the feeling of planning together rather than being hurried into immediate action. A feeling of being pushed into a decision rather than being helped to make one is detrimental to relationships as well as to sound planning.

It is important also that the determination of the family's plan be done in such a way as to encourage positive action. "Do you expect to go to the hospital as the doctor advised?" may lead to doubts and indecisions on the part of the patient or family as to the wisdom of following the medical advice at all. "Have you considered what you might do about hospital care?" assumes that positive action will be taken, yet leaves the patient or family free to discuss the matter further.

Through suggestions, directed conversation, or encouraging further talking-out by listening or reflecting the statements made, the nurse supplements the family's plan when it is incomplete or inadequate. The man who has been advised to enter the hospital for a thorough physical appraisal may say "I guess I'll go to the hospital," but may have no idea as to when or where he will go, or what preliminary preparations he should make. In such instances the nurse may supplement the plan by indicating additional things that should be done, or points that should be considered. She may suggest the types of clothing that will be needed in the hospital, procedures used in the various tests, or describe the daily hospital routine or regulations regarding visitors.

She may encourage the family to amplify its plan by raising pertinent questions such as "Have you decided how you will arrange for Jimmie's care when you go to the hospital with Mr. Smith?" or "Can you arrange to go while Jimmie is in school?" If the family seems to be considering private hospital care despite a limited income she might ask "Have you ever visited the County Hospital? Do you know what it is like?"

If the nurse is to be successful in assisting families with health plans she must prepare in advance of the visit or conference for the questions that must be answered or for action that should be suggested if it is not proposed by the family itself. Prior to a home visit to an injured industrial worker, for example, the nurse should be sure she has all the necessary information about private physician, clinic and hospital resources, including admission requirements and procedures. She should have a clear understanding of the compensation benefits this worker might expect, and what type of financial and social assistance he might receive from the company or from community agencies. However, these should be considered reserve supplies, not a ready-made program to sell to the family.

Occasionally the nurse may be required to take a large measure of responsibility in making plans. For example, if a patient is emotionally disturbed he may be temporarily quite dependent. This is apt to be true in emergency situations. The nurse may say to a badly injured industrial worker, "You must report to the doctor at once. We will send someone with you," realizing that the patient is unable to decide for himself at that point. Telling or leading the family to accept a plan already made by the nurse should be used only when it is not possible to achieve a more cooperative approach.

Setting up a Program of Action.   Once health needs have been established and accepted, and general plans have been outlined, a time schedule is needed for the various activities.

As a first step the family and the nurse will select areas for immediate action. Sometimes the most urgent needs are very obvious. A cardiac patient in great distress or an acutely ill child obviously needs immediate care; in such instances the first steps are very clear. In other situations the relative importance of various needs may not be so well defined. For example, a harassed parent may feel that some restraint of Sally's outbursts of temper is the most urgent family problem. Actually, the resolution of certain marital or household management problems that are creating an atmosphere of strain and tension may be much more important. The worker who is exposed to radioactive materials may fail to see the need for regular physical check-up, though to the nurse the need is obvious.

In selecting problems for immediate attention, personal as well as objective factors may need to be considered. In one case a nurse discovered a woman with evidence of toxemia grave enough to warrant immediate hospital care. The woman herself, however, felt that the most important thing to be done was to arrange for her husband's meals and care during the time she was away from home. This problem had assumed major proportions in the patient's mind, and she was unwilling to have the nurse proceed with plans to secure hospital care until it had been resolved. The nurse accordingly arranged with a neighbor to prepare the husband's evening meals and to care for the house while the wife was away. Only then did she proceed to talk with the husband and to arrange for hospital care. Except in situations where it might result in actual danger, the family's criterion of urgency should be used, giving first attention to those problems that the family considers most important.

Step-by-step plans for the details of health care may be constructed in a single unit or in several parts, depending upon the length of time health supervision will be necessary, the ability of the family to accept its problems as a whole, and the extent to which emotional trauma affects the planning ability of the family. Sometimes family health needs at a given time are relatively few and simple. Nurse and family can readily decide what needs to be done, and set up a plan for doing it.

In other instances the problems may be many and rather complex. It may not be possible to foresee developments that will affect the situation, or to judge just how much will need to be done. In such a case, those problems selected for immediate care would be discussed, and detailed plans be worked out only in those selected areas. In one family, for example, the record indicated that there was a child with scarlet fever, several members of the family in need of dental care, and an adolescent boy with marked behavior problems. The mother was postponing surgical care, and suffering from "weak spells." Although these needs were known to the family and accepted by them, the problems seemed so overwhelming that any attempt to meet them was frustrating. A detailed plan for care of the sick child was made, and discussion of the other problems was left for consideration at a later visit.

The specific program of action should be planned in small

enough units to avoid overwhelming the family and creating confusion. If the family has not fully accepted its health needs, it
may be necessary to proceed with small units of planning and
to hold some problems for discussion and action at a later date
when there may be greater motivation and interest.

In planning for spacing of nursing contacts, consideration
should be given to "high impact" points, and to the level of
anticipated independent action by the family. Certain points in
the course of a disease or special health condition will have high
impact value. The period just prior to hospital discharge, for
example, is a point at which the family of the tuberculosis or
psychiatric patient has high receptivity to help, and a recognized need for the nursing service. At this point, nursing service
would be much more effective than it would be two weeks after
discharge. The immediate preschool period is an effective one for
securing necessary preventive care for the young child; the period
about ten days after hospital discharge (as well as immediately
prior to discharge) is particularly effective in long-term illness.
At this point the intensive neighborly calls are beginning to thin
out, and the reality of the long hard pull ahead is more keenly
felt by the patient and the family. The level of independence
will also affect the spacing of nursing visits. The confident, relaxed prenatal patient may be seen at regularly spaced intervals,
while the dependent fearful young woman may require very
intensive visiting in the early phases of the service, until she has
gained greater independence.

In planning for a scarlet fever patient, for example, visits may
be scheduled immediately after diagnosis to teach care and help
with home adjustments and to interpret health department and
school regulations; in the second or third day to check nursing
care and isolation procedures; on the sixth or seventh day to
help in adjustment to increasing activity of the patient and help
with convalescent care; at the end of the third week to arrange
for terminal disinfection, follow-up care, and return to school.

Nursing visits should be scheduled with respect to health services the family is receiving from other sources. Prenatal visits,
for example, may be scheduled so they alternate with the patient's visits to the physician. In this way there is a maximum
amount of professional observation of the patient, and the family's
access to professional guidance is spaced more evenly. The same
procedure may be followed in scheduling visits to the family of
a diabetic patient so that clinic and home visits may be alter-

nated. In supervision of the preschool child the nursing visits may be arranged so that they follow closely upon the visit of the physician to provide for interpretation and effectuation of his appraisal and advice, with other visits arranged so that there will be periodic checks between medical appointments.

This step-by-step agenda for action should be specific and should indicate the approximate time at which things will be done. In planning for home care of the child with measles, family and nurse need to determine how to arrange for the sick child to sleep apart from his brothers and sisters. Perhaps it will be necessary to borrow a cot from a neighbor or from a community loan chest, to arrange for transportation of the cot through the use of the family car or a friend's truck. If plans are being made to increase the amount of milk in the family diet, such practical and specific items as the type of milk that will be bought, the meals at which additional milk might be introduced, the kinds of food and special dishes that will be presented to the family will need to be considered. Suggestions such as "Maybe you can try that tomorrow for lunch," or "Perhaps your husband can get the cot when he gets back from work, and you can have Johnny's room all ready for him tonight" will help to set time limits in planning.

PLANNING WITH OTHER AGENCIES

Planning with other agencies should not be confused with securing the approval of other agencies or with keeping them informed. Sometimes nurses speak of obtaining the cooperation of other agencies, by which they really mean getting the agency to agree to the plans already made. In contacts with physicians, nurses may call to request diagnosis and orders for care, feeling they have then engaged in joint planning. Nurse and physician should consult with one another about the total plan for family health care, not just the physical care and medical treatment of the sick person. Except with very simple and obvious problems, effective planning with other agencies requires consulting before plans have been crystallized. Such planning together for the total care of the family will promote maximum use of individual and community resources, and result in better care.

Joint planning may be done by any of these suggested methods or by any combination of them: (1) direct planning for the individual patient or family; (2) planning through establishment of "standing orders," "emergency orders" or "routine procedures"; or (3) participation in planning through exchange of information.

Individualized Planning by Worker-to-Worker.   In arranging for joint planning for a particular family or individual, the public health nurse may telephone, write or call upon the physician, teacher, social worker or other professional worker to discuss the plan for care. When the background information is extensive or complicated, an exchange of records or abstracts of care may precede the planning conference, so all workers can come to the conference with the necessary facts. In most cases there will be no need for such advance planning. The nurse may, for example, call the physician and plan with him for family nursing care in a very informal manner.

At the conferences, whether they are personal contacts, telephone calls or written reports, the nurse should have information regarding the situation available and organized for ready reference, with all significant factors clearly outlined. Planning conferences should be particularly frequent between the nurse, physician and family, since they comprise by far the most common team for health care.

Sometimes it is desirable to do physician-nurse planning on a group basis. The nurse may arrange with the physician for a conference, at which time the care may be reviewed and the plan made for several patients or families at once. The health officer or clinician in the health department may, for example, review tuberculosis or orthopedic cases with the public health nurse at regular intervals. The nurse brings the family records to the conference, discusses progress and new needs of the families, and consults with the physician about plans for future care. The rural nurse may visit the doctor's office occasionally to discuss with him those cases that she has under her care, and plan with him for future services.

Use of Case Conferences to Plan Family Care.   Sometimes family problems are extensive and complex, involving several agencies. In such cases, a case conference may be indicated. For example, in the care of a child with rheumatic heart disease, it may be wise to call the physician, teacher, parents, social worker and public health nurse together at one time in order to make a plan that will take into account the many aspects of the needs and resources for care. In planning care for a diabetic patient the nutritionist, family and public health nurse may meet together; in the case of a cardiac patient about to return to work the plant physician, section supervisor or personnel worker, public health nurse and industrial nurse may work out a coordinated plan.

Such case conferences, organized to plan for a specific family, may provide the basis for more general agreements. For example, in the care of a rheumatic fever patient, two or three case conferences may be scheduled, after which each agency will proceed in the care of other similar patients along the general outline of the specific plans which have been worked out.

Routine Procedures or Standing Orders. In some instances the need for inter-agency planning may be met on a group rather than upon an individual basis. For example, while every prenatal patient has individual needs, not all may need joint decision or action by the nurse and medical supervisor. It is not necessary to plan with the private physician for all aspects of care of his prenatal patients on an individual basis. The physician may provide directions regarding diet, special exercises, restriction of activities and so forth that he would like carried out for all but the exceptional patient. He may approve the content of teaching used by the nursing agency, or suggest special instruction. He may decide to divide with the nurse the responsibility for such diagnostic procedures as blood pressure determination or urine analysis. Such agreements for care of patients may be written, or may take the form of blanket approval of the usual procedures of the nursing agency. School health authorities may establish standing orders for the treatment of pediculosis, for exclusion on the basis of symptoms suggestive of communicable disease, for first-aid treatment of injuries. Routine procedures for treatment of dysmenorrhea, headache or other minor ills may be prescribed in industry.

Agreements may also be reached about division of responsibility or methods of referral and reporting that will affect planning. For example, a welfare agency may decide upon division of responsibility for such activities as instruction in nutrition or handling child behavior problems in families that are carried by both agencies.

Such agreements save time, assure more uniform and less confusing care for families and serve as an excellent means of maintaining cooperative relationships.

Standing or emergency orders should always have medical approval. Some agencies have worked out suggested standing orders in cooperation with the local medical association. In some states the State Health Department and the State Medical Association have approved standing orders on a statewide basis. In the latter case, the local medical group should also be asked to approve these.

Standing orders or emergency orders approved by the physician for use for his patients should always be written. If they include orders for care that go beyond the usual first aid that might be rendered by any nonmedical person, they should be signed by the physician. While it is important that standing orders be clearly understood, sometimes it does not seem wise to insist upon too formal an agreement. A letter "to confirm my understanding of our conclusions" will provide a written record of the agreement without too great formality.

Exchange of Information.   This is the most generalized of the methods suggested. Through some established clearance and reporting procedure, each agency notifies the other of services or developments in its contact with the family or its members that may affect the planning of the other agency. This facilitates planning because it places needed information in the hands of the nurse or cooperating agency at the time it is needed for planning. Such exchange of information may be effected by periodic review of records, exchange of reports or abstracts of care, or regularly scheduled telephone or personal conferences.

Sometimes it is sufficient to secure permission to review records as the need arises. The public health nurse may, for example, be given access to school guidance folders; the visiting nurse may be permitted to see health department records of cases that are carried by both the health department and the visiting nurse association; the industrial nurse may have access to personnel folders, and so forth. In other cases, information may be exchanged on a routine basis. The hospital may notify the public health nursing service of all patients discharged from the hospital when patient or physician have indicated previous contact with the service, or a desire for future service. Such referral procedures may be accompanied by information that is valuable in planning.

In small communities the periodic informal personal contact may prove very useful as a means of exchanging information about families. The nurse may plan to stop in at the doctor's office about once a month, and discuss his patients and their care at that time. Sometimes the nurse plans to have lunch occasionally with the teachers in her district, or with the welfare worker. "Friday lunch" in one small rural community was the occasion for teachers, librarian, social case worker and public health nurse to meet. While its primary expressed purpose was purely social, many plans for coordinated action grew out of this simple procedure.

Plans for exchange of information should be carefully worked out to avoid wasted effort or misunderstanding. If forms are used for exchanging information they should require a minimum of copy work, and be so arranged that any significant information is readily located. Office or clinic visits for the purpose of securing information should be scheduled so that they are convenient, and should be preceded by such advance preparation as is necessary to make the contact effective.[8]

Arranging for the Nursing Visit or Conference.   In addition to case planning, there is need to arrange for each visit or conference to assure maximum return. The family should, whenever possible, be prepared for the visit, being notified either by a postcard or phone call saying the nurse will call, or by having the doctor, clinic, or industrial nurse explain that the call will be made. Family reminders such as circling the date on the calendar or postcard reminders will help to cut down "not at home" calls when subsequent visits are to be widely spaced.

It is well to avoid times when family demands are at a peak if possible, such as mealtime, or the time at which children must be called for at school. Sometimes it is necessary to arrange for Saturday or evening visits to reach members of the family who are away from home during the work day. When such arrangements are made they should be cleared with the health officer or supervising nurse to be sure that there is no administrative reason for not planning in this way.

If the visit is to be in the nurse's office, arrangements should be made to assure privacy and informality. Since children must often accompany the patient to such conferences, provisions should be made to keep them occupied. A few children's books or toys kept in the office or clinic will provide distraction for the youngsters while parent and nurse confer. If office or clinic conferences are grouped so there are several in succession, a volunteer worker may be recruited to supervise the children's activities during the conference period.

Checking Understanding and Progress.   Throughout the nursing contact it is necessary to check the degree to which the family understands the problem and the projected action, and to appraise progress in acquiring knowledge and skill. The problem of evaluation is discussed in detail in Chapter XI. However, it is important to keep in mind that planning must include a clear-cut idea of just what is expected in the way of family understanding

8. Referral systems are discussed in Chapter XIV.

and skill, and a plan for the types of questions, applications or family demonstrations that will be necessary to test the degree to which these understandings and skills have been developed. Non-verbal indices of understanding are also significant—inattention, restlessness or a look of puzzlement may be very revealing.

This long and rather detailed discussion of developing a plan for care does not mean that service is postponed until the planning phases are over. Planning and service will proceed simultaneously.

Sound planning is essential to good service. Only as it is done in a broad way with full participation and self-determination of the family, with cognizance of the contributions of other professional workers and agencies and with full recognition of the depth and breadth of nursing itself can families get the most from the nursing services they receive.

CHAPTER IX

Giving and
Teaching Personal Care and
Therapeutic Procedures

A PRIMARY FUNCTION of public health nursing is to assure safe and adequate nursing care for those who are ill and not in a hospital. Whether given by the nurse herself, or by a practical nurse, aide, midwife or family member, the public health nurse has the final responsibility for seeing that the best possible care is given. Instruction and supervision as well as direct services are necessary to assure a reasonable quality of care.

Selecting the Type of Care.   The increasing use of a nursing team in public health agencies makes it important to determine not only what care is needed, but also the level of skill required. When several levels of nursing service are available in a community, such as practical nurses, nurses' aides, public health nurses and registered nurses without public health preparation, discrimination must be used in selecting the type of care that will be most satisfactory and economical.

Within the limits of available community resources, the public health nurse may establish one of the following patterns for provision of nursing care in a particular family:

1. Major care given by the public health nurse, with family providing supplementary care.
2. Nursing care given by the hospital, clinic or private practice

nurse with the public health nurse giving intermittent care in pre- and post-hospital periods.

3. Nursing care provided by the practical nurse, aide, or family member with the nurse providing instruction and continuing supervision.

4. Nursing care given by the family or by a subsidiary worker in the home or in a nursing home, without continuing supervision by the public health nurse.

Whatever the pattern, the nurse retains responsibility for seeing that the best possible care is provided. The nurse working in an agency that does not include home care of the sick in its program and where there is no other agency doing so, must still be concerned with this aspect of care. She will need to plan for teaching, coaching, instruction in home nursing or development of other school or community programs to meet the community need for home care of the sick as well as possible within the limits of agency policy and community resources.

The type of care afforded will depend largely upon the amount of public health nursing time available for this activity, the presence of other sources of care, and the policies and purposes of the community nursing agencies. Certain activities in public health nursing may represent obligations of the agency; for example, the department of health must act to control communicable disease. If these commitments are many and time-consuming, there may be little time available for care of the sick.

Patterns of care in hospitals, clinics and in nursing homes, the amounts of service offered by industrial nurses and the presence or absence of a visiting nurse service will affect the degree to which the nurse in the department of health becomes involved with home care of the sick. If the hospital operates a home care program, with extensive home visiting by social workers, physicians and nurses; if the outpatient service carries a large load of "repeater" services for injections or dressings; if the industrial nursing service includes home as well as plant visits with workers and their families, the work of the generalized public health nurse in relation to home care of the sick will be correspondingly decreased. If none of these services exists, the public health nurse's responsibility must increase.

When nursing time is limited and it is not possible to care for all who need it, careful selection of cases is important to place the service where it will make the most difference. If care is given by the hospital or other community agency, close cooperation is necessary to make available to it the resources of the public health nursing service, even though the nurse herself is not caring for the patient. For example, the hospital nurse may want to inform patients about community loan closets, or about the availability of wheel chairs that may be rented or loaned without charge. The private practice nurse might like to have some of the materials and procedures for home care as developed by the community agency, or to refer her patient's family to community classes in home care of the sick.

When care is taken over by the family or an auxiliary worker without continuing supervision by the nurse, the family should have the support that comes from knowing that the nurse can be called upon for advice or help if the situation should change.

The level of nursing care to be used will be determined by:

1. The degree to which professional skill and judgment are required in observation of symptoms and in carrying out treatments.

2. The need for emotional support or for services designed to change attitudes.

3. Family and community expectations.

4. Available resources.

Professional nursing care is obviously needed when the type of illness requires a high degree of judgment in estimating the importance of symptoms or changes in condition, or in administering treatments. Many hypodermic injections now given at home are apt to produce adverse symptoms, or to require a high degree of skill in administration. It is not possible to say arbitrarily that acute illness requires professional skill and that chronic or convalescent illness may be cared for by subsidiary workers or family members. Nursing care in the period immediately following diagnosis of diabetes requires a high degree of judgment and skill, since the treatment is being stabilized and the family and patient are making difficult psychologic adjustments. The need for highly skilled observation, teaching and support is great. Later in the course of the disease, care might well be given by the family or by the individual himself. Even then there will usually be social or emotional factors that require occasional professional service. Nor can the seriousness of the condition or the complexity of the care needed be the sole criterion. In some situations a relatively simple condition is accompanied by unusual emotional stress, and may demand professional-level care.

Sometimes the patient or family needs professional nursing care to provide reassurance that the nurse is concerned. Perhaps a family member or aide could give perfectly adequate care to a paraplegic patient, but, if the patient is feeling depressed or resentful about his condition, having the professional nurse provide direct service may say in effect "I *care*." This assurance may be as important to the paraplegic patient as is the "tender, loving care" we now recognize as such a significant factor in the nursing care of infants. Furthermore, in the long run, providing such care if it does result in a sense of assurance of concern on the part of the nurse may result in a lower rather than higher demand for nursing time. The patient, so reassured, may be able to move with higher motivation and greater despatch toward self-help if he is "over-nursed" a little in the early period of care. He may be less apt to develop a "what's the use" attitude if he knows the nurse is concerned and anxious to help him.

Sometimes, too, the family may be willing and able to give care to the long-term patient who is ill at home, but needs an occasional "relief" day when the nurse takes over to prevent discouragement, and to give the *family* a feeling of support. Such care is not "unnecessary." It may make the difference between a family feeling that they can keep the patient at home, and feeling that he must be placed in a hospital or nursing home. The benefits to the patient in home care as well as the savings to the community make this a worthwhile achievement.

The type of care provided will also have to be adjusted to family and community expectations and resources. Communities or families that resist the use of practical nurses or self-help may need some time to readjust their attitudes, and in the interim care may be given by the professional nurse even though it does not demand her full skill. If practical nurses are not available, or if those available are not well prepared, or if family members who might give care live at a distance or must be away from the home to work, the nurse may need to provide services that might otherwise be delegated. Precision in the use of nursing skills in accordance with the level of need may have to give way to the more fundamental principle of meeting human needs.

The nurse's own attitude toward providing personal care should also be taken into account. Poor attitudes toward bedside care— a feeling that it does not require the high degree of skill used in counseling or teaching—may cause the nurse to underestimate needs for care. Lack of recent experience in direct care of the sick may also be a deterrent. In some agencies which have not customarily provided such care, the nurse may become fearful of her competence in this type of service.

Functions and responsibilities of practical nurses and aides are usually spelled out in agency policy statements. They have also been considered in detail in recent publications.[1] The nurse should be familiar with such regulations, and bring to her supervisor or administrator new questions which are not clearly answered in existing policies, so a clarification can be made. In particular it is important to know just which of the bewildering number of drugs used in long-term illness can be administered by the practical nurse—a question which must be answered by the appropriate medical adviser or advisory committee of the agency.

It is important that the family and the physician understand the type of care being provided, and the limits of such care. When family members, practical nurses or aides are used, the nurse should as far as possible retain responsibility for over-all case management. In this way she is in a position to recognize and adapt to changes in the situation that might indicate a need for nursing service of a different type.

Providing Nursing Care in the Home. The principles of providing nursing care in the home do not, of course, differ from those of providing care in any other situation. There is the same need for dealing with the patient as a whole and in relation to his environment, as well as with his disease; the same need for skillful relief of distress and discomfort, and for treatments combined with selective and accurate observation of the patient's condition.

There are, however, some problems that arise from the locale of the service, and from the nature of illnesses that are cared for at home as compared to the hospital. These include:

1. Need to adapt nursing to a variety of patterns of medical care.
2. Need to adapt techniques to the facilities available in the home and to possible delegation to the family.
3. Need for intensive teaching, since the nurse is absent much of the day and must be concerned not only with the present condition, but also with other conditions found in the family.

1. Joint Committee on Practical Nurses and Auxiliary Workers in Nursing Services, *Practical Nurses in Nursing Services.* New York, American Nurses' Association, 1951.

4. Need to keep currently informed about an unusually wide range of conditions and diagnostic procedures.

5. Need to relate care to other family activities and responsibilities.

The public health nurse will be caring for people receiving medical care from several different private physicians, each with his own approach to care, and from many hospitals and clinics, each of which also has different procedures and routines for care. Since the public health nursing represents only one segment of the total care of the patient it must be integrally related to what others are doing. For instance, it is confusing to the family to have the nurse in the hospital suggest one method of bathing the baby, and then find the public health nurse suggesting another (equally good) method. Different medical advisers have quite different views about the degree to which the diabetic patient will be given responsibility for modifying the insulin dosage, or the degree of physical activity that should be encouraged for the post-hospital cardiac patient. For this reason it is necessary to clear carefully with the medical supervisor, to be sure the patients understand the care that would be given if standing orders are followed, and to clarify the relationships between hospital or physician's services and the public health nursing care. Observation of hospital care may help the nurse to make home and hospital care a more integrated unit. Careful case planning, discussed previously, is also basic.

Teaching as well as procedural content of service needs clearance—the physician should know what is being taught to pre-natal patients about exercise and fluid intake, and either approve what is being done or suggest modifications for his patients.

The public health nurse must constantly adapt procedures and techniques to the materials found in the home. One home may have a bath blanket, while another does not; in one home facilities for boiling equipment are good, while in a furnished room with "kitchen privileges" a different method of sterilization may be preferable; isolation in one home may mean a separate room and even a separate bath; in another home it may mean part of a room shared by several others. The agency may have a manual of suggested procedures, adjusted to the average home situation encountered, but these too will frequently need to be modified. Furthermore, the simple act of carrying out procedures in the home is in itself a teaching activity—family members will watch and try to copy what they see. For this reason, techniques must be adapted to what the family can do, as well as to the equipment they have.

Techniques should be:
1. Safe
2. Low in equipment and supply cost
3. Low in energy cost
4. High in teaching potential.

Assuring Safety of Techniques.   The techniques used by the nurse in care of the sick should be safe in terms of preventing possible spread of infection, and in avoiding any accident hazard and harm to the patient through exposure or overfatigue. Equipment should be properly cleansed to avoid contamination. Methods of cleaning thermometers, syringes and other equipment may be checked by bacteriologic study, to determine whether, after cleansing, equipment is free of harmful organisms. Such studies, similar to the study of disinfection of thermometers undertaken in one service, may be done by health department or university laboratory personnel.[2]

Methods of hand-washing also require study. The use of a hand-brush has generally proved unsatisfactory because of the difficulty of disinfecting the brush in the home. Sterilizing equipment in the home may prove less satisfactory than having equipment packed and sterilized in the hospital. The latter method may necessitate a slightly larger supply of equipment or materials, but the savings in time as well as the increased safety may more than compensate for this.

Epidemiologic study provides another check on the effectiveness of the techniques used. Obviously, evidence of cross-infection would indicate need for a thorough field check of the techniques in use. More frequently the techniques or procedures may be checked to make certain that they provide protection against the known methods of transmission of the diseases under care.[3, 4, 5]

For example, for diseases transmitted by secretions from the

2. Notter, Lucille E., Disinfection of Clinical Thermometers. *Nursing Outlook*, 1: 559–561, October, 1953.

3. *Control of Communicable Diseases in Man*, 8th ed., New York, American Public Health Association, 1955.

4. Anderson, Garlord and Margaret Arnstein, *Communicable Disease Control*, 3rd ed. New York, Macmillan Co., 1953. Chapters 7 and 8 provide detailed information regarding the role of the public health nurse and home care procedures.

5. Ibid., p. 140.

nose and throat, the technique used should be checked to see whether it at all points protects the exposed individual from any possible contamination with these materials either by direct contact, handling of equipment, or droplets. When discharges from the gastrointestinal tract are important in transmission of disease the technique should be checked carefully with this in mind. Recent increased interest in air-borne infections may well lead to some modifications in nursing procedure.

In evaluating techniques in terms of their conformity to known epidemiologic factors the points of emphasis, as well as the total content of the procedure, should be considered. For example, in teaching the family, the procedure should be so organized that the emphasis is placed on controlling the main sources of spread. A technique that includes a great many refinements may not produce as good results in control of the disease as a simpler procedure that teaches only the most important points, but teaches them more completely. While the nurse's personal technique must be strict since she goes from home to home, Anderson and Arnstein state that "it is neither practical nor necessary to teach a family to observe a strictly aseptic technique in the home."[6]

Techniques should be checked to make certain that they do not constitute an accident hazard, even when used by someone other than the nurse. For example, raising the height of the patient's bed by the use of bed blocks may make it easier to give care when the patient is in bed. However, if he is in bed for treatments or for a bed bath, but is able to get out and sit in a chair several times during the day, the hazard of moving the patient from the higher level of the bed may be of greater importance than the saving of energy of the nurse and homemaker when giving in-bed care. The place chosen for the baby's bath should be safe from danger of his rolling off if he is left for a moment. Methods suggested for administration and storage of drugs and medicines should be such that the danger of wrong dosage or incorrect use is minimized.

Finally, techniques should be such that the patient is protected from unnecessary fatigue or exposure. It may be better to give a partial bath rather than a full one if the patient tires easily; sometimes with home equipment the energy demand on the patient is greater than it would be with hospital equipment. Self-help procedures may have to be set up in quite a different

6. Ibid., p. 140.

manner for home use than in the hospital—giving one's own bath in a poorly heated home may be very taxing. Bathing may require special timing when the house is warmer, or use of a sponge bath in the kitchen rather than in the bedroom.

Low Equipment Cost.   Home techniques must make the greatest possible use of materials readily available in the home. Inprovised equipment may be needed if the disease is of short duration. The sickroom should be so placed that it permits reasonably constant patient supervision. An extra bed that may be placed within sight of the kitchen, and furniture arrangement that will permit isolation of a sick person are "musts" in a home with small children. For chronic care, time and nurse-saving equipment such as a bed table, extra basins for use in the sickroom and, if the bathroom is not near the sickroom, a commode contribute greatly to patient care. Most of such equipment can be bought inexpensively, improvised from available materials or borrowed. The public health nurse should be familiar with methods of improvising equipment for home care of the sick. Suggestions may be secured from home nursing textbooks.[7] The nurse should also find out where special equipment such as hospital beds, bedpans, or cellucotton can be obtained, and the approximate prices. When community loan closets are in operation the nurse should find out what is available, and under what conditions equipment is loaned.

Low Energy Cost.   Procedures for home care of the sick need to be carefully planned to conserve energy. Both the public health nurse and the home nurse will have many obligations in addition to the care of a particular patient. The procedures should be checked to see whether they minimize the number of steps and motions required. For instance, it takes fewer steps to make a bed if all necessary work is completed on one side of the bed before proceeding to the other; care of the in-bed patient is much simplified if the bed that is ordinarily pushed against the wall can be pulled out to provide access on both sides. Keeping supplies for care near the place of care also helps to save energy. A "baby tray" on which small equipment needed for the bath is kept makes for easier organization at bath time; use of the bathroom for the baby's bath may be indicated if the size of the room and equipment make it feasible.

The procedure used should also promote good body mechanics,

7. See, for example, American Red Cross, *Red Cross Home Nursing*. Philadelphia, Blakiston Co., 1951.

and avoid unnecessary strain. In getting the patient out of bed, for example, placement of the patient's chair, advance preparation of blankets, and height of the bed will affect the ease of managing the patient with a high degree of disability.

The nurse should be constantly on the watch for gadgets that promote better care at less energy cost; the terrycloth large bib for the patient with some paralysis who is apt to spill, the dry shampoo, the tilting table that may be used over the bed and at the patient's chair, cuffs and splints that help the patient to feed himself, and lifting helps such as pull ropes are examples.

High Teaching Potential.   The nurse's procedures should, wherever possible, be usable by the family without change. In this way teaching is enhanced. For example, it may be equally safe and require the same amount of effort to use either tincture of green soap or regular household soap in cleansing a thermometer. However, the teaching value differs considerably. If the household soap is used, the family sees a procedure using materials familiar to them every time they watch the nurse cleanse her thermometer. It is easy for them to adopt a similar procedure for their own use. In the hospital class where mothers are taught to bathe their babies, the use of a sponge bath is usually preferable to a spray bath since few families will find equipment for the spray bath in their own homes.

Equipment used by the nurse either in the nursing office or in the home should be easy to keep clean, effective in use, and when possible similar to family equipment to make teaching easier. Equipment carried in the nurse's bag should be light in weight and compact in design. The nurse should not carry equipment that is easily found in the home or is used infrequently.

TEACHING THE ESSENTIALS OF NURSING CARE

Even when the nurse provides the major share of care for the patient, it must be remembered that for a large part of the day the family will be responsible for the patient. Therefore, it is important that the basis on which care is provided, the relation of the treatments ordered to the total care pattern, and the supplementary care and observation the family will need to provide between nursing visits are understood.

The nurse may provide instruction in simple care of the sick to an individual family, demonstrating care and assisting with the home adjustments necessary for effective service.

Usually this is done by providing care during the acute phases of the disease or for a long enough period for demonstration, then gradually turning over this responsibility to someone else.

Teaching in groups may be indicated when there is a scarcity of nursing time and the type of care needed is the same for a number of families. For example, if there is an increasing incidence of measles in a community, and the public health nurse is unable to visit each reported patient in his home, she may arrange for mothers to meet at some central place for instruction in the recognition of measles, the need for medical care, and the methods by which home nursing care may be given effectively. Teaching midwives the essentials of modern maternity care, and holding grandmother's classes in baby care when there are many working mothers and the grandmothers serve as substitute mothers are other examples of group teaching applied to specific needs.

More formalized class teaching of home care of the sick is an invaluable aid, especially in situations where the scarcity of public health nurses makes delegation of nursing care imperative. Such classes may be organized under the auspices of the nursing service, or by the local chapter of the American Red Cross. Enrolled Red Cross nurses may also be recruited to assist with teaching. Such classes serve not only to teach family members to give care in their own homes, but also to develop a group of informed women who are alert to health problems and able to help their own and neighbor's families when necessary. Such group work may be the only way in which nurses can effectively meet their responsibility for insuring good care of those who are sick at home when the nurse's load is so great that it precludes giving nursing care herself. It also serves as one approach to the ever-mounting problem of nursing care for the chronically ill. Group methods are discussed in detail in Chapters XII and XIII.

Demonstration and Supervised Practice. One of the lessons learned in wartime training was that there is no substitute for realistic, controlled practice in learning skills. In teaching home nursing skills the same holds true. No amount of discussion or telling can accomplish what can be done by a combination of demonstration and supervised practice.

In demonstrating care in the home, it must be remembered that there may be competing interests for the homemaker's attention. The following steps might be suggested:

1. Be sure that the learner is comfortable, and can see what is being done. As far as possible minimize distractions—arrange for care of the children, etc.

2. Go through the procedure slowly, explaining each step and giving the reason why it is done as it is. For example, the enema can is held low to keep the force of the flow down, and so keep the patient more comfortable and make retention easier.

3. Repeat the key points in the procedure—the critical parts of the process that are most important in safeguarding the patient and in making the treatment more effective. Stress the principle.

4. Have the family nurse help with parts of the procedure when it is possible—she may make one corner of the bed after the nurse has demonstrated on the other corner.

5. On the next occasion for the treatment, have the family nurse do it, explaining each step as the nurse did, while the nurse observes, helps, and re-directs as necessary.

6. Observe a second time a few days later if necessary, correcting any errors that might have crept in. In very long-term illness it may be necessary to provide "booster" instruction or discussion of care occasionally.

In general, it is best to teach only one way to carry out a particular procedure to a particular family, even though there may be more than one acceptable method. Different families may be taught different methods to adapt to their own space, facilities or ways of working. But if several methods are taught, relying on the family member to recognize and apply the principle in several different ways, the time required for learning is greater and likelihood of error is increased. The family may be told that there are several ways to do the task (for instance, to sterilize hypodermic needles), but that just one of these will be taught.

The Intangibles of Care.   Reassuring the patient, taking account of his likes and dislikes, letting him decide how fast to go and waiting for him to do things for himself should be stressed as thoroughly as the technical or mechanical aspects of the procedure.

If the home nurse is anxious or awkward, it may be necessary to repeat the demonstration and supervised practice periods several times to give her greater security. Some home nurses like to have the steps written down as a reminder when they carry out the treatment. This may be a desirable safeguard if the treatment is done infrequently, or involves many steps in the preparation of equipment.

Throughout the demonstration, methods of conserving the energy and of safeguarding the health of the home nurse should also be stressed. Good body mechanics in lifting or moving the patient will minimize fatigue and strain, handling soiled bed-clothing without shaking or getting it into close contact with the face is important in protecting the home nurse caring for a communicable disease.

Professional Supervision and Guidance. In many cases, as in the care of the chronically ill, the professional nurse will need to provide continuing supervision and guidance to the family member or auxiliary worker caring for the patient.

Until skills are established, it may be necessary to plan nursing visits at a time when daily care or treatments are being given, to be sure that the care is safe and adequate, or to check the care given to the patient's skin or back. After the skills of the home nurse have been well established the visit may be arranged at another time so that there will be an opportunity to chat with the patient and family and to contribute to the less tangible aspects of care, such as meeting the emotional needs that grow out of chronic illness, or discussing possible help from community agencies that provide educational or friendly services.

The principles of working with aides and volunteer workers discussed in Chapter XIX apply equally well in supervising family members giving care.

Preparing the Family to Meet Future Needs. When care is delegated to the family or to an auxiliary worker the nurse should be certain that the responsible individual is prepared to recognize the need for future help, and equipped to secure such help without unnecessary delay.

The family should be familiarized with symptoms of possible complications, or reactions from treatment or drugs that may require medical or professional nursing care. Its members should know when and how to call for medical or nursing service.

The provision of adequate and safe nursing care is basic to public health nursing. The public health nurse must take leadership in making the best possible nursing care available to all who are ill at home, either by providing such care herself or by teaching and supervising others who do it.

CHAPTER X

Individual and Family Health Counseling and Teaching

COUNSELING HAS been defined in many and often conflicting ways. Many definitions do not distinguish clearly between counseling, education, guidance, or psychotherapy. For purposes of this discussion, therefore, we will assume a definition that places counseling and teaching on a continuum, with the differential attributed to the degree to which self-direction by the patient is possible. This is expressed graphically in Figure 12.

In nursing, counseling may be considered as the application of the professional nursing relationship and of professional knowledge and skill for the purpose of increasing the competence of individuals or families in defining and acting upon their own health problems.

Counseling in nursing may include activities varying all the way from telling individuals or families what they should do or know, to giving encouragement or support that provides a setting within which the patients or families can think through their own problems with virtually no direction from the nurse. The fundamental purpose of counseling is educational rather than manipulative—the purpose is not to "persuade" the family to do something, but to help its members to recognize what is needed, and to take such action as is necessary on the basis of the family's own decision. It is collaborative rather than coercive. It is based upon the conviction that people want to help themselves, and have both a drive toward solving their own problems, and a high degree of competence in doing so, provided they have help.

Counseling recognizes, however, that illness with its concomitant emotional stress may inhibit or delay self-sufficiency. There will be points where the individual and the family have a very real need to be dependent, and a right to assume that the professional workers responsible for their health care will respect

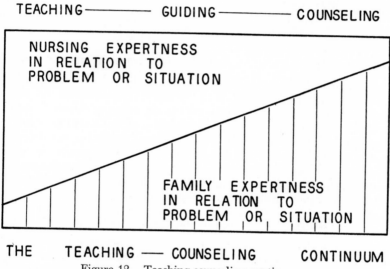

TEACHING——————— GUIDING ——————— COUNSELING

NURSING EXPERTNESS IN RELATION TO PROBLEM OR SITUATION

FAMILY EXPERTNESS IN RELATION TO PROBLEM OR SITUATION

THE TEACHING —— COUNSELING CONTINUUM

Figure 12. Teaching-counseling continuum.

and cope with this need. It recognizes, too, that in relation to health care certain expertness and factual or judgmental information reside in the nurse, and that there will be times when the nurse must stand in the relation of a teacher or an expert if the family is to have the information needed to make wise decisions.

For these reasons, counseling in nursing will fluctuate from a highly directional activity to one in which the family takes the lead, thinks through the problems and makes the necessary decisions without interference or control. While the more common pattern is to move from the more to the less directive approach, in many instances there will be need to move forward or backward as the type of problem or the experiential or personality background of the family in relation to a particular need varies. Counseling involves six major elements:

1. Establishing a professional relationship.
2. Motivating the family or individual.
3. Telling, explaining or directing action.
4. Releasing and guiding family or individual potentials for self-help.
5. Anticipating and combatting impediments to care.
6. Evaluating results.

Evaluation of results of counseling may be considered as a part of evaluation of the nursing service as a whole, which is discussed in Chapter XI.

ESTABLISHING AND MAINTAINING A PROFESSIONAL RELATIONSHIP

Good professional relationships are the foundation upon which good professional service must be built. The degree to which the nurse is able to establish and maintain associations that contribute positively to the accomplishment of her service, while at the same time promoting the maximum level of self-direction in the individual or family, will do much to influence the effectiveness of nursing care. Skills in inter-personal relationships are an important facet of nursing competence, and must be developed as other skills are developed by the nurse.

THE NATURE OF A PROFESSIONAL RELATIONSHIP

The ability to get along with people or to establish friendly contacts is no guarantee of ability to promote suitable professional relationships. Personal relationships are established for the purpose of meeting some personal need—perhaps to express love or affection, to promote easy social contacts or to gain attention or achieve a sense of power. In the terminal illness of a parent, for example, an individual may give unstintingly of time or money far beyond the amount which might be considered wise or justifiable from a purely rational point of view. Such action and the relationship which prompts it are both understandable and desirable; such deep emotional response represents one of the major experiences of life, and contributes much to the sum of one's happiness and security. It would, however, hardly be considered a desirable nurse-patient relationship. The family which is served by the public health nurse might be embarrassed or upset if the nurse's attitude were so emotionally charged, and the nurse herself would be unable to fulfill her many obligations if burdened by such feelings.

A relationship which is a satisfactory one to establish with a grocer or a neighbor cannot be expected to function equally well in a professional situation. In such social contacts, friendliness may be of paramount importance, and efforts to change the behavior of others might be considered unwarranted interference. A professional contact is expected to produce changes in behavior. If this is to be done, the need to establish a feeling of friendliness cannot interfere to the point that it destroys the nurse's capacity to be objective in approaching problems. Indeed, overanxiety about securing such approval may cause the nurse to ignore vitally important professional activities that cannot be consummated without accepting some degree of temporary disapproval or resentment.

A professional relationship demands a certain degree of putting aside of one's self and one's feelings and prejudices, to comprehend the values and feelings and perceptions of a family or individual without distortion by one's own values, feelings and perceptions. Rogers, describing the relationship of a counselor, says:

> "The counselor says in effect to be of assistance to you I will put aside myself—the self of ordinary interaction—and enter into your world of perception as completely as I am able. I will become in a sense another self for you . . . . a safe opportunity for you to discern yourself more clearly, to experience yourself more truly and deeply, to choose more significantly."[1]

While Rogers was speaking of counseling as a therapeutic procedure—a level of counseling not ordinarily undertaken by the public health nurse—the need to put aside one's self exists in helping people with simple problems as it does with the complex ones.

The service the nurse expects to render must include both contribution of her own expert knowledge and judgment and the encouragement of active participation of the patient or family. This dual pattern of expert instruction and self-directed problem-solving complicates the problem of relationships. It is not enough for the nurse to gain the confidence of the family; it must have confidence in itself as well as in the nurse. Nor is it always possible to rely on guiding the family to its own decision, when protection of the community is involved, or when factual or emotional disability limits the possibility of self-determination of self-help.

1. Rogers, Carl R., *Client Centered Therapy.* New York, Holt, 1951.

Furthermore, some public health services such as restrictions imposed to control communicable disease, may not be welcomed by the recipient or may be rejected in whole or in part.

A good relationship is one which allows the nurse to accomplish in the most effective manner the task for which she has come—to help the family or individual to meet its or his health problems constructively. This implies more than friendliness or acceptance, although both are essential for productive mutual effort.

Warmth. Probably the most vital characteristic of a professional helping relationship is warmth—an attitude that makes the family feel that the nurse is interested in its members as people, not just as a case or a problem. Families want and need to feel that the nurse is concerned with their problems, that she can share their happiness when a grandchild is expected, understand their disappointment when a far-away son or daughter doesn't write. If recognized by the nurse the bewilderment of a happy husband and wife when one or the other reacts to stress with irritable complaint, their pride in the achievements of their baby and their progress in home making—all matters of deep concern to the couple—build a bridge of understanding and acceptance that facilitates the job of counseling.

The warmth is shown in many ways—in the physical contact when the nurse places a hand on the child's head or shoulder. in cuddling the baby when teaching the new mother how to bathe him, remembering to ask for the news of a son off on military service and to refer to him by name. It is shown when giving care to the woman with arthritis by being willing to wait for her to handle her pain in moving, rather than hurrying as quickly as possible with the bath or treatment.

Of course, the best method of showing warmth is to feel it— to "feel with" the family enough to understand its problems, its values and the source of its joys. Thinking "how would I feel if this were my problem" may help. It may also be necessary— particularly if the nurse is herself a reserved person—to think consciously of ways to make clear to the individual or family that this feeling exists.

Recognition and Acceptance. Every individual has a need for status—to feel of value as a person. Illness, especially when associated with incapacity or guilt, may offer a real threat to this sense of worth. The nurse can contribute to the patient's satisfaction with himself by accepting him as he is without reference to differences in his values and hers, and by using nursing services as a channel to provide recognition of him as a person.

Ordinary courtesy is, of course, basic. Introducing one's self by name and organization, and refraining from undue familiarity in addressing patients and families demonstrate the same courtesy one would expect in any social situation.

A nonjudgmental attitude is equally important in a helping relationship.[2] It is not the job of nursing to decide whether the family is or is not to blame for its problems, or whether its attitude toward authority or the attitudes of its members toward one another is "good" or "bad," but rather to help the family to relate its own values and attitudes to the demands of the problems which it faces. The nurse must accept the family's fundamental human right to meet its basic human needs for security, affection, and recognition in the way it feels is best, provided this does not endanger others.

The key to achieving such an attitude rests in a thorough understanding of the human behavior roots of action—a knowledge that individuals become what they are because of the personal equipment they have and the environmental facilities that were available to them to meet their basic human needs.[3] The child brought up in a household characterized by drunkenness and neglect has a different problem in meeting his need for recognition and status than does the child brought up in a secure and loving home. Each will react differently as adults because of this early experience. It is understandable that one of these adults may react by hostility and aggression to all in authority or with a driving ambition to be a good parent and citizen that leads to repressive or anxious treatment of his own children, while the other is cooperative, helpful and relaxed in child care. The patient with venereal disease who reacts with lies and evasion has a *reason* for this behavior—a reason which he believes to be valid and necessary to maintain his integrity as a person.

It takes maturity to work effectively with those whose values are different from one's own, and to be accepting when the patient's or family's need to strike out at things—to get even with

2. Biestek, F. P., The Non-Judgmental Attitude. *Social Casework*, 34: 239, June, 1953.

3. Brown, E. L., The Social Sciences and Improvement of Patient Care. *American Journal of Nursing*, 56: 1148–1150, September, 1950.

life—takes the form of criticizing, blaming or resisting the nurse
or the health department. But looking at the reason rather than
the manifestation of the behavior can help.

Another essential in achieving nonjudgmental acceptance of
others is a thorough *understanding of one's self*. The nurse needs
to recognize those factors in her own background and experience
that will affect the way she feels, and the values she holds. She
should try to track down the reasons why she finds it hard to
like the bragging, "show-off" adolescent. Is it because he threatens
her confidence in her own "rightness"? Because her family culture placed a premium on quiet modesty and abhorred "show"?
Is it hard for her to be sympathetic with the terminal cancer
patient because she fears cancer herself, and doesn't like this
reminder of what it can do? How far is her feeling based on
prejudice, described by Powdermaker as attitudes reached without sufficient consideration of facts?[4]

The nurse must recognize that she, too, is acting in a way
that is consistent with meeting *her* needs for status, security and
affection; and that these actions may be in conflict with permitting patients or families to meet *their* needs effectively. For
example, the young public health nurse may meet her need for
recognition by a feeling that her professional knowledge is sound
and comprehensive. The patient may meet her need to express
resentment of an unwanted pregnancy by challenging or re-
fusing to accept the nurse's knowledge, saying that the only
way to know is to have the experience of motherhood. It takes
considerable maturity on the part of the nurse not to defend her
professional lore, or to label the patient as ignorant or uncooperative. Yet, unless she can find a way to maintain her own sense
of adequacy in relation to professional knowledge without denying to the patient the right to hostility or distress, the nurse's
capacity to help will be lessened.

There are many tangible ways in which the nurse can recognize the worth of an individual. She can comment on some
positive virtue—the mother's capacity to have fun with her children, even if her housekeeping ability is not as evident; the
affection an incapacitated patient has generated in children of
the household even though he feels he is making undue demands
on a son or daughter; the responsibility shown by an unmarried
pregnant girl in caring for her baby even though she feels she
has "let down" her family—and thus help to restore the balance

4. Powdermaker, Hortense, *Probing Our Prejudices*. New York, Harper &
Bros., 1944.

of self-respect. Asking for help or advice is another method; the request for a recipe for a national dish rich in protein or for a slip from a house plant for another patient, and asking one patient to help to orient a new patient to the routines of the well-baby clinic are examples of building recognition by letting the individual help. One nurse encouraged patients who had suffered a heart attack and made a good adjustment to write letters of encouragement to new patients with the same condition.

Offering advice modestly or tentatively may also give the patient or family a sense of being valued. "You probably already know——," or "Have you thought about——?" implies quite a different relationship than does "You should——."

Leadership and Confidence. In many of the areas included in health counseling the nurse will be in the position of an expert. Her knowledge and insight, because of her professional background of training and experience, will enable her to see problems or needs and possible action more fully than the family can. In relation to these facets of counseling content, the family must have confidence in the nurse's expertness and "know how" if it is to benefit fully from her services. At the same time, this expertness must be used in such a way as to encourage rather than inhibit the family's independence.

Usually families have full confidence in the nurse in matters relating to technical care. This is in the common perception of "nurses' training," and is enhanced if the nurse has an orderly, smooth way of carrying out procedures. However, in matters relating to family relationships or adjustments to illness, incapacity or the management of children, there may be less acceptance of her ability to help.

Families may lack confidence in the public health nurse because they feel she is young, or has not had enough practical experience to help them. They may need to be told where the nurse's information comes from—the nurse may say, "They studied a great many babies in the hospital and found that those who got tender loving care did better," rather than, "Babies do better if they are loved." She may relate her suggestions to what other patients or families have done—"One of my patients found she could get her husband to eat a better breakfast by . . ."— and thus recognize her reliance in those who have had experience comparable to that of the family being helped. As the family recognizes the sources of the nurse's expertness they develop confidence in her.

Sometimes the reverse is true—the family has the utmost

confidence in the nurse, but may be unwilling to take responsibility itself, turning to the nurse when decisions are to be made, asking her what to do in matters in which its own competence could well be called into play. In these instances the nurse has a delicate balancing job to perform—to supply the necessary support and information, yet at the same time to encourage the family to think out its own problems. She may say, "Of course I know what other families have done, but every child is different, don't you think? George is quite an individual. What do *you* think could get George to be more thoughtful with his younger brother?" The family may not be ready to think things out; it may be blocked by fatigue or irritation, in which case the nurse can suggest several alternatives, helping the family to see each in relation to its own feelings and personalities and facilities.

SERVICE—FOCUS

The demands of the situation, rather than personal factors, should be the focal point in all professional relationships. The delinquency of a clinic registrant is important because it interferes with his treatment, not because it interrupts the clinic schedule; immunization for diphtheria is important because it protects the child from disease, not because its accomplishment pleases the nurse; the industrial worker should wear goggles because the situation demands their use, not because the nurse tells him so, or because it is a rule of the company.

The recipient of nursing care, as well as the nurse, should recognize that the service rather than the worker is the determinant. The family who refuses to have "any nurse but Miss Brown" is demonstrating a relationship that is built upon personal trust and affection rather than upon the demands of the situation. The family has learned only to use the services of Miss Brown, not how to use the medical and nursing services provided by the community.

Furthermore, the nurse should be able to feel with the patient and family, yet not become emotionally involved to the point where she cannot cope with the realities of the situations with objectivity. For example, the nurse who is dealing with a situation in which an individual is facing the reality of a serious disabling condition hopes to guide the patient to a satisfactory adjustment. If she herself is filled with despair for the patient or with pity for the family, it is difficult for her to appreciate and present clearly the need for matter-of-fact acceptance of the disability by those in contact with the patient. An objective and rational approach does not preclude understanding or sympathy; it harnesses emotion to concentrate on what may be done, rather than upon the release of nonconstructive outlet. It may also, through the power of demonstration, enable the nurse to direct the family into a constructive use of its own emotions.

Recognition of Family-Centered Responsibility. An unidentified philosopher once said, "If you give a man a fish he satisfies his hunger for one day; if you teach him to fish he satisfies his hunger for many days." One of the objectives of nursing service is to promote the independence of the family in dealing with its own health problems. Obviously there will be instances in which the nurse cannot avoid making decisions because individuals or families concerned are intellectually or emotionally unable to make them at the time when action must be taken. In most instances, however, families or individuals should take responsibility for their own health decisions as soon as possible. The young, fearful mother whose husband is ill and whose parents are in a distant state may demand the reassurance of a relationship in which the nurse takes the major share of the responsibility. As the patient gains familiarity with the community and increased skill in the care of her child she should come to depend less and less upon the nurse. She should assume an increasing amount of independence in recognizing the need for medical or nursing care, and in locating suitable sources of information about health matters. The nurse who comes first as a teacher and guide may later become a counselor. A relationship based upon continuing dependency does not promote increasingly competent handling of health problems, nor does it usually utilize fully all of the available resources for family health care.

Levels of Participation. The degree to which family participation may be secured will vary with the capacity of the family, the demands of the situation and the skillfulness of the nurse. At the lowest level of participation the nurse may simply impose her own will or judgment upon patients or families and tell them what must be done. At the highest level, patient and nurse think and plan together, each aware of the particular contribution made by the other. At various times the nurse may be called upon to use any of the four levels of participation listed below, but it is assumed that the lower levels will be used only when the situation makes it impossible or dangerous to use a less authoritarian approach.

The lowest level of participation may be described as coercive.

Such a relationship may be necessary when a patient is unwilling or unable to cooperate in his care and is endangering himself or others. The patient who refuses to follow the procedures which will prevent infection of others may be forced to accept care in a hospital where control is possible; the hysterical or psychotic patient may be told that he MUST take treatment. This is usually not a very satisfactory relationship for patients or families since they are apt to resent such coercion, and may resent and resist future health services as a result.

Sometimes a "persuasive" approach is used, and the patient is inveigled into accepting treatment, or following advice, though he really doesn't want to and doesn't understand or accept the reasons for it, and a permissive or acquiescent relationship is established. For example, the young child who does not want to submit to immunization may be persuaded to do so, though he cannot appreciate the reason for the procedure or be taught to accept the treatment for its own sake. A mother may be urged to accept surgical treatment for which she sees no need, or to continue with her prenatal class because the nurse tells her it is the thing to do. In this type of relationship the nurse decides, and the family accepts but does not participate in the decision. Because the family accepts no responsibility in the decision, this approach if carried on for any length of time is apt to discourage initiative and independence of family action. The family may agree to a course of action in a given situation without seeing the implications for future health care. For example, a mother may be persuaded to accept vaccination for her child. If she isn't helped to make the decision on the basis of the reason for vaccination or the relationship to other preventive procedures, when another immunization program is launched she must be persuaded all over again.

More satisfactory is the relationship in which the patient and nurse share in discussion and in the planning, which may be called a participating relationship. Here the nurse maintains some control, but there is still opportunity for decision by the patient, or for limited participation in planning. The nurse controls the direction of the action, while the patient or family exercises some selection in methods or details. This approach may be effective with individuals who do not yet have enough facts to make independent decisions, but are able to decide minor points, raise questions or suggest possible applications. For example, in discussing the need for hospitalization for a severe psychiatric disorder the family may not be able to decide whether or not to accept such care; the nurse must be forceful enough to assure the reaching of that decision, but the family may decide when, where and how the patient will be admitted. The very young mother may not know enough about child development to decide without help what the needs of her baby are, but she can decide upon the household adjustments that might be made to meet these needs.

When the patient or family and the nurse are able to work jointly in the analysis and solution of problems, and each contributes to the fullest extent throughout the entire process, the relationship might be described as cooperative, or fully participative. Here nurse and family share responsibility, with the family deciding in consultation with the nurse just what action will be taken. For example, in discussing prenatal care, the family may want to discuss the merits of ward care as opposed to semi-private care in the hospital, or the attitudes that might be expected among the siblings upon the arrival of the new baby, and ways of promoting good sibling relationships. Nurse and family discuss the problem without the nurse being called upon to "guide" the family in one or the other direction, but simply to help the family clarify its thinking and see important relationships that will help in making the decision of what to do with wisdom and confidence.

In the course of professional service the level of relationship will shift in accordance with the nature of the problem and other modifying factors. However, the objective should be to secure the greatest possible family independence, and the trend should be toward more and more decision-making by the family, and less and less by the nurse.

MOTIVATING THE FAMILY OR INDIVIDUAL

Sometimes families have problems which they recognize fully or partially, but about which they are not stimulated to take any action. This inaction or lack of desire to learn or do something may arise from several factors. (1) Families may not realize fully the implications or importance of the problem. (2) They may feel that the required action threatens their sense of security or prestige. (3) They may see no need for the action, or give it a low priority, feeling that the problem is one to be accepted rather than ameliorated. (4) They may be fearful or discouraged, and feel that by putting off or failing to take action they can deny the harsh reality of the problem. It is an essential part of public health nursing to build in families a desire to do something about their health problems, and a conviction that they can and should take the necessary action. There are limitations to the degree of help that can be afforded by "doing for"—it is only as the family accepts responsibility and wants to solve its own problems that it can benefit fully from the nursing services.

This desire to do something is dependent not only on knowledge of the need, but it is also frequently affected by emotional or impulsive factors that may have nothing to do with the facts.

The nurse can do much to get families "steamed up" about health problems. She can:

1. Evoke dissatisfaction with the present situation.
2. Relate health action to existing goals and values.
3. Make specific goals in relation to the problem clear and reachable.
4. Recognize, respect and help to remove emotional blocks.
5. Appeal to the individual's best concept of himself.

Evoking Dissatisfaction.   The young wife who is caring for an incapacitated mother may be satisfied that this can be done only at the cost of her own excessive fatigue and some neglect of both husband and children. A parent may take pride in the bookworm who earns high grades without realizing the cost to him of withdrawing from his group, or may feel that "brains will triumph." A woman with a lump in her breast may feel that diagnosis is unimportant because she believes that there is no hope for cancer patients anyway. The industrial worker may not realize that his late home recreation and resultant fatigue and hangover affect his safety on a hazardous job.

The public health nurse may stir the family to a sense of dissatisfaction—to a recognition of a need for action. She may do this by raising questions, carefully designed so that they do not belittle the beliefs of the family or seem to place blame on its members, but do stimulate thinking along a new channel. For instance, she may ask how the good student and model child gets along with others of his own group whom he considers his best friends; or ask whether the industrial worker has seen accidents of other workers in his plant and how they happened, helping him to see the possible relationship between physical condition and accidents.

She may also provide information that makes the problem

more apparent. Stories of studies of successful men in many fields, for example, indicate the importance of ability to work with others or to relax as well as the value of knowledge and persistence. She may call upon the experience of others to point out the problem—indicating the trouble another parent had in securing a balanced life for a brilliant child, or calling on the reported experiences of parents of child prodigies.

Relating Action to Existing Goals or Values. Depending upon the individual's and family's concepts of values and life goals, the nurse may help to relate health action to them. The older man or woman may want to remain independent—not be a burden—which can be related to early diagnosis and care of chronic illness; the young mother wants a good life for her children, which can be related to the type of care provided for her ailing mother; the industrial worker may want to keep his job or get ahead, both related to wise scheduling of off-the-job activities. The object is to let the family see that "Will no action get you where you want to go?" is the question that must be answered.

Making the Problem Clear and Solvable. Sometimes people don't want to do anything about their problems because they appear so big or so hopeless that they seem insurmountable. The nurse can help by pacing her prodding to the family's readiness. When a diagnosis of rheumatic fever is first made in a child the parents are apt to be unready to look ahead to the need to safeguard the child's personality and independence, balancing his demands with those of other children in the family. At the moment, all they are interested in is getting this child well— everything else is temporarily pushed into the background. After a few weeks, when the reality of the situation has been accepted, the family may be ready to look at the long-range problem. The time will differ for each family. The public health nurse must be sensitive to these points of readiness—not push ahead so fast as to frighten or discourage the family, and yet not delay to the point that the family feels deserted and frustrated. The cues will be clear if the nurse is sensitized to them—for example, when the mother of the sick child arranges to have her hair done, or when the conversation begins to include concern about other members of the family, or about the child's problems when he returns to school.

Once the family is ready to look at the problem, it can be clarified by discussion between the nurse and family. The nurse must help the family to see the problem realistically, yet hopefully.

The nurse can make clear, also, that there are people and agencies who will help. Statements such as "We can work things out with the school," "We can talk with the doctor about that," and "I'm sure we can find a way to get a cot for Jack" reassure the family, make them feel they are not alone and that the problem is a solvable one.

Also important is to whittle down the problem to manageable proportions. "We can worry about that later," or "If we take care of this now that's all we can expect to do" will relieve the family of the stress that goes with revolving over and over the multitude of things that need doing.

False cheerfulness—"you'll be better in no time"—or evading the realities will not help. But an attitude of matter-of-fact confidence on the part of the nurse is essential.

Recognition of Emotional Blocks.   Unwillingness to act may be due to fear or unwillingness to face reality. Patients or families may feel that if they take no action they can escape facing the problem. The man with shortness of breath or chest pain may be reluctant to seek medical care, because, once he does, facing the fact that he has a heart impairment may be inescapable; if no action is taken he can push the disturbing fact back in his mind. Working to counteract the blocking emotion itself—the fear or immaturity or feeling of inadequacy—is the only way to get the individual or family to take necessary action willingly. Providing additional information or exhortation will have no effect, since neither is related to the reason for lack of motivations. Methods of dealing with emotional blocks and action are discussed later in this chapter.

Expecting Positive Action.   Most people react in the ways that are expected of them. If the public health nurse assumes that an expectant mother must be persuaded to accept medical supervision the patient may well react with resistance. Expressing confidence that the patient or family *wants* to act in the best way that is consistent with basic human needs as well as with the health situation often has a powerful motivational effect. For example, it is not reasonable to expect every expectant mother to *want* her baby. But whether or not the baby is wanted, the reasons for seeking care are so compelling that it is reasonable to assume that it will be sought. Fairness to the baby and obligation for protection of one's own health *can* be expected because it is logical to assume that people are basically decent and fair, whatever their feelings are.

Implying that such basic values exist will often elicit them. By assuming the patient's willingness to "do the right thing," health services can contribute much to safeguarding the personality of the individual who is threatened. A manner that takes for granted that the man with gonorrhea will want to help others from whom he got the infection and to whom he may have given it implies a quality of responsibility and generosity which may counteract his destructive feelings about himself, as well as stir him to action.

Very rarely, patients may have to be stimulated to action by fear of the consequences of nonaction. Despite the advantages of a positive approach, fear may be a powerful stimulus to action; fear of legal action if the careless tuberculosis patient does not accept hospitalization, fear of death or disability if one goes to a nonmedical abortionist, or fear of public disapproval if children or parents are neglected may be the only way of securing the necessary condition to initiate necessary action.[5] However, this approach has many disadvantages. First, it has limited carry-over value—the patient will go to the hospital to escape legal action, but this will not help him to cope with other aspects of care of his disease, nor will it encourage him to use health department facilities for other health problems which occur later. Secondly, it often leaves the patient feeling "pushed around" and resentful, so that his adjustment to his situation is impeded rather than enhanced. For these reasons, fear as a motivational force should be used very sparingly, only when the situation is sufficiently serious to demand it, and only when a more positive approach has proved ineffective.

Getting the family ready to do something takes skill and patience. But without this readiness to act, only partial returns may be expected from the services provided.

TELLING, EXPLAINING, DIRECTING

An important aspect of counseling by the public health nurse is that of providing information or direction in matters in which the family does not have and cannot get easily the necessary facts or skills to proceed, and in which the nurse is expert. In telling, explaining or directing families the nurse needs to or-

5. Kleinschmidt, H. E. and Savel Zimand, *Public Health Education.* New York, Macmillan Co., 1953.

ganize and present materials in accordance with the present knowledge of the family, and in such a way that the facts are clearly understood and acceptable.

Instruction Should be Based on Present Knowledge and Desires of the Family.   It is important to know just how much and what information the family has, as well as the way it feels about the health situation, before starting to give information or direction. Teaching that repeats what is already known dissipates the interest and attention of the patient, so that even when new information is introduced there is no response. By encouraging the patient to express what he already knows, the nurse can judge by the way the patient expresses himself at what level to place instruction, so she neither talks down to him nor goes over his head. "What did the doctor say?" or "What do you expect to do?" opens the way for the patient to indicate what knowledge he already has.

The family members may have had previous instruction in school, in a home nursing class, in the hospital or in previous nursing service that will provide a base for new material. It is important to know what the patient or family *want* to know as well as what is already known, and this is usually made apparent if the nurse listens for a bit after raising some general questions. Being willing to sit through a few moments of silence, or offering a reflecting remark, rather than raising another question or proffering advice too promptly, usually encourages the patient to discuss his feelings more fully.

Sometimes related information is important—the taxi driver who is accustomed to keeping a manifest may find keeping a record of his temperature and treatment results quite similar; the former secretary who has had experience getting along with a difficult boss or planning her work will find that a good basis for the human relations and planning skills needed in family management.

Present Information Clearly and Acceptably.   Information must be intelligible to the family. To many families the statement "It's a communicable disease" will be perfectly understandable; to one whose language skill or education is scanty it may be clearer if the term "catching disease" is used. Words like "infectious material," "contaminated," or "pediculosis," familiar to the nurse, may confuse the family. If the nurse observes the patient or family member carefully as she provides such information she will notice when confusion is revealed, and will be able to restate the information so that it is understood.

In attempting to be understandable, however, the nurse must be careful not to swing too far in the direction of simplification, and seem to belittle the intelligence of the patient or family. No one likes to be "talked down to." Medical terms may already be part of the family's vocabulary, or could be learned quickly. For example, the prenatal patient may have learned to use the word "uterus" rather than "womb." Because the more scientific terms may be used with greater accuracy and impersonality, they are usually more acceptable to the patient. The nurse should proceed at the higher vocabulary level when the family is ready for it, and, in some instances, should teach families to use the more descriptive technical terminology.

Information should be presented in sufficient detail to avoid misunderstanding. For example, in explaining the significance of a positive tuberculin reaction, great care must be exercised in differentiating between infection with the tubercle bacillus and the existence of clinical tuberculosis. Too brief an explanation may lead to misinterpretation by the family, or arouse unnecessary fear or indifference. At the same time, too great a degree of refinement or interpretation of details that are not of central importance may make learning more difficult for those whose experience and training have given them little skill in identifying significant factors among many others. An individual who is being taught the available resources for diagnosis of cancer need not know all of the detail and relative dependability of the many experimental diagnostic procedures—she *does* need to know how frequently she should secure a check-up, the tests in current use and the importance of related physical symptoms as well as laboratory tests in diagnosis. The patient who has a broader background of information and more extensive academic experience will probably want and accept more detailed or complicated information.

Information should be given in such a way that it is acceptable to the patient or family. Condescension or professional snobbishness may be imputed to the nurse if she seems to lecture as she gives information. One young nurse, visiting a mother of three, began her prenatal conference by saying, "Now, Mrs. Smith, I want to tell you how babies develop and are born." The mother, who actually did need further information about intrauterine development and the physiology of labor, and who had the reputation of being a difficult patient during delivery, answered "I

think I should tell you about that—after all, I've had three!" If
the nurse had recognized the mother's experience and approached
the imparting of knowledge with greater humility, it would probably have been entirely acceptable or even welcomed. An informal
approach to the exercises for improving muscular tone might
have led to questions and to opportunities for recognizing and
giving credit to the mother's past experience while still leaving
the way clear to add to her information.

In correcting misinformation, too, care must be exercised to
avoid embarrassing the patient. To the mother who made the
statement that every doctor should give his patients analgesics
during the delivery, the reply "Oh, no, that's not right" would
be apt to build a desire to defend a position already taken, or
produce embarrassment for being mistaken. "Many people used
to think that, too, but now doctors have learned a lot about what
an individual thing it is to have a baby, and how differently every
person reacts to this experience. I've just read a book you might
like to see . . . ." Such an approach will give the impression that
the patient can learn—along with doctors and nurses—about new
things.

Use Specific Applications to Clarify Generalization.   The
ability to generalize or to act on the basis of a generalization will
vary from family to family. In teaching, the nurse should be sure
to express the specific applications clearly while relating them
to the principle or generalization. Discussion of the specific basic
protective foods and of ways of including them in the usual food
purchasing and meal pattern of *this particular family* is more apt
to produce a change in food habits than is a discussion of proteins
and minerals and their importance to health. However, the principle also must be stressed that most protective foods must be
taken regularly, and that even large quantities of protective foods
taken spasmodically will not produce the same result.

Statements such as "You need annual examinations after 40"
and "You should have an eye examination by an oculist" should
be substantiated by the reasons that lie behind this need. The
reason *why* should be stressed constantly, so that the family learns
to recognize the principle, and through repeated specific applications learns to apply the principle in new situations.

Emphasize Important Points by Repeating or Marking.   Because the nurse's contact with families is limited in time, and
constant supervision following instruction is not possible, it is
imperative that a clear distinction be made between the points

presented that are of major significance and those that are less so. In this way, the family is helped to remember.

Emphasis may be secured by repetition of a point—by saying the same thing two or three times, perhaps with some change in wording. It may be secured by using visual aids—a picture, or a demonstration, or a sketch that makes the point clear. For example, the importance of rest for the tuberculosis patient may be emphasized by showing a graph of the respiration rate for the patient at rest and when engaged in different types of activity; or the growth pattern of babies may be emphasized by showing silhouette pictures of infants at different stages of physical growth. Providing practical applications is perhaps one of the most effective methods of emphasis. For example, in discussing growth and development, the ways in which parents may cope with negativism or adolescent awkwardness will emphasize the normality of the developmental pattern.

Just calling attention to a particular point—saying "This is really the most important thing to remember"—will also make it stand out.

Pace the Instruction to Suit the Family. Families will vary in relation to the speed at which they can assimilate new ideas or information. If ideas are presented too rapidly or in too short a time the family may feel inadequate or overwhelmed, and so not benefit from the instruction provided. Learning is facilitated if there is time to think about and apply a few ideas before moving on to new material.

During a visit or conference, too, it is important to allow time for the patient to react to the materials or the suggestions that are made, or to ask questions. Just waiting will usually secure some response, or saying "This must seem rather confusing to you" or "It's a lot to learn at once, isn't it?" will pave the way for questions or requests for additional explanation.

Check Understanding. The result desired in telling is understanding rather than recall—the ability to see the information in relation to its practical applications and in a variety of situations. Therefore, it is important to be sure that the family has grasped the meaning, rather than just remembered the words. For example, a mother may be able to answer the question "How much milk does Johnny need?" correctly without really understanding why it is important, or how she will actually provide for it in her daily meal-planning. Or the anxious woman suffering from menopausal symptoms may agree to a suggestion without any concept of what it really means—for example, agree that one should not worry, and should obtain sufficient rest, without translating this into the methods by which they are achieved when one is tense and disturbed.

The nurse can often get clues to lack of understanding without any need for words; a puzzled or blank expression, or lack of attention or interest may provide the clue. Discussing with the patient how he will apply the information—for example, just what play arrangements may be made for a small child to decrease the home accident risk, or in which room a post-hospital patient will go for rest during the day, or what approach the patient with newly acquired syphilis will use in talking to someone he may have infected about coming in for diagnosis—may correct misinformation and fortify learning.

Follow Through.   The results of instruction should be checked after an interval if possible to determine what was *done* as a result of the information given. If it is not possible to re-visit, the nurse may ask the patient to phone, or phone him to see how he is getting along, or she may ask him to complete and mail a post card report indicating whether he has gone to a physician or clinic (or taken other suggested action).

Only as instruction is reflected in changed practice is it possible to know to what extent there has been understanding and acceptance.

RELEASING AND GUIDING FAMILY POTENTIALS FOR SELF-HELP

An essential component, and perhaps the most significant facet of counseling, is releasing and guiding families to help themselves as contrasted to helping them. In this phase of counseling the nurse's primary tools are not her technical skills and know how, but the relationship she has established with the family. Her position as an recognized expert and at the same time a friendly, nonjudgmental supporter, makes the nurse a significant factor in the situation.

The nature of a professional relationship as it pertains to public health nursing and the methods by which such a relationship may be developed have been discussed previously. The following discussion is directed toward the ways in which this relationship in the family-nurse contact is put to work to help the family to cope with its health problems.

The Setting.   Essential to the knowing and disciplined use of a relationship for the attainment of a professional service goal is an emotional climate that allows the relationship to function. The nurse must bridge the gap between her own background and experience and those of the patient, identifying common interests and concerns that supersede differences in values, educational status, or culture. This may be done by general conversation to indicate this mutuality of interest—discussing the house plants, the baby's resemblance to one or the other parent, the newspaper headlines, or any other generalized subject that says in effect "We are both interested in the same thing."

The physical setting may also have importance in establishing this climate. If the conference is held in the nurse's office, she should be free from telephone calls or interruptions, and make clear that for the period of the conference all else has been put aside. There should be provision for privacy, so that the family member can feel free to discuss matters of personal or confidential nature if they are pertinent. The seating arrangement should contribute to the idea of cooperative discussion rather than the giving of professional advice; if the nurse sits behind her desk and the patient in a chair nearby, the effect is at once of a difference in responsibility—the position itself emphasizes the nurse's expert status as contrasted to her helping, supportive status. This effect is reversed if both patient and nurse sit in chairs away from the desk, for the desk is a symbol of authority or expertness.

As in teaching, vocabulary may help or interfere with communication. Words must be considered, not only in relation to their preciseness in carrying an idea, but also in relation to the feeling tones they may convey. "Compromise" to an active labor union member may mean "giving in temporarily" and be associated with a struggle for power not inherent in the meaning of the work itself; a "good milk producer" may convey to a young mother the idea of a cow-like attribute; use of a lay terminology with the individual who knows the technical terms may convey a sense of condescension. Careful observation—especially of the nonverbal expressions of reaction—will enable the nurse to identify and avoid these "red flag" words.

The nurse's demeanor is also a significant factor. A relaxed, unhurried attitude may be conveyed by the nurse's posture or facial expression as well as by the time allocated for the interview or conference. Stacks of records or other undone work may make the patient feel that the nurse is pressed for time, and cause him to feel guilty about taking the time necessary for discussion.

Clearing the desk of undone work may have a beneficial effect in creating a relaxed approach to discussion of problems.

If the conference has a time limit, it is well to make this clear at the outset so that both the patient and nurse can have it in mind without undue concern.

Within this setting, then, and with the knowledge that the job is to direct the inter-personal relationship of nurse and patient toward the solution of a problem which is of concern to both, the nurse proceeds. The objectives of this activity are fourfold:

1. Facing the problem.
2. Building family confidence in its ability to handle the problem.
3. Modifying destructive emotional states.
4. Securing forward movement in thinking and action.

Facing the Problem.   A prerequisite to wise action is a clear concept and acceptance of the problem. Often problems are seen unrealistically or partially. Because of the emotional stress and threat to the individual that so often accompanies health problems, there may be a tendency to deny the problems altogether, or to see them either overhopefully or overpessimistically. For example, a young woman with symptoms of gonorrhea may refuse to admit she has any symptoms, or to ascribe them to menstrual difficulty or fatigue. The man who has had a coronary occlusion may assume that his problem is how to live as a permanently incapacitated person. These misconceptions or evasions are not always based on lack of information, but rather upon habits of escape from reality, or emotional blocks. It is important to obtain a realistic acceptance of the problem so that plans and action to cope with it may be set up in a productive manner.

To help the family face a health problem, the nurse must be aware of its concept of the problem. Often what the family says may not reflect what it really believes. The relatedness of what is said or done yields the clue; what is *meant* as well as what is said has significance. The successful business man, going for a cancer check, may say, "Well, it can't scare me; I've had a full life and faced dying many times when I was in the army." While he says that he is not concerned, what he means is that he *is* concerned—that he fears what may be disclosed in the examination. The young mother may say, "I didn't want another baby so soon, but, now he's here, of course I love him." But overmeticulous attention to every detail of his care, unusual concern over every minor symptom, a conviction that he is "more delicate" than his older sister may suggest that the verbal and social acceptance of the new baby has not yet reached the mother's heart, and her *personal* acceptance is not yet complete. Encouraging the family to talk, listening with interest, posing statements or questions that may produce clue responses will help to direct the discussion so as to clarify the family's concept of the problem. Nonverbal behavior will yield many clues—the way in which the home nurse turns the bed patient, or the method of holding the baby may contradict a verbally expressed concern. It is important to remember, as has been stated previously, that the same situation may produce different problems with different families or with the same family at different times. Long-term illness that may present a minimum of emotional stress when the family is stabilized and doing well may precipitate a crisis and threaten the integrity of the family as a whole if it comes when there is unemployment of the wage earner, or marital distress. The fact that the family's concept of the problem differs from that of the nurse does not mean that its concept is either unrealistic or inaccurate; both concepts need to be considered in the light of the factors that cause the difference.

In helping the family to face its health problems there is need to allow time for adjustment. Not everyone can or should move immediately into a stern facing of all of the facts. This does not mean that the nurse should withhold information from the family if requested, but rather that it may be desirable to postpone any effort to stimulate the family to look at the situation in its entirety until its members are ready. For instance, the period of shock that follows diagnosis of psychiatric illness may be a poor point at which to discuss prognosis. It may be better to put off such discussion until the immediate needs have been taken care of, and the family has had time to realize that it is not alone—that the community forces are behind it and ready to give support. Then the prognosis can be considered in the light of its effect on family decisions and action.

There are occasions when the individual or family persists in failing to recognize the realities of the situation. The devoted son may refuse to consider anything but private hospital care for his parent with psychiatric illness that is expected to be of long duration, to the point of sapping family financial resources and borrowing, because he is unwilling to face the situation objectively. In such cases the nurse can be helpful through pa-

tient unhurried conferences with the family, providing an opportunity to talk out the situation. This may help its members
to see the effects of the action planned, without denying their
right to do as they wish. The nurse may raise questions as to
the physician's appraisal of the situation and suggest that they
talk with him. She may ask whether they have seen and know
about the governmental hospital and its facilities, suggesting that
they might like to visit so that they may understand the choice.
By her own unemotional, matter-of-fact approach to questions
and by refraining from trying to impose her own ideas and
values on others she can convey the feeling that this situation is
not unique; by recognizing and encouraging the son to express
his feelings of love and concern for his parent she can show
that she recognizes the difficulty of accepting an unpleasant fact.
By giving the son time to talk about his feelings of concern for
other members of his family and perhaps his job, she can give
him an opportunity to come to a realistic appraisal and re-
direction of plans himself.

When the reality of the situation demands acceptance of authority—as when health regulations require a food handler to
stop work for a time or even to change his employment—the
source of the authority should be clear and the family should
understand that it is impersonal. For example, it is not the nurse
who is responsible for the obligation of not working when so
doing may endanger others, it is the need of the community as
expressed in its laws; it is the authority of the school and not
of the school nurse or principal that makes it necessary for the
child who cannot adjust, and who disturbs others, to stay away
from school unless he can be helped to change his behavior.

Building Family Self-confidence. The family must have
confidence in its own ability to cope with problems, and sometimes this self-confidence needs to be developed and built up
patiently. To develop confidence, most families need to know
that there is someone standing by to help—that they can call
the nurse or the doctor or the clinic if anything goes wrong.
They may need also to have the assurance that comes when the
help *is* given—in other words, the dependency needs of families
must be met fully before they are ready to move on to independence. The woman with arthritis, for example, may need
to have the nurse, rather than a family member, give her personal care for a while until she is sure she can depend on this
source of help. Then, gradually the family and the patient

herself can be brought to take on more and more of the care, permitting practice in the nurse's presence, to call upon her for advice, or in other ways obtain additional help for as long as necessary. One of the important factors in making home care programs effective seems to be the knowledge that if things get too difficult the patient will be readmitted to the hospital. The knowledge that this can be done often gives the family members confidence to undertake care which otherwise they would not feel that they could even start.

Demonstrating confidence in families may also help them toward independence. This is often a matter of intangible little things—the tone of voice that implies expecting the patient giving his own insulin to try and to succeed, yet makes the possibility of failure nothing to fear or be ashamed of; the touch on the shoulder that tells the child about to use crutches on his own for the first time that you know it takes courage, but know he has it; the recognition of general ability may also help—suggesting that the man who could organize an office can organize his daily life for the complex and difficult job of physical rehabilitation, which requires study and scheduling, and planning when and how to use the help of others and when to get along alone.

In suggesting what families can do, and so building their confidence, it is important not to belittle what they are already doing or have done. This should be recognized as an achievement that sets the stage for greater progress.

Being sure that the mechanical aspects of care are fully mastered before placing the patient on his own is also important. If the boy using crutches is fully competent in using them, and has learned to maneuver under the watchful eye of the nurse, and then of a family member, he is more able to face the problem of the social adjustments he must make in outdoor contacts with other children. Having given insulin for several times under supervision, the family member is confident of this aspect of care and so more able to manage the other problems in care of the diabetic. Anticipating and playing out emergencies or problems that may arise also gives the family confidence. For example, discussing with the child who must use crutches the initial awkwardness the other children may feel with him gives him advance help.

Modifying Destructive Emotional States. Fear and guilt are frequent causes of failure to carry out plans for health action.

Fear is often unexpressed, or demonstrated in compensatory behavior. It may be revealed in extreme argumentativeness, failure to believe the doctor's diagnosis, delaying action that will confirm the fear, or by failure to show any strong response to a situation that is overwhelming. For example, a young woman who has many fears associated with her pregnancy may reveal them by always finding a reason for not going to the doctor, or she may seem unconcerned and almost disinterested in her condition. Until it is possible to deal with the mother's fears of death, of pain, of violation of modesty, of economic disaster, of diminished attractiveness, of inadequacy or of a host of other conjured consequences of maternity, it will be impossible to secure positive health action.

When fear is an impediment to action, the public health nurse may help counteract it by (1) finding the basis of the fear, (2) providing simple reassurance, (3) providing facts when the fear is based on inadequate information, and (4) projecting attention to the post-action period.

Establishing the basis of fear may require skill and patience. Sometimes the individual will state his fear freely and discuss it willingly. In other cases, only the most delicate and painstaking search will reveal the cause. Questions, relating the experiences and worries of other patients (unidentified, of course) who have faced similar problems, or "trial runs" with information that may be in the trouble area may bring the fear into the open. When the nurse suspects an unadmitted fear she must be particularly leisurely and reassuring in her investigation, and alert to the slightest changes in expression or to overconfident statements and attempts to change the direction of the conversation that may provide a clue as to the cause of the fear.

Reassurance may be given directly and positively, or indirectly. In giving direct reassurance it is important to place it at the right time. Reassurance given too early may cause the patient to repress his fear. For example, if the nurse says at once "There's no reason at all to worry because you found this lump in the breast early" the patient will find it hard to say "But I do worry." Reassurance comes best after the fear has been fully ventilated. Reassurance should also be both truthful and positive. One nurse, intending to reassure the mother who had expressed the fear that she wouldn't live through her fifth pregnancy said, "After all, only one out of every thousand mothers die in childbirth in this state." The result was, of course, that the mother was convinced that she would be the one. Talking out, followed by discussion pointing out that the mother's previous pregnancies had been uneventful, that the mother's physical impairments were slight and under careful medical control, that her doctor and her hospital were the best to be had, and that fatigue and physiologic changes associated with pregnancy sometimes produce unfounded fears would have strengthened the mother's feeling of security.

Indirect reassurance may be provided by the nurse's own attitude and by the way in which she plans with the family. The nurse's attitude must be genuinely positive if she is to help. If she reveals her feelings by sympathizing with "those poor devils" who are patients in the syphilis clinic, she may find it difficult to convince a young patient that it is not a catastrophe but a communicable disease that is susceptible to treatment that brings him to the clinic. Emphasis upon the good fortune of the individual to have discovered the disease early, and a calm and matter-of-fact approach will do much to reassure him. One nurse used to make it a practice to comment informally to each new patient that the clinic had lost two (or three or one) of its nicest patients that week, because the patients had been successfully treated and dismissed from care. It was characteristic of this nurse that she always felt she did have the "nicest patients!" Refraining from an overprotective or oversympathetic attitude will also help to reassure the patient.

When fears are based on inadequate information or old wives' tales the nurse can do much to substitute facts for fear. Information should be carefully presented. When possible, printed materials should be used so that the individual may read them later and thus reinforce the information given by the nurse. Sometimes charts or graphs are helpful, as in explaining the process of labor or the effects of rest therapy in tuberculosis.

The sources of the information provided should be stressed. The individual can have more confidence in the information offered if he realizes that it is based on long and carefully controlled clinical study, on laboratory research or on the judgment of the physician who has gained that judgment through long training and experience.

Directing the individual's attention to the post-action period may also help to minimize fear. The mother who is thinking about the lovely baby she is going to have, of his clothes and guidance, of his father's pride in him will have less time to worry about her fear of pain at delivery. Talking of the post-hospital period with the tuberculosis patient and his family places the hospital in its proper perspective as an interlude in treatment. As such it loses much of its awesomeness. One nurse, dealing with a discouraged patient and trying to get him to look ahead to his discharge from the hospital was told by the patient that he couldn't plan that far ahead. She suggested that he think of a period six months prior to this visit, and realize what a short time it seemed. With this encouragement, he was able to plan more optimistically. The object of this projection is to keep the goal of the care in the place of primary importance—to help the individual think in terms of what he hopes to accomplish through the suggested health action, rather than in terms of the action itself.

Fear is a destructive force to the individual as well as a deterrent to action. The nurse who guides her patients toward a cheerful, positive and courageous attitude toward health care not only secures a larger measure of success in meeting health needs, but she may also make a significant contribution to the development of the individual as well.

Guilt or shame may be equally strong impediments to desirable health action. The unmarried girl who is pregnant may prefer to leave her town or neighborhood and conceal her condition as long as possible, rather than let others know of her pregnancy. Similarly, individuals afflicted with tuberculosis or with mental illness may feel that there is a stigma attached to the disease and want to hide all evidence of their illness, or syphilitics may refuse to bring contacts in for examination because they are ashamed to acknowledge their condition.

If the feelings of guilt and shame are brought into the open much may be done to combat their negative effects. The individual will be more apt to reveal his feelings if it is possible to provide for privacy during the conference with the nurse. An interested but untroubled manner on the part of the nurse may also encourage frank discussion.

The nurse should accept the patient's guilt and shame as both natural and important. She should, however, also help him to direct the forces that motivate his feeling of unworthiness into constructive rather than resistive channels. For example, the man who has contracted a venereal disease through extramarital adventure may be very much ashamed of his defection. He may demonstrate this in refusal to talk with his wife about his condition, and failure to bring her to the clinic for diagnostic tests. He must be helped to see that concern for his wife and affection for her are basic to his attitude; if he didn't care it wouldn't matter what he told her. This concern may then be turned toward helping to protect his wife, and thus to compensate for his previous fault.

Building self-esteem of the individual will also help him to overcome the negative effects of guilt and shame. The personal worth of the individual must be recognized in every possible way. For example, calling individuals by their names or making a special effort to greet each person individually as he comes to the office lends dignity to the contact between patient and nurse.

Reinforcing positive or commendable behavior also contributes to the building of self-esteem. Pointing out that the husband showed his sense of responsibility by coming in for treatment, that he did not expose his wife to infection intentionally, that he is a good provider and a kind father, or a good spender, or mentioning some other commendable quality that may have been demonstrated, helps to restore a feeling of personal value that is essential in conquering shame and fear.

Sometimes the individual needs help in meeting the practical problems of admitting or explaining the situation to others. The public health nurse may help the young girl to decide upon the specific approach she will use in making the difficult confession of extramarital pregnancy to her parents. Giving the woman who has venereal disease an opportunity to talk with the individual who is the source of her infection, and discussing the ways in which she can interpret the condition and the need for care will give her confidence, and will make it easier for her to take appropriate action.

The public health nurse should recognize emotional problems requiring more expert care than she is able to give. Evidences of deep-rooted emotional maladjustment should be referred for social work or psychiatric care.

Immaturity may also play a part in preventing appropriate health action. Maturity is described by Friedenberg as four-faceted—awareness to know and take account of what is going on around and within us, objectivity to see things as they are and not just as we would like them to be, emotional responsiveness and civility.[6] Not all individuals achieve the independence,

6. Friedenberg, Edgar Z., The Mature Attitude. *Adult Leadership*, 5: 248–250, February, 1957.

competence and responsibility that should be characteristic of their chronologic age group. They may choose to be dependent, saying "Let the health department make me do it" when urged to accept hospital care for tuberculosis, or "Tell me what I should do" when discussing the care of the preschool child, moving ahead only when someone else provides the motivating force. Other evidences of immature behavior may be revealed in the mother who never develops competence in recognizing symptoms of illness, who refuses to learn to take a temperature or to evaluate the general condition of her children's health, is afraid to learn to give insulin to a sick member of the family, or gets sick at the thought of changing a surgical dressing.

Irresponsible actions may also characterize the immature individual. The milkman who tries to conceal the fact that a member of his family has typhoid fever and risks exposing a large number of people to the disease; the prenatal patient who refuses to modify extravagant physical activities and as a result has a miscarriage; the young industrial worker who is absent on the day physical examinations are to be given because he has had symptoms that he believes are characteristic of tuberculosis and doesn't want it to be discovered—all are exhibiting lack of mature and responsible action.

The public health nurse must work within the maturity limits of the family, realizing that individuals and families will vary widely in this respect. She must also recognize that maturity is a configuration of traits, and that an individual may be relatively mature in some aspects of his behavior and shockingly immature in others. By encouragement, support, and by strengthening competences and by teaching, the individual may be helped to achieve the highest degree of maturity of which he is capable.

Coping with Social and Cultural Impediments to Care. Superstitions or fallacious health beliefs may be harmful in themselves. More often they are harmful because they prevent or delay the acceptance of sound health care.

Superstitions do not yield easily to argument or denial of their validity. They are rooted in group culture which changes slowly, and believers can always find "proofs" of the potency of a particular belief. The ineffectiveness of reason as a deterrent to superstitious belief can be demonstrated by noticing the number of intelligent people who pick up pins for good luck, who say "bread and butter" to forestall disappointment, or who knock on wood to ward off evil!

Sometimes it is wise to ignore superstitious action temporarily. If a nurse sees a patient for the first time when she is in labor, and finds an axe under the bed "to cut the pains" she might well proceed without comment, planning to instruct the family at some later time about the process of labor and the cause of the pains.

When attempting to counteract superstition it is important to avoid seeming to patronize or to lecture. It may be possible to explain how the superstition arose, how well it was adjusted to the situation in which it arose, and the changes that make the superstition untenable now.

Sometimes natural leaders in the community are focal points of superstitious belief. If these leaders can be convinced, they may exercise great effect upon community thinking. It may be possible to appeal to the pride of the local "granny" or kindly neighbor who is "a great one to help in sickness," encouraging her to obtain up-to-date information, and to use her influence to get others to seek suitable care. One woman, an unlettered midwife of forty years' experience, told the nurse, "None of my ma's has a knife under the pillow. I tell 'em I know from that course I took with the doctors." Her leadership has been turned to positive uses through her pride in having knowledge above that of her neighbors.

Social customs may also cause resistance to health action. For example, in a group where it is customary for the man of the family to take responsibility for all decisions, action may never be taken if the nurse talks only with the mother of the family. Standards of housekeeping or traditional patterns of homemaking may also present a problem. The woman who has always dried dishes may find it hard to get used to letting them drain dry; the woman who takes great pride in her ability to bake pies and cakes may find it difficult to change dietary habits so that the family diet is more balanced; the family that puts great stress on "good" children may find it hard to encourage independence and allow sufficient freedom to develop initiative and judgment.

Sometimes group pressures will determine individual action. A high school crowd may think it is "sissified" to drink milk, so all will drink "pop" or coffee. A group of girls working in industry may decide it is smart to wear clothing that is safe and sensible on the job, with the result that the individual members conform to the group pattern and safety is promoted.

When group pressures exert a negative influence it may be necessary to change the attitude of the whole group before substantial results can be obtained with individuals. Seeking out and instructing natural leaders in such groups may enable the nurse to influence group attitudes more readily than by working with the group as a whole. Other professional workers may be particularly helpful here; teachers, social workers, recreational directors, or members of the clergy can often help as an incidental part of their own services.

Securing Forward Movements in Thinking and Action. Sometimes a family-nurse contact is very pleasant and active, but does not move forward. It may be that general friendly discussion, intended to create a relaxed and friendly atmosphere, continues until it becomes the whole visit, or leads to social rather than professional overtures. The family may move toward providing tea for the nurse, rather than discussing the problems for which she is prepared to help. The nurse will need to:

1. guide conversation to the objective of the visit or conference;
2. re-direct conversation when it becomes nonproductive;
3. "clinch" decisions and plans for action;
4. combat forgetting or procrastination.

While preliminary conversation is necessary to establish an identity of interests and create a feeling of appreciation for the individual, it should not be prolonged to such an extent that the call becomes a social rather than a professional visit. Getting down to the business of the visit within a reasonable time fosters a business-like attitude which helps to move the discussion to productive channels.

Transitional conversation, which will direct the visit from introductory stage-setting remarks to the real purpose of the visit, accomplishes this purpose smoothly, and forestalls offers of excessive hospitality which would consume time without producing results. A little conscious attention will produce any number of key phrases such as "He is a cute baby," followed by such transitional remarks as "I expect you find his care quite a change from office work," which may lead to discussion of daily programs; "I imagine his father is proud of him" to a discussion of parental relationships; "Is he always this good?" to a discussion of emotional hygiene.

At times conversation may get to the point where it is no longer concerned with the object of the visit, or has been reduced to a repetition of problems or ideas about which the family or individual is not ready to take any action, and which might better be put in "cold storage" for a later time. Discussion of anticipated neighbor reactions to the return of the hospitalized psychiatric patient may become a recital of neighborhood gossip, or the family member may say over and over "It's going to be rough, we'll all feel so ashamed" without being willing to talk about *why* they feel ashamed or what might be done about it.

When this happens, the nurse will want to re-direct the conversation, or perhaps put off the discussion entirely until a later time. This may be done by making a terminal summary remark that will shut off discussion—for example, "Yes, when you know a lot about families it's easy to see how important our home life is in determining our attitudes," or "It's true that no matter how much we tell ourselves about mental illness, it's hard not to feel embarrassed about it," or by a delaying remark, such as "I know how much this must be on your mind—maybe we'd better let it rest a bit. I'll be coming in Tuesday and we can talk about it then."

It takes fine distinction and judgment to know when to encourage and when to shut off conversation. With the new worker it is usually a good rule not to shut off conversation unless the worker feels that it is actually harmful, or that the family will regret it later, and so not want to see the nurse and be reminded of its indiscretion. But the nurse is with the family for a purpose, and the conversation should be contributing to the clarification or understanding of the problem, or to the development of relationships between the nurse and the patient that will enable them to work with one another in the solution of the problems that are present. When it does not contribute in this way, an effort should be made to get back on the track.

Sometimes discussion goes round and round, with the family reiterating that some recommended action is not possible, or proposing a plan that the nurse knows to be impractical or undesirable. For example, the family may propose that the incapacitated chronically ill grandfather be moved to the living room, so he "has the best." Actually the advantage of making it easier for callers, and providing a street view for the sick person may be much less than the disadvantage of having no place where the children can entertain their friends, and no central place for the family to congregate for socialization when the sick member is resting.

The nurse might re-direct thinking toward a new sickroom

by an oblique suggestion: "Have you thought of turning over
the dining room for this?" or by raising questions about where
the children will meet their friends. If there is a recreation room,
the family's answer may be perfectly acceptable. She may also
remind the family that what works for a short time may be a
difficult problem for a long term, again raising the question that
will help the family to see the problem rather than telling them
about it. Or she may suggest that it may be possible to move the
patient to the living room for short periods.

Sometimes just relating the other possible alternatives is desirable, pitching the statements so as to recognize the value of
the family's thinking and suggesting rather than advising. For
instance, "I've seen one family that used the dining room. They
found it much easier because the children weren't put out of the
living room. They ate in the kitchen, and when they had company for meals they used card tables in the living room."

When the family has reached a decision or decided upon a
particular course of action, this needs to be "clinched" so the
way can be cleared for moving on to new things. This can be
done by helping the individual or family to state exactly what
has been decided, by asking a question, or asking whether you've
understood correctly what has been decided. Tying the decision
to time, place and specific action also helps—what day the patient will go to the doctor, at which meals it is planned to introduce the additional milk, where the family will shop for the cot
on which the tuberculosis patient will sleep.

"Now let's see what we're going to do" provides a good opening
for a summary.

It is very easy to put off action when the health situation is
not an explosive or urgent one. The family may intend to secure
a physical examination, change food habits or seek immunization, but not get around to doing it. The wise public health nurse
finds ways to help families to overcome this human tendency to
delay action.

Sometimes a system of reminders will help, such as putting
a note on the kitchen calendar, sending a reminder postcard a
few days before a clinic visit has been scheduled, or checking
by telephone to see whether the family expects to be able to go
ahead with the plans made. Writing down what is to be done
day by day may also help. For example, the home nurse may
write down a series of daily activities for the chronically ill patient, or the mother of a small child may set up a daily timetable
that includes all aspects of care.

Setting a time limit may encourage action when the situation itself does not convey a sense of urgency. Setting a definite day and time for the clinic visit, deciding to try two new foods during the coming week, and planning to have the physical examination before the next nursing visit are examples of devices that may be used to set a time limit for the proposed action.

A request that the family report action may also stimulate prompt follow-up. When the nurse does not plan to revisit the family, or when the next visit is scheduled quite far ahead, the family may be asked to report by stopping in at the nurse's office or sending a postcard.

Action may be encouraged by making it easy to follow through with the plans made. Doing things in groups or with someone else may be easier than doing them alone. Suggesting that the high school student go to the dentist when his friend is going, or arranging for a new member of a parents' class to go with an older member may overcome procrastination.

Circumventing the impersonality and complexity of admission procedures of the modern medical center may also overcome a tendency to put off attendance. A detailed description of admission procedures and clinic or hospital routines will give the patient or family a sense of familiarity and security that makes attendance easier. Referral to a particular doctor or worker will also make the referral seem more personal, and harder to disregard or postpone.

It is in the realm of counseling and teaching that the nurse has the greatest possible leeway for creative approaches, for highly individualized judgments and for subtle combinations of methods and services. Counseling cannot be reduced to a "how to do it" analysis; it is learned by doing, by discussion with others, especially with those in a supervisory or consultant capacity, by self-appraisal and by constantly trying new ways and evaluating the old ones. No two nurses will function in the same way, or find satisfactions from the same types of relationship. Whatever the approach or the personal adaptations that are made in relationships, the use of one's professional self, that combination of technical expertness, ministration and motivational and guiding force, is a potent factor in improving family and individual health.

CHAPTER XI

Judging Progress

A PERIODIC CHECK on progress made by the family in health care is essential for case planning. It is equally important as a clue to the effectiveness of the methods used by the nurse in providing service. To secure such a check it is necessary to have:

1. A baseline
2. A clear statement of desired outcomes
3. A measure of change or status
4. An analysis of factors contributing to or retarding progress.

GETTING A BASELINE

Emphasis has already been placed on the need for an evaluation of the status of the family in relation to health knowledge, skills and attitudes as a base for designing the pattern of nursing care. For judging progress it is important that there be a clear description of the status at the time service was instituted or at the beginning of the period being considered. Questions such as the following should be raised.

1. To what extent does the family recognize its health problems? Are there problems which are unrecognized by the family? Is the family concept of the problem incomplete or inaccurate?
2. To what degree is the family response to the problem responsible? self-directing? socially oriented? based on facts? influenced by superstition or prejudice?
3. Is the family response to nursing care welcoming? neutral? demanding? resistive?
4. What are the physical needs of the patient for personal care? treatment?

5. In what areas of health care is the health information of the family adequate? partial? very inadequate?
6. How does the family use its own resources? Is it dominated by one or two members? Do family members work as a team to help one another?
7. Does the family know and use community health resources? some? few? virtually none?
8. What does the family know about the disease or condition under care? method of spread, if communicable? anticipated course or progress of the disease? symptoms that should be observed? emotional or personality factors associated with the disease or condition?
9. What does the family know about home nursing skills? What previous experience has it had with illness? Can some member of the family read a thermometer? bathe a sick person? give a simple enema?
10. What does the family know about general hygienic practices? nutrition? rest, relaxation, sleep? previous medical care? personal hygiene? growth and development? accident prevention? intra-family relationships?

A record notation should be made early in the course of care, or at periodic intervals if the case is carried for a long time, incorporating the salient information regarding the status of the family's health information, skill and behavior. This provides a baseline for later evaluation of progress.

Sometimes it is helpful to check the level of family health performance on a performance scale similar to the one suggested in Figure 13. This permits the nurse to estimate the level of family performance at intervals, and provides a graphic record of progress made. While the use of such a scale would hardly be justified for every case, for problem cases, or those carried over a long period of time it might be useful. It is also useful as a method of sharpening one's own judgments about family progress, or as a base for discussion about service improvement. The nurse might, for instance, complete several such estimates in anticipation of a supervisory visit, and use them as a basis for the supervisor-nurse conference; or they might be useful as a point of departure for a case presentation as part of the staff education program.

EXPECTED SERVICE OUTCOMES

In each family situation there will be certain things which it seems reasonable and desirable to accomplish—the expectant

Name_____ Nurse_____

Address_____ Date_____

Performance Area	Excellent	Above Average	Average	Below Average	Poor
Family nutrition	Food well selected, well prepared, wisely purchased, properly stored				Gross nutritional deficiencies, meals irregular, buying erratic, uneconomical
	1 2 3 4 5 6 7 8 9 10 Note:				
Intra-family relationships	Relaxed, mutually supportive, warm, shared responsibility				Tense, quarrelsome, little unity, competitive
	1 2 3 4 5 6 7 8 9 10 Note:				
Home accident prevention	No observable hazard, safety habits good				Untidy, lack of protection for gas or electric outlets, stairs dark, etc.
	1 2 3 4 5 6 7 8 9 10 Note:				
Care of sick person	Comfortable in giving care, procedures adapted to family, home nurse protected, emotional support given				Tense, awkward, overprotective, underconcerned. Home nurse overtired, resentful, care disorganized
	1 2 3 4 5 6 7 8 9 10 Note:				

Etc. etc. The areas and descriptions are suggestive only.

Directions: Fill out one sheet at beginning of service and another at completion of care or at six-month intervals.

Figure 13. Suggested form for family health performance scale.

mother may be expected to register with a physician or clinic, the tense daughter to become more relaxed in the care of a senile parent, the housewife's knowledge of and interest in use of inexpensive foods increased, the cardiac patient's participation in family and community activities broadened.

These should be clearly in mind at the time when progress is being measured. The objective is to measure progress in relation to this family's needs, competence and expected performance, not to measure how close performance comes to some ideal goal.

MEASURES OF PROGRESS

Some measures of progress are simple—the patient does or does not go to the clinic or hospital; the family nurse does or does not read the thermometer correctly; the patient does or does not take the medication or treatment prescribed. Other measures are far less tangible. For example, how can one measure an increase in maternal confidence and competence, the relaxation of intra-family tensions, the degree of rest actually achieved by the patient who is staying in bed but troubled and anxious, or understanding of the concept of preventive medical care? Observation of definite, uncomplicated occurrences provide "yes" or "no" answers to some important indices of progress. For others it will be necessary to rely on one's own or another's judgment of change.

Certain observable behavior may be revealing in itself, such as the confidence with which a mother holds or bathes her baby, the appearance of the patient after the home nurse has given him his daily care, the completeness of the record kept for the doctor. Sometimes observable results of learning have significance only in relation to other behavior. For example, the home nurse may have progressed very well in relation to understanding the physical and medical care of a child with rheumatic fever, but have increased rather than decreased her own and her husband's anxiety about the care.

Sometimes there is a tendency to use a "halo" judgment of progress. If the family has been friendly and receptive it is easy to mistake agreement or temporary adjustment to the nurse's way of doing things for more fundamental progress. For this reason, it is desirable to seek out as many as possible objectively observable changes in behavior that may indicate changes in skills or in attitudes or feelings in relation to health care.

In seeking evidence of change or progress, the fundamental

question to be answered is "What difference did nursing make?" Despite the fact that many of the indices of change are not clearly defined or easily measured, it is necessary to approximate as closely as possible an objective approach. In doing this the nurse may use a variety of methods singly or in combination, including:

1. Record review and summary evaluation note at conclusion of the nursing service.
2. A written analysis of the problems of the family, evidence of progress, and relation of progress to nursing care.
3. Case discussion with supervisory or consultant or other staff personnel, with or without a joint field visit.
4. A process record (or tape recording).

Record Review and Evaluation Summary. It should be standard practice to review each record at the conclusion of service, or if the case is carried for a long time at regular intervals, and to indicate the degree to which the objectives of service have been met. A summary note, placed in the record and so marked that it is readily located, indicates what progress the family has made. This serves the double purpose of providing a base for planning if the case is reopened, and of focusing attention on the degree to which nursing is in fact serving its function.

Such a review need not take a great deal of time, but should be undertaken thoughtfully in an effort to indicate as clearly as possible what was actually accomplished. When factors outside the family nursing situation appear to have affected progress, an interpretative note may be included for clarification. For example, indicating that a young mother has made only slight progress toward independent action, the nurse might note that the patient's mother and husband both "baby" her, and that they appear happy with such a dependent relationship. On indicating unusual progress in self-discipline and in understanding and following a prescribed routine of care by a teen-ager with diabetes, the nurse might note that during this period the patient's vocational objectives were clarified, and new impetus was given to his formerly wavering concern for health.

The summary note should indicate when necessary things were not done, and why. For example, the nurse might write that owing to pressure of other work a young mother received too little instruction in infant care, and came to rely too much on neighbors' and her mother's advice.

This presents an opportunity, too, to say "How well did I do?" Often the progress or lack of it may seem to be affected by nurs-

Family: <u>Smith, Edgar, Mary, Susie and John</u> Nurse <u>A. Black</u>

Address <u>2241 Crestwood Lane</u> Date <u>November 18</u>

Needs	*Evidence of Progress*	*Comments*
Prenatal medical supervision (mother says she knows this)	Attended Mem. Hosp. Clinic, but missed many appointments	Motivation inadequate? Was preparation for clinic sufficient? Does she know the reasons?
Increase intake of milk and green vegetables in diet	Both husband and patient report that whole family taking more milk. Made tapioca with evaporated milk which was well accepted. Talked of recipe in woman's magazine that used milk. "Trying" with vegetables	Appear to recognize need and are trying to change habits
Prepare Susie for new baby	Susie talks of new baby, helped mother pack bag for hospital, has a "just like mother's" bathinette, so she can bathe doll as mother bathes baby. Mother gives Susie much recognition	
Information regarding Susie's growth and development for both parents	Verbally recognizes Susie's need for independence, but still requires considerable physical restriction—"Sit still and be a good girl." Good recognition of Susie's need to feel wanted and loved, and to adjust to new baby. Did not attend parents' discussion group as was suggested	Probably this is not possible because of many household demands for time. May be able to do in six months—keep inactive 'til then, and ask another member to come with them
etc.	etc.	etc.

Figure 14. Family progress work sheet.

ing care. Perhaps the patient needing a cancer check-up has said, "You're too young to understand," or in retrospect it may be apparent that advice given was presented too fast and so not understood or accepted fully, or that a feeling of free communication was never fully achieved. At this point, too, it may appear that the family's needs were not adequately recognized, or that the goals set were not realistic. The nurse can thus locate deficiencies in her own performance and plan for improvement.

Written Analysis of Progress.   A more formal analysis of family progress in relation to health care may be helpful in pinpointing the factors associated with success or failure in modifying behavior. A work sheet such as the one illustrated in Figure 14 provides a guide for a more intensive look at a situation. It might be used for a sampling of the cases carried (for example, every tenth clinic case), or for a particular service area in which the nurse has a special interest or need for improvement, or which may be under consideration for "de-emphasis" (for example, all moderate or low-priority prenatal cases). Such a review may show that families who seem to have benefited much from nursing service have, in fact, changed very little.

In using such a progress analysis work sheet it is important to distinguish between evidence of progress (what the family has done) and *estimate* of progress (the nurse's opinion or judgment of changes that have occurred without observable or reported behavior change). It must be remembered that "evidence" or change which hinges on the family's statement of what changes have been made should be considered in the light of the reliability of such sources of information. Some families will want to please the nurse by saying what they think she wants to hear, rather than present a true appraisal, while others will be quite frank. Much depends on the communication established between family and nurse, and the nurse-family pattern of working together on problems.

Sometimes the progress of the family is not easily observable, and the nurse may want to try a purely subjective type of evaluation based on a multitude of small observations and on her opinion of the status of this family in comparison with that of other families she knows. The health performance scale referred to previously, or a narrative description of the family's health behavior as the nurse sees it, filled in at completion of the service may indicate progress or lack of it. When judgment alone is the basis for estimating change it is particularly helpful to have the assistance of a supervisor or consultant in deciding on what basis the judgments may be made.

There can be many variations of this "sit-down" kind of analysis, depending on the objectives of the services carried and the types of problems or needs prevalent in the community.

Case Consultation with Supervisor or Consultant. Informal case discussion, which may be preceded by a field observation by the supervisor or consultant, will also be helpful in judging family progress. The supervisor may see indices of behavior that the nurse would miss because of her lesser experience or sometimes because she is too close to the situation. For example, the supervisor may point out that while the home nurse providing care for an aged and bedridden parent complains just as bitterly to the nurse about the injustice of having this task to do as she formerly did, she also shows considerable pride in a rearrangement of the sick room that makes care easier, or that she shows increasing rather than decreasing patience with the patient's confused attempts at communication. The home nurse's need for a safety valve of complaint rather than a true unwillingness to help may be the key factor in appraising progress. Talking over cases with other staff nurses or other professional workers such as a caseworker or teacher who knows the family well may also help in securing a more accurate picture of progress made.

Process Record. The use of a process record in supervision has been described by Walker and McQuillen.[1]

A process record may be used equally well by the staff nurse herself in an effort to understand more fully the nurse-family relationship and its effect on family behavior. It is most useful for this purpose when there is a baseline record made early, and a later one produced when the relationship has matured and strengthened.

A process record is essentially a running account of what happened in the course of a service contact, including what was done, what was said and indications of feelings of the patient or family and of the nurse.

For example, recording a home visit to a tuberculosis patient a nurse wrote in part, after describing her entry to the home

1. Walker, Janet and Mary McQuillen, Process Recording in Public Health Nursing. *Public Health Nursing*, 44: 542–547, October, 1952.

and some preliminary conversation, "I asked him whether he had been surprised when the doctor told him his diagnosis, or whether he had rather expected it. He looked out of the window with what appeared to be indifference, and said he wasn't really surprised, but had hoped it wouldn't be so. I waited for him to take the lead, and after a minute or so he said he supposed I'd come to tell him he had to go to the 'san,' but that he didn't intend to go 'unless somebody makes me.' I made no comment, but wondered whether deep down he was wishing someone *would* 'make' him go. I waited again for him to take the lead. He seemed reluctant to talk about it any more, so I said it was a big decision to make, and probably it would take him a little time to figure out how he could get the necessary care. He said 'Yes, I guess it's up to me.' I felt a little guilty somehow, as though it was very easy for me to talk because I didn't really have his problem to face. I asked if he'd like me to come back the next day. He said he didn't think that I could help, but he'd be glad to see me. As he said this he relaxed a little in his chair—I felt he was glad I hadn't let him say 'no' too definitely. I felt a little anxious myself, however, as though perhaps if I had been more skillful he would not have been so hesitant about accepting hospital care."

Writing a process record is a lengthy job, but undertaken occasionally it may sharpen the nurse's perception of what is happening between herself and the patient.

Obviously, it takes judgment to observe and to listen with sufficient comprehension to give a complete and undistorted account; and also to interpret the meaning of what was seen and heard. However, using the help of a supervisor, as necessary, this method can be very helpful to the nurse in judging progress of the family, particularly progress in its capacity to use the nurse's help.

Sometimes tape recordings of visits serve the same purpose of providing an account of an inter-personal activity that can later be reviewed, studied and evaluated without the interference of the demands of the service situation.

ANALYSIS OF FACTORS CONTRIBUTING TO OR RETARDING PROGRESS

It is of little use for future planning to know what progress has been made unless there is an effort also to see what factors were operative in hastening or delaying the change.

These may include factors in the *family*, such as previous experience or health services which lead the family members to feel that public health nursing is for "the poor," or that nurses are being "bossy" or lacking in understanding. Or the deep religious feelings of a family may have enabled its members to adjust rapidly and easily to a terminal illness.

The quality of the inter-personal relationship established between nurse and family may also have affected the direction and rate of progress. If confidence in the nurse builds up slowly, progress might also be somewhat slowed; if the patient's relationship was one of total respect for the authority of the nurse and of dependence upon her, the level of self-help achieved may be relatively low.

Sometimes progress is hampered or helped by community factors. The neighbors who understand and welcome back the discharged psychiatric patient make a real contribution to his rehabilitation; a community with a high rate of delinquency and crime may deter the venereal disease patient from sticking to the necessary follow-up regimen.

Often there is some indication that the method of providing nursing service may have had a positive or negative effect on progress. Poor timing of visits, overteaching, or failure to be sufficiently specific or to repeat instruction sufficiently to assure understanding may reduce the patient's progress toward understanding. Group work used at exactly the right time may cause a real spurt of development.

The modification of service to provide better facilitation of family progress in health care must depend on what was important in determining the rate and direction of the progress. It is as important to know why progress was good as to know why it was slow. The nurse must be prepared to take time to think through the evidence she has collected, to see its implications for the family, for herself as a professional worker, and for the agency and community.

Thoughtful periodic checks on family progress are essential for effective public health nursing service.

CHAPTER XII

Group Work:
Organization Phases

Nᴇᴡ ᴋɴᴏᴡʟᴇᴅɢᴇ of the effectiveness of group experience in teaching and in changing attitudes places classes and discussion groups as major approaches to public health nursing. Home care of the sick may be taught in home nursing classes in schools or community; child growth and development may be interpreted to parents through demonstration and discussion; patients with syphilis may learn about their disease and its care and be helped toward a positive attitude in relation to treatment by group work in the hospital or clinic. Such group work may save nursing time, but its major value rests in the opportunity it provides for people to learn from one another, and to gain support and stimulation in coping with their problems.

There are many types of group work ranging from a series of lectures or demonstrations through varying levels of group participation, such as skill practice, problem identification and discussions to the "unstructured" group in which its members decide what will be discussed, and direct the course of the sessions with complete freedom. The nurse as leader of group work may, with advice from a committee or consultant, take full responsibility for setting content and direction of the work or may, at the other end of the scale, serve as a resource and facilitator as the group directs itself. Figure 15 shows the relative nature of leader-group responsibility.

The public health nurse needs an understanding of the techniques necessary to organize and manage group activities, and to use group approaches in teaching and in counseling.

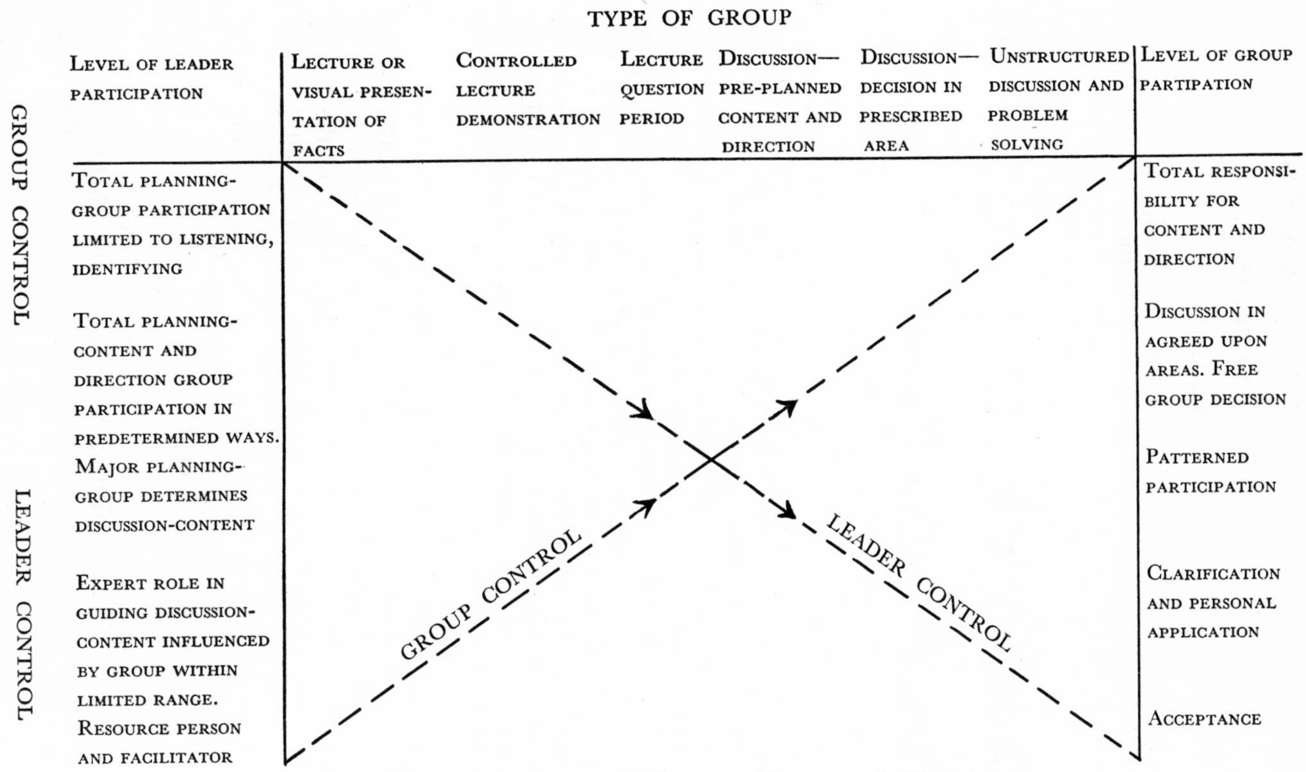

TYPE OF GROUP

LECTURE OR VISUAL PRESENTATION OF FACTS	CONTROLLED LECTURE DEMONSTRATION	LECTURE QUESTION PERIOD	DISCUSSION— PRE-PLANNED CONTENT AND DIRECTION	DISCUSSION— DECISION IN PRESCRIBED AREA	UNSTRUCTURED DISCUSSION AND PROBLEM SOLVING	LEVEL OF GROUP PARTITIPATION
						TOTAL RESPONSIBILITY FOR CONTENT AND DIRECTION
						DISCUSSION IN AGREED UPON AREAS. FREE GROUP DECISION
						PATTERNED PARTICIPATION
						CLARIFICATION AND PERSONAL APPLICATION
						ACCEPTANCE

LEADER CONTROL

GROUP CONTROL

LEVEL OF LEADER PARTICIPATION

TOTAL PLANNING-GROUP PARTICIPATION LIMITED TO LISTENING, IDENTIFYING

TOTAL PLANNING-CONTENT AND DIRECTION GROUP PARTICIPATION IN PREDETERMINED WAYS.

MAJOR PLANNING-GROUP DETERMINES DISCUSSION-CONTENT

EXPERT ROLE IN GUIDING DISCUSSION-CONTENT INFLUENCED BY GROUP WITHIN LIMITED RANGE. RESOURCE PERSON AND FACILITATOR

GROUP CONTROL   LEADER CONTROL

Figure 15. Relative group leader control in groups of different types.

ORGANIZATION OF GROUPS

READY-MADE GROUPS

One method of organizing groups for health instruction is simply to use existing groups in which there is interest. A church group, a group of clinic patients, a woman's club, a future nurses' club, and an industrial health committee are examples of groups in which there may be interest in and need for health instruction that comes within the scope of the public health nurse's competence. This cuts down on the nursing time required for organization phases of the work, but has the disadvantage that it may not always reach those most in need of the service.

Sometimes another agency will organize new groups for a special purpose. The Civil Defense Committee or the American Red Cross may organize groups for instruction in emergency nursing care, home nursing or care of mothers and babies. A parent-teacher association may organize groups for instruction in home care of communicable disease, accident prevention or for discussion of behavior problems of school-age children. Use of such groups saves nursing time in organization and it may serve a desirable public relations purpose. For example, a P.T.A. organized class in health problems of the school-age child may be the springboard for extensive volunteer participation of P.T.A. members in the school health program. It may also have the advantage of bringing in new sources of help—the Civil Defense Organization or Red Cross may recruit new support or volunteer help for the program.

NEWLY ORGANIZED GROUPS

The public health nurse may be responsible for initiating the organization of groups herself. She may work closely with the health educator, if one is employed by the agency, or the health educator may take major responsibility for the organizational phases of group work. In either case, it will be necessary to:

1. Secure necessary administrative clearances and coordination.
2. Organize a planning or helping committee to:
   a. Define the purpose of the activity
   b. Decide upon the groups to be reached
   c. Arrange for necessary promotional activities
   d. Help with administrative arrangements—finding meeting places, arranging for services such as cleaning and laundry.

3. With the help of the committee, decide on:
   a. Group size and composition
   b. Scheduling of classes
   c. Records, forms, etc., to be used
   d. Follow-up activities.

Administrative Clearance and Coordination. When group work is planned it should be an integral part of the over-all nursing agency and community health programs. The nurse should clear with her supervisor (or health officer, if she works directly with him) to be sure that the plan will not conflict with other agency activities, and to plan for coordination with other aspects of the on-going program. The public health nurse planning a series of group meetings for hospital clinic patients will want to know how this would contribute to the clinic's plan for patient instruction and to the health department's activities in maternal and child health services. The hospital may be stressing "rooming in," and want the instruction geared to this point, or the health department may be planning an all-out poliomyelitis immunization program, and prefer that the proposed class not be initiated at the same time, but postponed for a few weeks.

Sometimes clearances of a courtesy nature are important in maintaining understanding and good will. The local medical association, or practicing physicians, might be asked for support and approval of the group-teaching venture, even though there is no administrative necessity for clearance.

Establishing a Planning Committee. Committee organization and management are discussed in Chapter XVIII.

The establishment of a planning (or advisory) committee will relieve the public health nurse of responsibility for much of the detail associated with organization of groups, and, if properly constituted, will serve as an important channel of communication to other groups and to the community.

The size and composition of the planning committee will vary with the scope of the project. If a single prenatal class is being organized in a city area under existing policy and as a part of a long-established program, two or three volunteer workers may suffice. If the project involves reaching a substantial proportion of the population over a period of time with home nursing instruction as a part of the over-all civil defense planning, the committee would need more professional representation and would need to be larger. In such a case the Red Cross, the Civil Defense

Committee, and members representing different organized groups (such as industry, agricultural organizations) would be needed and there may be need for a system of subcommittees to work on segments of the program, or in different localities.

Defining the Purpose.   The purposes of a particular program in group work need to be defined, since many purposes may be served by this method. Among the purposes might be:

1. To develop skill in particular techniques or procedures, such as giving insulin, giving a bed bath or observing symptoms of illness.
2. To develop attitudes favorable to positive health action, such as acceptance of physical limitations by cardiac patients, a relaxed and accepting feeling toward children, or a sense of personal responsibility for curing one's self and protecting the community from tuberculosis.
3. To provide a medium for sharing experiences and practical methods of handling problems, such as methods of caring for the incontinent elderly patient, or recipes that use protective foods, or handling problems of disobedience in children.
4. To provide a factual base for health action, such as presenting the major causes of home accidents, or describing the rationale of drug therapy in schizophrenia, or explaining the routines of the hospital or clinic to which the patients expect to go.
5. To provide an opportunity for group thinking and problem solving, such as determining ways in which parents might help to decrease accidents among preschool and school-age children, or deciding how the long-term patient in the hospital can be helped to maintain the feeling that he is still a part of the family, or how a group of experienced patients could help those just beginning rehabilitative treatment.

Sometimes there are important secondary purposes in organizing a group—perhaps to encourage neighbor-to-neighbor help in a housing development, or to promote better understanding among different cultural, racial or economic groups. Group work may also serve a public relations purpose, providing a way for nursing service to become known among people who have not used the service extensively.

Determining the Groups to be Reached.   There is wide difference between offering group service and planning for it as a part of an over-all program. There is a tendency for those who need help least to be the most conscientious about seeking it. Hence, if prenatal classes are offered the indifferent or fearful mother may not attend, while the relatively well-informed and responsible patient never misses an opportunity. Group work should be planned with a definite target in mind, consistent with the needs of the community and the purposes of the activity. For example, group work in relation to home care of the long-term patient may be geared to reaching the middle and upper groups because they do not use the hospital for custodial care as much as do their less privileged neighbors, or because these groups have not been accustomed to using nursing services; prenatal classes may be directed primarily toward lower economic groups or racial or nationality groups that have a higher incidence of morbidity and mortality associated with child bearing or toward groups that have cultural patterns that lead to overprotectiveness. If a new program is starting, "natural leaders" may be the target, with the thought that they will influence others as well as benefit themselves from the work.

Promotional Activities. Promotional activities may include informing workers in agencies, hospitals and welfare organizations of availability of services to their clients; announcements placed in newspapers or distributed to groups, such as home-makers' clubs, schools, church associations; personal invitations, person-to-person promotion. In general, the more personal the approach the better the yield will be, and the greater is the possibility of reaching those who need care most. A personal letter will probably be more effective than a mimeographed announcement. Announcement and implied approval by a community leader to a group (such as by a priest or minister to his congregation, or the Parent-Teacher Association president to the members, or the physician to his patients) will be even more effective. In one city, classes in child care were "prescribed" by physicians reaching a middle and upper economic group who had not taken advantage of such services before.

Visits to homes or groups to explain the purpose and give the essential information about the group work may be justified if the program is much needed, or to reach groups in the community that might not be reached through other channels.

Whatever the promotional device, the approach should indicate clearly exactly what is involved—the number and possible location of meetings, costs, equipment, textbooks needed, and so forth.

Such promotional work will be time-consuming. Since it does

not require nursing skill, as far as possible the work should be delegated to volunteers. The nurse's function would be to provide the necessary information and briefing, and to bring to the volunteer group the help of the health educator.

Administrative Arrangements.   The committee may also help to arrange for suitable meeting places—convenient to transportation, and of proper size and equipment to handle the group. Seating should be adequate; and, if group discussion is part of the procedure, movable chairs with writing arms or small tables around which the group may sit encourage discussion. Equipment may need to be borrowed, purchased or transported to the meeting place. Arrangements may need to be made regarding such housekeeping details as laundry, cleaning, moving of chairs or furniture. Sometimes it is necessary to have hostess activities to welcome and introduce new group members, or to take responsibility for preparing and serving refreshments. Arrangements should be made for someone or for a group to prepare the meeting place for each meeting.

Group Size and Composition.   Effective group size will vary depending on the purpose of the meeting and the methods adopted. It will be influenced by the following factors:

1. Accessibility to equipment for practice. If a major purpose is to teach skills, practice under supervision is highly desirable.[1] The group needs to be sufficiently small to permit every member to be active during demonstration periods— either observing or checking fellow students or practicing the skill. The American Red Cross has found that ten to fifteen makes a suitable number for instruction in home nursing.[2]

2. Amount and type of learner discussion necessary. If the purpose of the session is to explain or tell something—for instance, to explain the poliomyelitis vaccination program— the method might well be one of a talk followed by a question-and-answer period. In this instance, size is not an important factor.[3] Some individuals will be shy about asking questions if the group is large, but the chances are good that someone else will raise the same point. The lecturer, too, may foresee and stimulate questions on the basis of his knowledge of the things that usually trouble families.

1. American National Red Cross, *Home Care of the Sick, Instructors Guide.* Washington, D.C., American National Red Cross, 1950.

2. Ibid., p. 10.

3. *Adult Leadership,* 1: 2–32, December, 1952. Several articles on conducting large meetings.

If general discussion for purposes of clarification is essential—if, for example, there is need to talk out the reasons why children behave in ways that are troublesome to parents and teachers—the group must be sufficiently small to permit everyone to participate, and to encourage free discussion. If group decisions are to be reached—for example, if the group is to decide what action parents will take regarding school and home safety—or if it is important to change attitudes and to permit airing of feelings, even smaller groups are indicated. For the latter type, ten or fewer has been suggested as desirable and for the more general discussion, not over twenty. Sometimes a large group is assembled, provided with general information basic to thinking, then reorganized on the spot into small discussion groups for problem study and decision. This method was used in the midcentury White House Conference on Education in 1955, when almost 2000 delegates were present.[4]

Group composition is also an important factor in effectiveness. If the purpose is information giving, composition has little influence unless there are cultural barriers to meeting together. If discussion is required, however, the composition must be such as not to inhibit free interchange of ideas. If problem solving and community understanding are the goal, composition that reflects a variety of backgrounds and types of competence will be best. For example, in a civil defense training program when a group meeting is held to explain the organization of civil defense organization it might be a large group open to anyone. When self-help and neighbor-help skills are taught it may be important to have small groups selected to represent different socioeconomic groups. Thus this provides for adequate practice and at the same time promotes an easy, mutually respectful relationship. The banker's wife will probably not be more skillful than the janitor in bandaging, and the janitor may be the air raid warden to whom she would report. Inter-group acceptance is vital, and is best developed by mutual efforts in advance of the time action.

There are many other ways in which group composition in and of itself can work for the public health nurse. A group made up of young expectant mothers may support and understand one another in an urban situation, feeling that members of the older prenatal group do not see prospective motherhood as a gay adventure. Young women away from home on an army post, however,

4. *Suggested Homework for the Participants in the White House Conference on Education.* Washington, D.C., Dept. of Health, Education, and Welfare, 1955, Back cover.

might gain much security from having more experienced mothers in the group; or in changing neighborhoods the experienced mother may help the inexperienced one to know how to use community facilities. When child care is the subject, much may be gained by having both fathers and mothers present because each will have a different contribution to make. It is important to anticipate ways in which group members will influence and help one another, and to prepare to use this force for the purposes of the group.

Scheduling. In general, attendance at group sessions tends to be better when there is a definite starting and ending point for the work. Classes available on a continuing basis at any time may encourage potential members to put off going, or to attend irregularly, whereas a series of five or six meetings in a course establishes limits which may serve as a motivating force in securing regular attendance. In discussion and decision groups in particular, where the maturing of the group itself is a factor in effectiveness, regularity of attendance is extremely important.

Using the same day of the week or month for meetings makes it more easily remembered and planned for. Attaching the meeting to another required activity, such as a clinic visit, provides an easy method of group assembly.

If sessions are held infrequently, postcard reminders may be necessary, timed to arrived not more than a week in advance. Schedules should be announced sufficiently far in advance to permit planning—not so far ahead that the matter gets cold before the meetings are to start.

Records. A record of attendance, and of subject matter covered, should be maintained for group work. For large groups where it is not feasible to count those present, attendance should be estimated and the estimate recorded.

Reports for individual members may be incorporated into the family folder if the group work is a part of over-all care for a health situation, such as a prenatal class.

Attendance certificates may be given to the participants as a recognition for completion of class activities, to encourage prompt and regular attendance. When certificates are given it is important that they be awarded only on the basis of attendance at a stated number of sessions or the completion of specific assignments. If certification is based on competence of the individual, proper measurement devices must be constructed to ascertain that the recipient is in fact proficient in the material taught. For example, if a certificate is given for completion of a course in first aid or home care of the sick, it should be awarded only after the individual has demonstrated his ability to perform the skills taught. If certification depends upon attendance and participation at the given number of sessions, the public health nurse must make plans in advance for make-up work or equivalent activities for those who must miss some of the sessions. Any plan for awarding attendance certificates should have administrative approval.

Sometimes it is desirable to have a brief summary of the session recorded. When the purpose is to change attitudes, solve problems, or arrive at group, or individual in a group, decisions, more intensive recording of group action may be desirable, with use of a recorder, observer or other means of reporting. The record may then be studied at leisure to estimate the effectiveness of the approaches used and to appraise the changes that occur in participants.

Follow-up.   Provision must be made for certain follow-up activities:

1. Checking with absentees regarding their attendance.
2. Locating needs and planning service for individual or family problems that are brought to light in group meetings but are not within the purposes of the group itself.
3. Evaluating the group work (this is discussed in Chapter XIII).

The organization of groups requires thoughtful preparation in the light of purposes of the group and availability of facilities. Most of the work of organization and administration should be done by someone other than the nurse, preferably by members of the group themselves. In all group work the nurse can receive invaluable assistance from the health educator. When there is none available she may find help in local educational institutions —a college professor in social organization, group dynamics or human relations—or in voluntary health agencies such as the National Tuberculosis Association. Occasionally, industrial firms have training personnel with experience in group work who may be willing to provide advice on matters such as class size, approach or evaluation.

CHAPTER XIII

Group Instruction and Group Discussion— Problem Solving

G<small>ROUP</small> <small>INSTRUCTION</small> differs from group problem solving in that its purpose is to teach skills or give information that is known to the instructor but not to any degree to the group members. Group discussion or group problem solving has as its purpose the identification of problems common to the group, and mobilization of the thinking experience and skills of the members to arrive at ways of coping with the problems. In group instruction, the nurse functions primarily as an expert and as a teacher; in group discussion and problem solving, she serves as stimulator, facilitator and occasional informational resource. In practice, most group work will include both types of approach to some degree, often within a single session. However, since the methodology differs the two types are discussed separately here. The practitioner must combine and arrange her approach to use whichever is suited to the purposes of the activity, the nature of the subject matter and the temper of the group.

GROUP INSTRUCTION

Group instruction must be carefully planned and related to subsequent as well as immediate action by the participants. Usually the purpose implies that people will *do* something about what they have heard, discussed or practiced. Knowing how to examine the breast for symptoms of cancer in itself has little value—it is only as the knowledge is translated into periodic self-check that it serves its purpose.

Planning in Relation to a Baseline. Before instruction can be planned it is necessary to determine as far as possible what is already known by the group, and what the interests and needs of the members are. Sometimes it is possible to have those attending indicate in advance what they feel they can do or what they would especially like to have discussed, at the time they indicate they plan to attend the group meeting. For some groups an "intent-to-enroll" blank can be used in which group members can check their special needs or interests. For example, a member of a group to discuss care of the disabled patient might indicate just what type of patient is being cared for; whether or not she has had instruction in reading a thermometer, making a bed or bathing a sick person; and what she considers her major problems in giving care. Sometimes simple pre-tests may be set up to determine what factual information or skills the group members have. These may be paper-and-pencil tests or could be set up as a verbal check on information or skill. Information may be obtained in the first session, by discussing with the group as a whole or in individual conferences scheduled apart from the group, in what areas of content the group feels secure, and in what areas it feels the need of help. Whatever the method, it is important to know:

1. The needs as seen by the group in relation to the nurse's concept of its needs.
2. Special interests or problems felt to be important by the group.
3. The educational level and cultural background of the group.
4. Prior experiences, exposure to instruction and knowledge or skills now possessed.

In an attempt to find needs that are common to all members of the group, it is important not to generalize the content or problem to the point that it loses its immediate usefulness. For instance, if one member reports as a problem handling a "cross" patient and another an apathetic one, these problems might be grouped as those of attitude. However, the group might gain more from discussing one or the other specifically.

Arranging and Presenting Content. Content to be covered should be selected in accordance with the needs of the group as estimated by the nurse and by the group itself. Sometimes there is a tendency to go beyond group needs, and develop an over-full or too theoretical plan for content without allowing adequate time for discussion, clarification, and "clinching" by applications, practice or repetition.

The nurse will need to collect more information and prepare more material than she expects to use, in order to be prepared to answers questions, or to amplify a point if interest of the group seems high in a particular area.

The material should be prepared in advance of the sessions, and those skills, ideas or concepts that are of particular importance should be selected, clearly indicated and marked for emphasis.

Arrangement or sequence of presenting material should be orderly, and wherever possible directed first toward those areas in which the group has an expressed interest or known need. For instance, if the major problem presented by a group learning to give better rehabilitation care to patients with arthritis is one of "feeling weighed down," "never getting away from it" or resenting continued demands even though the reason is understood the over-all aspects of planning for home care, protection of the home nurse and use of family and community resources might come before a discussion of the nature of the disease and rationale of rehabilitation therapy.

The nurse will be concerned with five phases in such a presentation:

1. Telling the facts or describing the procedure. Simple words and nontechnical language should be used for ready communication of ideas, and when possible wording should be pre-tested by having a nonprofessional person read the material and indicate points that are not clear or words that are not understood. For example, "utilize" should not be used where "use" will serve; "thinking how the other person feels" communicates more to most groups than does "empathy."

2. Emphasizing essential principles by giving illustrative examples, or by repeating the same idea in different words. A three-time re-statement is not too much. Showing different applications while stressing the principle is an excellent method. For example, placement of the sick child's bed in three different home situations would show different placement, but demonstrate application of the same principles.

3. Giving the "why" as well as the "how" of all procedures.

4. Using the blackboard or substitute, slides, charts, pictures,

graphs or other visual aids to emphasize the essential points. Whatever is used should actually contribute to the presentation. Visual materials are not good of themselves; it is possible that some materials might, in fact, detract rather than add, as when they represent tangential information, or an aspect of the material that is overcomplex for the group. For example, a prenatal group might be interested in the relative safety of delivery today. However, showing slides of trends in maternal mortality might be confusing and not helpful since the *major* purpose is to teach *care*, not the statistical picture. Furthermore, many audiences, unfamiliar with mortality rates, will interpret rate expressed in terms of thousands or ten thousands of the population as though it were a percent, with startling results, or may concentrate on the fact that there is a possibility of death.

5. Checking for and correcting misinformation. This may be done by asking questions, or asking group members to describe their understanding of a particular procedure or concept in their own terms. Such questions need careful advance preparation so they are not threatening to the group, and are directed toward the most essential learning points. For example, a group might respond with some anxiety to requests to repeat verbal concepts such as "What are the essentials for the sick room?" Response to "How could you do it in your home?" might lead to more fruitful and easy discussion which permits stressing the principle involved.

6. Stressing ways in which the knowledge may be applied. For example, the nurse may indicate that the disabled patient may be made to feel less isolated if he is given small household tasks to perform, such as preparing vegetables, or mending or sorting and pairing children's socks; or if minor household problems are discussed with him, such as what kind of pie to have, or whether Johnnie's snow suit should be a Christmas gift or be given to the child in advance. These "take-home" ideas encourage use of the information or skills.

Demonstrating and Supervising Practice. The exigencies of war produced much work in speeded-up teaching of skills needed for industrial and military effort, some of which has influenced nursing procedures. In general, it has been found that teaching a single way to carry out a procedure rather than many possible ways, and placing emphasis on a small number of "key" points are the fastest methods and the least apt to produce misinformation when time is limited. However, teaching the principles on which a procedure is based maintains its importance. As an example, one might teach how to hold a baby by delineating the principles: the position should assure that the baby both is and feels secure; it should be neither awkward nor tiring for the parent and should permit a feeling of warmth and cuddling. Then several possible holds might be described, with each person deciding which he wants to use. Or a *single* method may be chosen for demonstration and practice. Sometimes this method and a step-by-step procedure are developed into a teaching manual, such as that evolved by the National League for Nursing and the United States Public Health Service for the training of nurses' aides.[1] Demonstrations should be so set up that each of the procedures is visible to everyone in the group. Equipment should as far as possible duplicate that which patients themselves will be apt to have. In Guam, for example, it is more effective to use gourds as containers in care of the sick than to use pitchers; for apartment dwellers it is better to wrap contaminated food scraps for incinerator disposal rather than for burning in the stove.

In demonstration, a combination of telling and doing is more effective than is doing alone. The steps followed will vary with different instructors, but the ensuing might be considered a fairly typical sample:

1. Explain the purpose of the procedure and the basic principles involved.
2. Go through each step of the procedure slowly, telling what is being done and emphasizing why it is done this way. Repeat each *key point* at least once—twice is better!
3. Go through each step of the procedure again, asking the group to tell what is being done and why.
4. Have group members, under the instructor's guidance, observe and check each other in the procedure, telling what they are doing in each step. Every member should have an opportunity to practice each essential procedure.
5. Correct errors that are observed, emphasizing reason *why* they are wrong.
6. Test for understanding by asking questions.

Handling Questions and Discussion.   Time should be allowed

1. *Division of Nursing Resources, U.S. Dept. of Health, Education and Welfare, Public Health Service, Nursing Aide Instructor's Guide.* Washington, D.C., Government Printing Office, 1953.

for questions or discussion following a talk or demonstration. If a request for questions brings no response, participation may be encouraged by asking a member of the group who is known to be fairly self-confident to interpret a point or tell how he would apply it, or by saying, "A question often raised is——————." This may open the way for unsolicited questions or contributions. If the person to whom the question was directed does not know the answer, it is important to him and others in the group that he be made comfortable about not knowing the answer, otherwise future participation may be lessened. The nurse might say, "That really is a hard one to answer" or "Even pretty experienced people have trouble sometimes answering that." Or she may shift responsibility to herself saying, "I was afraid I hadn't made that point clear."

Questions which are obviously of individual rather than group concern or are inappropriate may be postponed until after the meeting, although if the reply is a brief one it may be given immediately. If it is not appropriate for the nurse to answer, the reason should be given; for example, nurses could not say what teachers should do about "problem" children in school, or what orders the physician should give for care.

Clinching "Take-Home" Ideas or Values.   The steps in presentation and demonstration involving illustration and application are one way of clinching with the group the things they might use at home.

Sometimes it is helpful to have mimeographed reminder sheets, or notebooks in which each member can record the points of importance for later use.

Asking members whether they have used information or material from a previous session may produce some testimonials which help to stress the usefulness of the content, or in some cases bring up the need for further discussion of application in the home situation.

Evaluation of the progress and understanding of members during each session helps to estimate the degree to which they may be expected to use what has been presented. Sometimes a review discussion or written evaluation may be helpful. Such an evaluation may be around *how* the individual will use the information or apply the skill rather than simple recall. For example, drawing a rough plan of one's own home and indicating where a long-term patient might be placed and giving the reasons why are apt to be more revealing than is asking for repetition of the criteria for selecting a sick room.

The greatest possible informality should be secured in any such testing procedure. An "information please" type of program in which teams of members vie with one another, or a class-developed skit of home care applications as a kind of graduation fun, may elicit much more information than will a formal test.

GROUP-DIRECTED DISCUSSION AND PROBLEM SOLVING

Group-directed or unstructured activity is felt by many to have unusual potentials for influencing behavior.[2, 3] These basic concepts underlie such group work:

1. There is a force generated by the association of individuals in group situations that can be turned to self-help and to the help of others.
2. People in groups have the capacity to understand and work through many of their own problems if they are in a situation which encourages free exploration, problem analysis and evaluative consideration of possible action.
3. Within each group there will be found several who have the necessary expertness, ability or personal equipment to assume leadership in relation to some phases of the group's work.
4. Members of a group will assume different roles at different times—sometimes being leader, sometimes summarizer, sometimes peace maker or clarifier, and so forth.
5. There is need and a methodology developed for freeing people to express and work on their own problems.
6. The group leader's job is not to direct the course of thinking or to determine answers, but to free the group to direct itself, and to assist the group in securing basic information necessary for understanding or decision.
7. The group may delegate the leader to carry out its own decisions regarding the conduct of the group—for example, to stop discussion at a certain time, to rule out extraneous contributions, to direct the group's attention to the decisions it has agreed to make.

In public health nursing the use of group-directed discussion and problem solving is particularly useful in changing attitudes toward health care, and in promoting an independent confident

2. Bond, E., *Group Discussion Decision.* Minneapolis, Minnesota State Department of Health, 1956.

3. Gordon, Thomas, *Group Centered Leadership.* Boston, Houghton Mifflin Co., 1955.

approach among patients in working out their own health problems. For example, group-directed discussion among people with newly diagnosed tuberculosis might be expected to bring into the open some of the fears and anxieties each one has. Discussion with others whose problems are similar helps make these fears and anxieties seem respectable, and at the same time may help to provide the courage to work out problems and to learn from what others are feeling and planning. Instructing such a group would provide them with the necessary informational background and might motivate action that is socially approved, the "right thing" to do. It would be essential for the patient to know these facts and society's expectations as a basis for his decision. But the way he *feels* about the decision he makes, and his capacity to accept and to cope with his problem without undue stress are more apt to be influenced by his own action and decision as expressed through his group experience.

Planning and conducting such group sessions requires no less preparation and planning on the part of the leader than does the more controlled situation, even though the major responsibility for decision and direction rests with the group. Because the direction of the discussion cannot be predicted, the nurse must be prepared with a broad range of information relating to the general topic, not to be presented to the group, but to enable her to participate by raising questions or suggesting new areas for discussion to assure a sound basis for decisions the group may make. She also needs to study the group with exceptional care, and to plan how to encourage each member to contribute fully.

Group-directed discussion can be conducted with the use of very specialized skills, as, for instance, when there is deep probing for personal psychologic problems or as part of group psychiatric therapy. The assumption here is that the nurse will not be concerned with such deep-seated or complex problems, and that a relatively simple approach will produce effective group work within the areas of public health nursing concerns.

Setting the Stage. The physical and social environment in which group work functions has much to do with its success. It is necessary to:

1. Provide a setting in which members of the group can see and talk to one another easily. Movable chairs arranged in a circle or around a table (with no special place reserved for the "teacher") make it easy to talk back and forth with informality.

2. Encourage informality and identity with the group; the use of first names and name tags helps, as do recreational activities, such as a coffee break or group singing. Having each member of the group introduced—by himself or his neighbor—with some indication of his interests and background also helps to establish a sense of belonging and knowing one another.
3. Have available basic information for which the need could be anticipated.
4. Make clear the potential within the group itself for working on the problems, relating leader's contribution to that of the others in such a way as to indicate the shared responsibility of leader and group for the action to be taken.

Assuring Participation and Involvement. To be fully effective, group work should actively involve every one of its members. Each should feel that he has a stake in the group, a responsibility for its actions and a concern with its outcomes. Each should feel that his participation in the group has importance, and that he is free to say what he thinks or feels. Involvement of members will be promoted by the following steps:

1. Getting the group to express its own problems in a specific way and to decide which it wants to discuss. Discourage indefinite problems like "wanting to be a better parent" in favor of more tangible ones stated by the group—"how to get the kids to behave without slapping them down all the time." Some problems will be very similar to others and might be considered together; others may be of concern to only one or two in the group and can be held out for individual handling. Even when only those problems pertinent to the whole group have been selected, it may be necessary to select one or two for discussion because of limits of time. Problems should be expressed in the words of the group, and written on a blackboard or on large paper sheets as a guide to the group.
2. Encouraging shy members to contribute in ways in which they can feel confident; remarks such as "Mrs. Smith, I noticed you use your bulletin board for children's jobs at home—how does it work?" make it easy for even a very shy person to respond. The overtalkative member may be enlisted to help you to get others to participate.
3. Having a member of the group serve as an observer, and note which members of the group participate and in what

way. A simple form for recording such information might
provide for a check system, or chart, to indicate who raised
a question, made a statement or related an experience, or
who backed up one questioner or clarified someone else's
idea. Figure 16 suggests a simple form that might be used.
The observer could also report behavior (such as listening
intently) that indicated nonverbal participation. Through

Member	Asked a Question	Made a Suggestion or Gave an Example	Backed up Someone Else	Disagreed or Objected	Summarized	Comments
Joe	1	1	1 1		1	
Alice				1 1 1		
Jean		1 1			1	
Frank	1 1	1				
Grace	1				1	
Evelyn						Didn't participate but looked interested throughout the session
Jim	1	1 1 1	1	1 1		

Figure 16. Participation record for group discussion.

reporting back the group becomes aware of the distribution
of its participation. If this is not practicable, the nurse herself or a volunteer or student helper may keep such a notation, and encourage those who are inactive to participate by
directing questions to them, or suggesting that they may
have had experiences pertaining to the discussion.
4. Avoiding a "teacher" attitude, by encouraging members of
   the group to take the lead in areas where their knowledge,
   skill or experience exceeds that of the others, or letting group
   members call the group to order.
5. If members become irritated or hostile toward one another,
   try to draw the subject back to yourself to relieve the tension.
   For example, if one member says another reacts as he does
   because of his religious belief, and the comment appears to
   upset the group, the remark could be picked up as a gener-

ality and broadened to include cultural factors other than
religion by a remark such as "It is true, isn't it, that our
upbringing makes a difference in the way we look at things;
my New England background makes me blind to the justifi-
cation for a relaxed attitude toward life—it gets mixed up
with being lazy!"

Using Resources.   The nurse will find that often the group
will turn to her for an authoritative answer—for example, "What
should we do when a child is overdemanding?" Part of the nurse's
job, then, is to turn the group back to its own resources, or perhaps to other resources outside the group itself. She might say,
"What do *you* think makes children overdemanding?" or suggest
that the members consider some of the possible reasons based on
their own experience. Or she might say, "Did any of you find
any suggestions about that in the pamphlets we had to read?" or,
"Perhaps we could ask Dr. Perkins [the psychologist] to talk with
us about how this kind of behavior gets started."

When she has information that is needed it should be given as
far as possible without reference to implied action, leaving the
group to make the inference for itself. For example, she might say
that overdemand may grow out of insecurity or anxiety, expecting
the group itself to work through its implications for parent behavior and to relate this to the things that can be done to combat
the basic causes, and also to emphasize the fact that behavior is a
response to human needs.

A resource person brought into the group only for a short period
should be briefed as to reason for being there, the nature and
present status of the group, and the special interests as they relate
to the resource person's field of specialization. Otherwise, his contribution may be limited or may be pitched too high or too low
to be wholly acceptable to the group.

Sorting Out Ideas, Agreements, etc.   Occasional summary
during the course of discussion is essential to keep some sense of
progress and direction. The leader may do this, or it may be done
by a member of the group serving as a recorder. The recorder
keeps an account of the action and decisions of the group.

Writing out suggestions on the blackboard sometimes clarifies
the areas of agreement or may show the basic similarity of ideas
proposed.

Sometimes it helps to keep a running record on the blackboard,
which may be organized in some way to make for easy reference.
For example, the blackboard may be lined off in three columns

labeled "Problems," "Suggestions," "Agreements" or a single problem may be written on the board with suggested action placed below it, modified as the group proceeds.

---

1. How clear were we about what we wanted to do?
   (1) Did we have some definite questions or problems to which we wanted an answer?
   (2) Were the questions or problems ones in which all of us were interested?
   (3) Did we really choose items ourselves, or did our leader push us into them?
   (4) Were they questions or problems about which we could do something?

2. How well did we work together?
   (1) Did every member of the group contribute in some way?
   (2) Was the group free from domination by one or two members?
   (3) Were we willing to talk about our feelings as well as about our knowledge?
   (4) Were questions directed to various members of the group rather than only or mostly to the leader?
   (5) Did we all take responsibility or did we wait for the leader or for one or two members to do things?

3. Were we productive as a group?
   (1) Did we achieve some definite agreements or suggestions for action?
   (2) Were the ideas we got to take home practical ones?
   (3) Do most of us feel confident we can do the things we learned?

4. Did we improve ourselves as individuals through this experience?
   (1) Did we learn how to say what we mean more clearly?
   (2) Did we learn to understand one another better?

Figure 17.   Suggested outline for evaluation of group activity.

Evaluation.   In group-directed activities, evaluation as well as planning conduct of the sessions is the responsibility of the group.

Evaluation of the group sessions should help members to see what they got out of it, how they felt about the group work, and what if anything they intend to do as a result of it. Figure 17 suggests a possible outline for evaluation of group sessions.

Sometimes a delayed evaluation, secured several weeks or months after the sessions have ended, may be more revealing than one done immediately at the conclusion of the series. In this case it is possible to ask what has been done, or done differently, as a result of the group work.

Group instruction and group-directed discussion and problem solving are useful adjuncts to nursing programs. The nurse who works through groups expands her potential influence, and through practice develops a potent professional tool.

SUGGESTED READINGS

PART II

Alfino, Genrose J., What Rapport Means to Me. *Nursing Outlook*, 3: 326–327, June, 1955.

Allport, Gordon W., The Teaching-Learning Situation. *Public Health Reports*, 68: 875–879, September, 1953.

American Public Health Association, *Nutrition Practices: a Guide for Public Health Administrators*. New York, The Association, 1955.

Anderson, E. Loretta, The Patients Talked It Over. *Nursing Outlook*, 1: 294–296, May, 1953.

Anderson, G. W. and Margaret Arnstein, *Communicable Disease Control*, 3rd ed. New York, Macmillan Co., 1953.

Bard, Morton, The Sequence of Emotional Reactions in Radical Mastectomy Cases. *Public Health Reports*, 67: 1144–1148, November, 1952.

Benne, K. and others, *The Improvement of Practical Intelligence*. New York, Harper & Bros., 1950.

Berengarten, S., When Nurses Interview Patients. *American Journal of Nursing*, 50: 10–15, January, 1950.

Berlien, Ivan C., Growth As Related to Mental Health. *American Journal of Nursing*, 56: 1142–1145, September, 1956.

Biestek, F. P., The Non-Judgmental Attitude. *Social Casework*, 34:239, June, 1953.

Brown, Esther L., The Social Sciences and Improvement of Patient Care. *American Journal of Nursing*, 56: 1148–1150, September, 1950.

Caplan, Gerald, The Mental Hygiene Role of the Nurse in Maternal and Child Care. *Nursing Outlook*, 2: 14–19, January, 1954.

Cline, Nora, How the Public Health Nurse Uses Mental Health Concepts. *Public Health Nursing*, 44: 83–87, February, 1952.

Coleman, Jules V., Attitudes of Professional Personnel in the Treatment of the Tuberculosis Patient. *American Journal of Public Health*, 45: 849–854, July, 1955.

Coulter, Pearl, *The Nurse in the Public Health Program*. New York, G. P. Putnam's Sons, 1954.

Erickson, C. E., *The Counseling Interview*. New York, Prentice Hall, 1950.

Dunbar, Helen Flanders, *Mind and Body*. New York, Random House, 1947.

Fawkes, Barbara and others, How Skillful Is Our Communication? *American Journal of Nursing*, 55: 448–450, April, 1955.

Fenlason, Anne, F., *Essentials in Interviewing*. New York, Harper Bros., 1952.

Freeman, Ruth, The Nurse As a Family Health Counselor. *American Journal of Public Health*, 42: 1379–1387, November, 1952.

Garrett, Anette, *Interviewing: Its Principles and Methods*. New York, Family Welfare Association of America, 1942.

Gilbert, Ruth, *The Public Health Nurse and Her Patient*, 2nd ed. Cambridge, Harvard University Press, 1951.

Ginsburg, Ethel, *Public Health Is People*. New York, Commonwealth Fund, 1950.

Gregg, Dorothy, Reassurance. *American Journal of Nursing*, 55: 171–174, February, 1955.

Greenhill, M. H., Interviewing with a Purpose. *American Journal of Nursing*, 56: 1259–1262, October, 1956.

Harlow, Elizabeth, A District Nursing Association Changes Its Sterilization Techniques. *Public Health Nursing*, 43: 129–131, March, 1951.

Hartigan, Helen, Nursing Responsibilities in Rehabilitation. *Nursing Outlook*, 2: 649–651, December, 1954.

Hearn, Gordon, A Social-Psychological View of Nursing Service. *Nursing Outlook*, 1: 632–634, November, 1953.

Hoffsommer, H., The Health Culture Patterns of Rural People. *Public Health Nursing*, 44: 307, June, 1952.

Lemkau, Paul, *Mental Hygiene in Public Health*, 2nd ed. New York: McGraw-Hill Book Co., Inc., 1955.

Lesser, Marion S. and Vera R. Keane, *Nurse-Patient Relationships in a Hospital Maternity Service*. St. Louis, C. V. Mosby Co., 1956.

Levy, D. M., Observations of Attitudes and Behavior in the Child Health Center, *American Journal of Public Health*, 41: 182–190, February, 1951.

Lucas, Ann F., Guidance and Counseling. *Nursing Outlook*, 4: 319–321, June, 1956.

McFadden, Daisy and Evelyn Walsh, The Nurse's Conference in a Child Health Station. *Nursing Outlook*, 4: 392–395, July, 1956.

Montague, Ashley, The Meaning of Cooperation. *Nursing Outlook*, 1: 98–100, February, 1953.

National Organization for Public Health Nursing, *Public Health Nursing Care of the Sick*. New York, National League for Nursing, 1943.

Neal, Ernest E., Health Is What You Think It Is. *Nursing Outlook*, 2: 478–480, September, 1954.

Notter, Lucille E., Disinfection of Clinical Thermometers. *Nursing Outlook*, 1: 569–561, October, 1953.

Oliva, Anthony T., Personality Factors in Human Relations. *Nursing Outlook*, 2: 578–579, November, 1954.

Owens, Charlotte, Concepts of Interviewing. *Nursing Outlook*, 1: 577–580, October, 1953.

Paul, Benjamin, and Miller, W. B., *Health, Culture and Community*. New York, Russell Sage Foundation, 1955.

Pendall, R. J., Speaking with People. *Nursing Outlook*, 2: 96–97, February, 1954.

Phillips, Elizabeth C., *Nursing Aspects in Rehabilitation and Care of the Chronically Ill*, League Exchange No. 12. New York, National League for Nursing, 1956.

Randall, Ollie A., Helen E. Hested, and Lucille Larson, Problems of Extended Illness and Old Age. *American Journal of Nursing*, 54: 1220–1225, October, 1954.

Richardson, H. B., *Patients Have Families*. New York, Commonwealth Fund, 1945.

Roberts, Doris, The Positive Approach to a Tuberculosis Nursing Program. *Public Health Reports*, 68: 338–340, March, 1953.

Roberts, Helen L., J. E. Gordon and A. Fiore, Epidemiological Techniques in Home Accident Prevention. *Public Health Reports*, 67: 547–551, June, 1952.

Rogers, Carl, A Counseling Approach to Human Problems. *American Journal of Nursing*, 56: 994–997, August, 1956.

Ross, Mabel, The Nurse in Family Counseling. *Public Health Nursing*, 41: 485–488, September, 1949.

Rusk, H., Implications for Nursing in Rehabilitation. *American Journal of Nursing*, 48: 74–79, 1948.

Schantz, Georgia, Judge Not. *Nursing Outlook*, 4: 524–525, September, 1956.

Selected References on Cardiovascular Disease, Public Health Bibliography series #15. Washington, D.C., U.S. Government Printing Office, 1956.

Shortal, Hazel and Estelle Hunt, Epidemiology: A Joint Activity of the Private Physician and the Public Health Nurse. *Nursing Outlook*, 1: 468–470, August, 1953.

Speroff, B. J., Empathy Is Important in Nursing. *Nursing Outlook*, 4: 326–328, June, 1956.

Strang, Ruth M., Motivation in Health Education. *Public Health Nursing*, 40: 11–14, January, 1948.

Stuart, H. C., Meeting the Health Needs of the Child. *Public Health Reports*, 67: 1076–1079, November, 1952.

Sutherland, Arthur, Psychological Impact of Cancer Surgery. *Public Health Reports*, 67: 1139–1143, November, 1952.

Tabershaw, I. R., and Margaret Hargreaves, Functions of Standing Orders in Industry. *American Journal of Public Health*, 37: 1430–1434, November, 1947.

Towle, Charlotte, Helping the Client to Use His Capacities and Resources. Part II in *Proceedings of the National Conference of Social Work*, 1948. New York, Columbia University Press, 1949.

Travis, Georgia, Social Considerations in Patient Management. *Public Health Reports*, 70: 1155–1160, December, 1955.

Upham, Frances, *A Dynamic Approach to Illness*. New York, Family Association of America, 1949.

Voiland, A. M., M. L. Gundelach, and M. Conner, *Developing Insight in Initial Interviews.* New York, Family Service Association, 1947.

Whitehorn, John C., The Development of Mature Individuals. *Adult Leadership,* 5: 206–208, January, 1957.

Winkley, Ruth, When a Child Must Go to the Hospital. *Child,* 17: 34–36, November, 1952.

Witmer, H. L. and R. Kotinsky, *Personality in the Making.* New York, Harper & Bros., 1952.

Wolff, Ilse, Mothers' Views on Breast Feeding. *Nursing Outlook,* 1: 145–148, March, 1953.

Wright, Elizabeth, Interpersonal Relations in Nursing. *Nursing Outlook,* 1: 451–454, August, 1953.

GROUP WORK

Bakst, H. J. and E. F. Morra, Experience with Home Care for Cardiac Patients. *American Journal of Public Health,* 45: 444–450, April, 1955.

Bond, Betty Wells, *Group Discussion-Decision.* Minneapolis, Minnesota Department of Health, 1956.

Bradford, Leland, Who Has a Question? *American Journal of Nursing,* 55: 181–184, February, 1955.

Chapman, A. L., An Experiment with Group Conference for Weight Reduction. *Public Health Reports,* 68: 439–440, April, 1953.

Chase, Stuart, *Roads to Agreement.* New York, Harper & Bros., 1951.

Gordon, Thomas, Leadership: Shall It Reside in the Leader or in the Group? *American Journal of Nursing,* 54: 1087–1088, September, 1954.

Guntert, M. and E. Henry, The Diabetic Goes to School. *Public Health Nursing,* 44: 335–337, June, 1952.

Lewin, Kurt, *Resolving Social Conflicts.* New York, Harper & Bros., 1948.

Workshop: Helping Adults Change Attitudes. A Series of Five Articles in *Adult Leadership,* 5: 241–259, February, 1957.

Supervisory and Management Responsibilities

CHAPTER XIV

Participation
in Agency and
Community Planning

A MAJOR CONTRIBUTION that public health nursing makes to community health is bringing to planning and executive groups the point of view and the special knowledges and competences of nursing. The nurse will have information about the potentials and patterns of nursing in agencies other than her own and how these affect plans under consideration. She has special skills in counseling and community organization that may help to judge possible service outcomes. She is close to people and apt to know the temper of the community and the readiness for a particular type of program. She knows what the nursing care demands are apt to be. For example, if a plan is under study to extend home care for tuberculosis patients, the nurse will know much that is of importance in determining the final program. She will know what teaching is done in the hospital by nurses, the adequacy of nursing staff there in relation to patient needs, and the level of coordination. She can estimate the readiness and probable response of families for this program, how well equipped they are to assume the necessary responsibility, and the probable use of private medical care as compared to health agency facilities for designated services. She will know about how much and what kind of related services will be required in new cases, for in families in which there is a patient with tuberculosis there will also be pregnancies, child-behavior problems, minor ills and a multitude of other situations requiring nursing time, and not to be ignored if the family is under care. If many new families are to be reached, allowances must be made in estimating the time required not only for the accomplishment of the primary program objectives of the tuberculosis service, but for the incidental nursing care which must also be provided.

The public health nurse may participate in agency and community planning directly, as a member of an agency or community planning group. She may be a member of the school health committee or of an agency committee on maternal and child health services; or a member of a medical resources unit in the community civil defense organization. In large agencies, the nurse may participate more frequently through someone else— a supervisor, or a staff representative. She will in this case make suggestions, help in reviewing tentative plans, work in small discussion groups, obtain ideas from others to submit to the planning committee or council. In the latter case, the nurse's *responsibility* to participate in planning is no less fundamental—it is just channeled differently. Three areas of responsibility may be identified:

1. Relating individual experiences to the problems of the whole agency or community.
2. Functioning as an effective member of committees, councils or other planning groups.
3. Establishing communication systems with other agency workers.

RELATING INDIVIDUAL EXPERIENCE TO THE WHOLE

The ability to participate in agency and community planning depends upon the capacity to see one's own experience in the light of the whole agency and community program. For example, the nurse may see the enormous need for counseling services for actual or potential juvenile delinquents in a particular area. If she knows to what extent this is a problem of the whole community or of a particular section, the range and limits of counseling services, the availability of trained counselors in schools and in other agencies, her suggestions can be more helpful. If she recognizes the relationship between this problem and programs in housing or slum clearance, or welfare problems due to the migratory character of the population, her observations will be more perceptive. Needs for increased nursing staff, too, must be seen in the light of the whole. Nursing, even in adequate amounts, will not be effective if no medical direction is available, or if facilities for coping with the additional problems that may be uncovered by extended nursing service do not exist.

Sometimes awareness of over-all planning and action will direct the nurse's observations in new ways. For example, the knowledge that schools are sponsoring an extensive accident prevention program might lead her to observe more carefully the effect of school instruction on parental behavior, the pertinence of the instruction given and the practicality of suggestions made. The possibility of home-care programs for mentally ill patients may lead her to look more closely at the competence of families to cope with emotional situations.

Realism in facing the compromises that must be made between the "ideal" and the "possible" is also necessary in planning without losing faith in the power of imagination and the seeking of new ways to do more for less. It is not helpful to suggest that nothing less than a fully prepared public health nurse can provide family service if there is no prospect of finding such a staff in the foreseeable future, or that nothing less than the recommended number of nurses can be considered. It may help enormously, though, to differentiate between the expected competences of nurses with or without special preparation in public health and the possibility of self-help by families or community groups. In this way, the program can be developed around the competences that may be expected to be available, and may be extended even though there is not ideal preparation or concentration of nursing staff.

Equally important is the capacity to avoid "guild consciousness"—the tendency to support nursing at all costs, without relevance to the needs and contributions of other disciplines. Nursing, as well as the nurse's own experience, must be seen in relation to the whole effort and its potential impact on human welfare. At certain points, for instance, sanitarians or health educators may be needed more urgently than other workers, and the nurse on the planning group should be prepared to see and support this need even at the expense of nursing.

Committee Membership. More and more there is a tendency to have staff (field) nurse representation on planning and decision groups. It is felt that this "fresh-from-the-field" point of view has real value in thinking through possible activities and arriving at sound decisions.

Being a committee member implies certain obligations—to prepare one's self for the work of the committee, to communicate one's ideas and feelings to others with effectiveness and to think with others in a productive group-focussed manner. As a committee member, the nurse can do many things. She may suggest new problems or new approaches arising from her experience; she may gather information or opinions of others that have significance for the direction of her own work; she may provide information or judgments that are important to clarification or decision making; or test ideas of others against her own field knowledge. In addition, she can do much to encourage others in the group to contribute, by referring to their experience or asking for their opinions or for clarification of their ideas. She may present the point of view of her agency or group as a staff representative.

Preparing for Committee Activity.   Prior to committee meetings, each member should review the purposes and previous actions of the committee as shown in the minutes, and look through the agenda a few days in advance to gain a clear concept of what is expected of this particular meeting. Often it will become apparent that the nurse has or can get information that would add to the understanding of the problems or clarify the issues to be discussed.

If there is to be discussion of the maternal and child health program, for example, it may be necessary to find out what proportion of the population at risk are actually under public health nursing supervision, what problems are presented, how many visits are being made per patient and whether there are substantial differences in needs and in the services provided in relation to age, neighborhood, cultural group, or other factors. This may involve only information readily obtained from the nurse's own case load, or it may entail asking others of their experience and for their help in obtaining the necessary facts. For example, the nurse who is a representative on a community planning committee for maternal and child health may ask other nurses on the staff for information from their case load.

Some advance thinking about the possible differences of interest and direction of thinking of committee members may be helpful in anticipating the issues that may be raised and the course of discussion. It is then possible to think through in advance the issues that are important and the stand that might be taken. It may be well, if policy matters are apt to come up, to obtain a policy statement from the administrator or supervisor.

It is also important to be prepared to function as a productive group member—to recognize that one's own interests will overlap but not duplicate those of other members and may have to be subordinated to group needs. A committee member should not feel that time is wasted when items outside her immediate interest are being discussed. At the same time it is important to interpret clearly one's particular area of interest, so that it too is incorporated into the whole in an effective way.

If membership is as an agency representative, preparation should include thorough grounding in the philosophy and history of the agency, in its activities and in declared plans for the future. There should also be a clear understanding as to the degree to which it is permissible to make commitments for the agency. For example, it might be quite appropriate for a member of a referral committee concerned with methods of securing better correlation of hospital and home care to agree to methods of notification to be used among the various agencies concerned, but not to a redistribution of responsibility for different aspects of patient care. If membership is on a representative basis, as when one nurse represents all field nurses, it may be well to canvass the group represented in regard to the issues to be raised. The representative has an obligation to reflect the opinions and thinking of her group, and is not free to represent only her own thinking, or to act contrary to the desire of those she represents. This does not mean that the representative cannot move ahead to decisions without going back to her group; it means that she should act in a way consistent with her group's ideas.

Participation in Meetings and Conferences. During committee activities it is important to:

1. Try to express ideas clearly and briefly.
2. Avoid monopolizing the discussion.
3. Listen carefully to get the implications of others' contributions for the total program. It is impossible to listen well if all attention is going to the effort to be heard one's self.
4. Avoid argument—seek out and build on areas of agreement rather than rely on argument to win a point.
5. Be willing to change or compromise if the facts or the realities of the situation demand it. There is no point in sticking to a plan to have all maternity patients referred for public health nursing follow-up if the medical group prefers not to have this done.

6. Look for the "instead of"—avoid "either/or." For example, one participant may feel that the doctor should approve referral of patients to the VNA and another that it is essentially a nursing responsibility to arrange referral. In the first case, nursing care would be integrated with the total medical care—obviously a desirable condition. In the latter case, referral would be expedited and probably better judgment used in relation to what community nursing services could offer. Better than either might be the decision to have the physician approve referral for groups of patients, upon certain designated conditions, but not be obliged to approve each referral. In this way the benefits of both methods could be achieved.

7. Be willing to wait sometimes for someone else to say what seems obvious to you. For example, the nurse member of a committee to discuss home care of psychiatric patients may see that certain things now done by hospital personnel could be done by public health nurses in the home with greater patient satisfaction. However, if by waiting rather than putting forth this idea at once, a psychiatrist or social worker brings out this idea, the basis for development is sounder since there can then be no suspicion of professional bias or "empire building."

8. Do your share to move the committee along by asking for clarification, bringing out essential agreements, pointing out issues involved, or summarizing when this seems appropriate.

Committee activities can make a real contribution to the professional growth of the nurse, while at the same time providing an opportunity for her to make a unique contribution to the work of the committee. Membership should be approached thoughtfully and used fully for promoting better total service, by relating the knowledge and experience of the nurse to that of others and directing both toward reaching sound answers to service problems.

AGENCY AND COMMUNITY COMMUNICATIONS

Communication between the nurse and others in her agency or with other agencies and the community is a combination of general public relations activities and the more specific interchange that goes on through clearance, exchange of information and referral. The report of a recent conference on communications gives in considerable detail aspects of coordinating nursing services.[1]

General Public Relations Aspects. Public relations represent a potential hidden asset in every nursing activity.[2] The way in which a prenatal visit is made may affect the way many people think and feel about the nursing services. The patient's doctor, her husband, her friends (and nurse's potential clients) and others may gain their impression of the usefulness and character of public health nursing from the nurse's incidental comments about her experience. The approach used in requesting medical orders from a physician may be limited to getting orders for a specific patient or may encompass the broader aspect of increasing his understanding and support of the agency's program, and appreciating its potential service in relation to private medical care.

The value of occasional personal contacts with others who provide care cannot be overemphasized. The nurse who provides morbidity services and who is new in a community should, for example, plan a personal visit to the physicians in that community early in her experience. This provides an opportunity to assure the physician of the desire to help, and to indicate in a general way the services available. The emphasis should be on mutual concerns and opportunities for joint effort, not on "selling" the service to him.

Other community workers—teachers, principals, social workers, probation officers, ministers, workers in voluntary agencies such as the American Red Cross and the National Tuberculosis Association—should also be visited as soon as possible, preferably in conjunction with a specific problem. Efforts should be made to gauge the degree of satisfaction users of the nursing service feel and to explain when dissatisfaction occurs. If the physician feels that nursing service is not adequate in amount, for example, the nurse should make every effort to interpret the reasons for limitations on service and the basis for case selection.

Printed materials, newspaper announcements, talks to groups and reports may be used to disseminate information about the service. Such publicity efforts supplement, but do not replace, the face-to-face contact and the impact of the service itself. The

1. Department of Public Health Nursing, National League for Nursing, *Communications between Nursing Services*. New York, The League, 1957.

2. Wensley, Edith, *The Community and Public Health Nursing*. New York, Macmillan Co., 1950.

public health nurse should be alert to the public relations implications of her work, and constantly promote good relations between her agency and the public.

Exchanging Information.   Within the all-nursing agency,
such as the visiting nurse service, intra-agency communication
is usually easily effected through staff meetings and informal
personal interchange. When the agency has a multi-discipline
staff there may be need for a procedure for interchange of information and joint planning. When the report of a visit to a
rural school reveals sanitation problems in relation to food preparation or need for pupil instruction about protection of individual
home water supplies, the nurse may request a conference or
send a copy of her report (with a personal forwarding note for
warmth!) to the sanitarian or engineer who is also concerned
with that particular district. If there is no regular program of
periodic conference with the health officer in a one-nurse unit,
the nurse may request a conference when she is developing her
service plan, or to review a group of tuberculosis cases to be sure
the care given is in the right direction. When a mobile orthopedic clinic is going to a community, consultation with the health
educator about previous community organization, activities or
special problems will save time and avoid duplication of effort.

Consultation with and referral to private physicians make an
important contribution to cohesive patient care. In most instances
the responsible medical officer (or chairman of the medical advisory committee in the visiting nurse service) will have made
some general contacts with the local medical society, and publicity materials will have been sent to individual physicians by
the public relations officer or committee of the agency. Thus the
individual nurse working with the physician in patient care has
a base on which to build her relationships with him.

Some kind of arrangement needs to be made to facilitate referral of cases by the nurse to other agencies or individual
workers and by other agencies to the nurse. Whatever the method
adopted, it should meet the following criteria:

  1. It should be *fast* enough to avoid a lapse in care.
  2. It should be *personal* enough to make the transfer easy for
     family and agency.
  3. It should be *simple* enough to avoid unnecessary paper work,
     yet provide such information as is necessary to avoid mis-
     directed efforts.

Telephone referral has the advantage of speed and personalization, and it also provides an opportunity to clarify or explain the situation when necessary. It provides no permanent record of the transfer.

A referral form may be developed and used on a community-wide basis. This permits transfer of essential information with a minimum of error, provides a permanent record and, unless it becomes very complex, may take less time than the telephone contact. It may also be possible to use clerical or volunteer assistance more easily than with a telephone referral. When

```
Name                    Number
Address                 Phone
Referred to
- - - - - - - - - - - - - - - - - - - - - - - - - - - - -   ← Perforation

Diagnosis:
Treatment:
Remarks:                          This half on gummed pa-
                                  per to be attached to
                                  receiving agency record
Referred by:
```

Figure 18.   Suggested referral form.

fast referral is necessary, and it is not possible to know in advance when the transfer to another service will take place, dependence on a mailed report may result in the public health nurse missing the opportunity to make a visit at the most productive time.

Referral forms in use vary greatly from extensive records with copious notes about patient and family conditions, attitudes and response to service, to a relatively simple one with a sentence or two for information that is deemed essential beyond the necessary identifying data. Careful thought, and use of the telephone or conference as an adjunct for the really complex situations, probably weigh the scales in favor of brevity, though there is considerable disagreement regarding this. The National League for Nursing Report on Communications suggests report forms.[3]

3. Loc. cit.

A brief form is suggested in Figure 18. The longer referral form may serve an educational as well as a service purpose when professional students in medicine, nursing or social work participate in care.

If comprehensive information is required—for instance, if the nurse is sending a full report of each prenatal visit to the private physician—a form that will permit use of a carbon copy of the nurse's visit rather than a separate report may save time.

A routine case pick-up is sometimes indicated. For example, the nurse in a rural area who visits a village on a weekly or less frequent schedule may go to the physician's office to check whether he has patients who need to be seen. If hospital and health department are in the same building or nearby, the nurse may check periodically to find out which patients are to be discharged and read the hospital record, rather than depend upon a harassed hospital nurse to abstract the essential points. If an agency—for instance, a private or chronic disease hospital—is just starting to use the public health nursing service, such a personal visit may be indicated for a while until the necessary mutual understandings have been fully developed. During the personal contact period there will be time to discuss what types of cases might be referred, the limits of community service available, and timing of hospital discharges in relation to home-care facilities. Such a procedure is sometimes useful in tuberculosis hospitals where one member of the public health nursing staff helps to make referrals and arranges case planning or case discharge conferences with staff nurses and hospital personnel when necessary.

Patient Care-Planning Conferences.   When patient care involves the concurrent action of several professional workers, or intermittent care by more than one agency, it may require more individualized planning than is indicated in the foregoing. A patient care-planning conference, in which physician, hospital nurse, community nurse, social worker and family member are included, may be scheduled for the tuberculosis patient about to be transferred from hospital to home care under conditions different from that of the majority of patients. This provides an opportunity for joint appraisal of patient and family needs, coordination of instruction, agreement on the general conditions of care and the areas of responsibility of community nurse, hospital, and family. Such planning conferences provide an excellent opportunity for extending mutual understanding among agencies, and consideration of a specific patient may be used as a means of working through general agreements about other patients. Such multi-discipline or multi-agency conferences are expensive. However, they are justified:

1. For patients whose care is complex and will extend over a long period with frequent interchange of responsibility among agencies.
2. When new programs are being developed, as a basis for identifying the relative responsibility of each agency and establishing a pattern of care that can later be applied—with necessary individual adjustments—to groups of patients.
3. When the conference is used as a method of educating students in basic professional schools, or for in-service education of personnel.

Clearances and Approvals. Sometimes it is necessary to secure approval from physicians, social workers or other hospital workers prior to referral to community agencies. Securing such approval and routing all referrals through a single hospital public health nurse may secure great uniformity, and may encourage more selective use of community resources. It has, however, a potential danger in terms of slowing down the actual transfer of information, so the community agency may secure the request for care too late for effective planning and service.

In general, it is better to rely on approval of referral for *groups* of patients or of *criteria* for referral rather than upon individual clearance. Once this is done, referral can be made on a nurse-to-nurse basis. Ideally, the nurse primarily responsible for the comprehensive nursing care of the patient in the hospital or in the home should assume responsibility for referral as an integral part of family care, and develop the competence to handle it.

The public health nurse has an important part to play in agency and community planning. Through relating her own service to the whole she discusses and transmits information to planning groups; through committee activity she adds values of her particular professional skill and field "know how" to the group solution of agency and community problems; through careful selective procedures for communication with other individuals and agencies concerned with patient care she helps to conserve and intensify not only her own professional contribution to family health care, but that of other groups as well.

CHAPTER XV

Planning the
Nursing Program

THE PUBLIC health nurse's responsibility for program planning will vary in accordance with the size of the agency, the diversity of the program and the availability of supervision. In the large urban agency the nurse's planning responsibility may be limited to management of her own case load, and offering suggestions regarding community needs in relation to the nursing program as a whole. In the sparsely populated community the public health nurse will have to make many more decisions regarding activities to be included in the program, delegation of responsibility to others, and scheduling work in relation to most effective intervals between nursing contacts when there is no possibility of being available on a daily basis to the communities served. Whatever the scope of planning the nurse must do, she will be concerned with:

1. Establishing the objectives of the service.
2. Conferring, clearing and planning with other workers and agencies.
3. Selecting activities.
4. Scheduling activities.

In general it is desirable to have a written plan for service, since this provides the impetus for thoughtful and specific thinking through of the problem, and the basis for discussion of the merits of the plan with supervisory or administrative personnel.

ESTABLISHING OBJECTIVES

Basic to planning is a clearly defined statement of what is to be done. These objectives must be properly related to the purposes of the agency, and to the needs of the community as a whole, since in public health the community is the patient. For example, the purposes of a visiting nurse service might be to offer services on a humanitarian basis, without regard for their preventive potential; a health department, on the other hand, may be committed to preventing death or disability. The effect of such differences is apparent when one considers nursing service in civil defense activities in time of war. The needs of the patient, in terms of his degree of illness, are not a major factor in deciding who should receive care, but rather whether or not his life can be saved. The very sick patient may receive minimal or no care if it seems certain he cannot survive in any case. This basis of selection would be quite different in peacetime, when the community would feel an obligation to help and relieve the very sick person, even though death from the condition is inevitable.

There is often a tendency to consider the present case load rather than the community as a whole as the basis for planning. For example, it may be that maternity patients under nursing supervision do not include those who are receiving medical care from a private physician. In deciding what is to be done, the question should be raised as to whether the needs of this group are being met or whether their needs might be as great or even greater than those of the families now included in the case load. The objectives for maternity nursing services must be related to the community as a whole. When maternal and infant mortality were high, economic factors and educational background which tend to be less favorable among those using community rather than private facilities for care were a reasonable basis for assuming lesser need among those attended by private physicians. However, in a period of full employment and extending public education, and in the presence of a favorable maternal and infant death rate, more attention might be given to emotional factors and general maternal competence. It may be that the career-woman-turned-wife-and-mother has a much greater problem of adjustment to child bearing and rearing than does the woman of limited educational background and lower economic status who faces no conflict when she relinquishes her repetitive factory job for the job of homemaker. Services not now included in the program may not be considered in planning, "because we're not even doing our present job well." However, new services may represent a greater need in the community than do those already carried.

Studying Community Needs.   Basic to establishing objectives for nursing service is an estimate of the total health needs of the community, and its relation to public health nursing needs. It is important to know:

1. Characteristics of the population that would influence needs for care.
2. Prevalence and incidence of illness as revealed by vital statistics or surveys.
3. Environmental factors that create health needs.
4. Patterns of care—proportion of care given by hospitals or other institutions.

The *character of the population* will greatly influence the amount and type of public health nursing service needed, and the direction the program should take. The following factors have particular significance for public health nursing:

1. Trend in population as a whole. Is the community expanding rapidly, or decreasing in size? Is the growth or decline slow or explosive? For instance, in a new community growing up around a newly located industrial plant or military installation, or in a "retirement community" sponsored by a real estate development, the increase in population may be sudden. This increases the strain on the usual community facilities and creates nursing needs for counseling and referral. The type of population change, as well as the rate of change, is also important. If, as in the retirement community or in areas where the climate is favorable, the influx is heavily weighted with older people the nursing needs would be different from those in the community in which the influx is largely young workers. If the change introduces a different cultural group—as when the new community members are of a different race, or when New England factories move south and bring with them many of their employees, or if the influx is largely laborers or factory hands coming to what was formerly a quiet village—the needs will again shift.
2. Age distribution. This is a strong determinant of needs. The suburban community with its burgeoning young population places special demands on school health, since the

school-child group is large in numbers in the population, and the development of new schools with new faculty means special needs for teacher orientation. The military post dependent population will also be weighted with young people, many requiring maternity care.

Indices of *general vitality* of the population are also revealing. The birth rate and infant mortality or fetal wastage rate provide direct information relating to the potential need for maternity care. Death rates and causes of death are also helpful. However, it is necessary to be careful not to overestimate the importance of mortality rates as a criterion for program determination. The patient with arthritis or schizophrenia may not die of it, yet her nursing needs are high. Need for tuberculosis nursing care may actually be increased rather than decreased as the mortality rate declines, since the need for care may be increased to the degree that patients who formerly died are now kept alive and require treatment and education. The need for care in mental illness, which will greatly influence public health nursing needs, is not reflected in mortality rates.

Racial distribution as it affects health needs should also be considered. Some health conditions such as tuberculosis are more prevalent among certain racial groups. While it is possible that the differential incidence is due to socioeconomic rather than racial factors, for planning purposes the nurse recognizes that the demand for certain types of care will change with the racial configuration of the community.

Socioeconomic factors will also make a difference. Incidence of illness tends to be higher in the low economic groups, and the medical care less intensive.[1] Need for nutritional guidance, planning for care of children of working mothers, and general morbidity services might be expected to be higher.

The striving community—in which there is a strong effort to move upward in the economic scale—will also produce an unusually high ratio of needs, though in a different direction. Stress, anxiety and tension produce emotional problems; parents who overwork need help in parent-child adjustments and in the prevention of fatigue.

Accurate estimates of morbidity are not generally available for planning. Studies such as the National Health Survey of

1. Falk, L. S., M. Klein and Nathan Sinai, *The Incidence of Illness and Receipt and Costs of Care among Representative Families.* Chicago, University of Chicago Press, 1933.

1935-36, and the more recent studies of incidence of chronic disease give some indication of what might be expected. The recently authorized National Health Survey Program of the Public Health Service will undoubtedly provide a much more substantial planning base than was formerly available.[2, 3, 4]

In the absence of accurate statistical data, some idea of the prevalence or incidence of illness may be gained from a review of hospital discharged cases, from past records of the agency, and from reportable disease records.

Environmental factors will also modify programs in public health nursing. In rural areas with many small milk producers, undulant fever may present problems; in urban areas with inadequate playgrounds, prevention of accidents among children may assume major importance. Excessive nitrate content in the soil may produce problems of safeguarding water supplies; hookworm may be associated with areas in which the climate combined with inadequate sanitary provisions favors its spread; or widespread anemia may be manifest where food supplies are limited.

Patterns of medical care will differ widely, and place quite different demands on public health nursing personnel. If the great majority of deliveries is in the hospital the maternity program in public health nursing must be adjusted to what is essentially a pre- and post-hospital care service; when home delivery by midwives is the pattern the content of patient supervision is broadened, and in addition there is need to plan for midwife supervision and training.

Most people in North America receive care from private physicians who are in general practice. When this is the case, there may be quite a different pattern of sharing responsibility between physician and nurse than when the care is given in special clinics or in the medical specialist's office.

The length of hospital stay has tended in recent years to become shorter, especially for acute illness, surgical care and ma-

2. Division of Public Health Methods, National Institutes of Health, *National Health Survey 1935–1936.* Bulletin No. 1, An Estimate of the Amount of Disabling Illness in the Country As a Whole. Washington, D.C., Government Printing Office, 1939.

3. *Chronic Illness in a Rural Area,* and *Chronic Illness in a Large City,* to be published as Volumes 3 and 4 in a series "Chronic Illness in the United States" by the Commonwealth Fund.

4. National Health Survey Act, 1956. *Public Law 652,* 84th Congress.

ternity care.[5] This means that many patients are released from the hospital when they are still in need of considerable guidance and often need treatments or dressings. There is still much variation in practice from community to community, and between private and governmental hospitals.

In thus considering the needs and characteristics of the community, the public health nurse needs to see the total health needs, the nursing needs within this total, and finally the public health nursing needs with which she must be prepared to cope.

Establishing Priorities. Since it is rarely possible to undertake every nursing activity that seems desirable, it is necessary to establish some system of priorities that will guide the nurse in setting her service objectives. In this way it is possible to concentrate upon those activities that are most apt to make a difference in the total community health. If, for example, the need for nursing supervision during the maternity cycle is considered, it becomes apparent that some patients have needs that are greater than those of others, or needs that are more likely to cause serious trouble if they are ignored. Young has indicated that maternity patients may be graded in relation to the degree of risk involved, based on previous obstetrical history, medical history, physical examination and other findings.[6] Those with a high degree of risk would obviously have priority when public health nursing time is limited. It may be assumed that primiparas have greater need of public health nursing than do multiparas with negative obstetrical and medical history. Similarly, certain services within nursing may take precedence over others, such as the care of sputum-positive tuberculosis patients who might expose others to infection. For each service the nurse may list in order of importance those groups of patients for whom care should be provided, so that in adjustment of program and setting objectives the most important groups will certainly be covered. For example, in prenatal care she may include as top priorities prenatal patients with a history of complications or premature delivery on previous pregnancies, primiparas, especially those in the under eighteen and over thirty-five age group, multiparas with more than six children closely spaced, those with poor nutritional status, especially when there is evidence of anemia or

5. *Facts About Nursing*, 1955–56 Edition. New York, American Nurses' Association, p. 167.

6. Young, Robert F., A Scientific Approach to Fetal Wastage in Halifax County, North Carolina. *Public Health Reports*, 71: 1065–1068, November, 1956.

nutritional patterns that would make anemia likely. In the tuberculosis service, those with positive sputum, those in households with small children, and those receiving treatment at home would rank high in priority.

The establishment of such priorities must be done in conjunction with the medical group responsible for the care of patients. The selection of groups for care should be based on the questions: "What difference might nursing care be expected to make in this situation? Is it more or less than would be expected in other groups?"

Priorities should be based on:

1. Preventive potential. The degree to which nursing care might be expected to help to prevent death, disability or recurrence or exacerbation of illness.

2. Emphasis in the agency program as a whole. Program development and emphasis will change from time to time. If accident prevention is being stressed in the total agency program, nursing participation will also be increased; if chronic disease diagnostic services are being instituted, nursing-follow up is essential to effectuate the diagnostic program.

3. Community expectations and interests. If community interest in mental hygiene is high, and the constituents expect their community nursing service to provide services to the mentally ill and counseling services for prevention of behavior difficulties, this should bear weight in establishing priorities, since community support and understanding will be encouraged as the needs as seen are met.

Writing the Objectives.   With the background of knowledge of community needs and priorities of service, the nurse may proceed to outline the objectives of service. In writing these it is important that they meet the following criteria:

1. Objectives should be realistically achievable. There is little use in planning to provide care for prenatal patients under care of a private physician if the nursing time is inadequate to do so; if the habit of the community is firmly against use of nursing care for any but the underprivileged; or if the medical group is opposed to any community service by the health department other than communicable disease control. The objectives should be within the competence of the nurse as well as within the available time potential; to take on a program of home care for psychiatric patients

released from the hospital on drug therapy may be unrealistic unless there is an opportunity for the nurse to
equip herself to provide such care, or has already had the
necessary preparation.

2. Objectives should be specifically stated. "To decrease deaths
from tuberculosis" is a laudable goal for all community
organizations concerned with care of tuberculosis, but would
provide little guidance for a nursing program. The objectives might include such as the provision of guidance to the
family in care of the discharged hospital patient, the provision of pre-hospital consultation to help with family adjustments to hospital care, etc.

3. Objectives should be flexible enough to allow for change.
For instance, to have as an objective the extension of group
counseling for families with chronically ill members under
home care permits fairly wide range in deciding for how
many groups and under what circumstances such counseling
will be provided. To indicate substitution of group counseling for individual home visits before the feasibility of such
a move has been proved sets up an objective that may prove
impossible to achieve, or that may prove to be undesirable.

4. Objectives for nursing service should be closely coordinated
with those of the agency as a whole.

PLANNING WITH OTHERS

Reference has already been made to the importance of coordination of plans for nursing service with those of others involved in
the total care of the patient. The nurse will plan at all times carefully with the nursing supervisor who stands in the position of a
generalized professional consultant. In addition, and in varying
degrees, the nurse will plan with the health officer, private physicians individually or with a medical association, the industrial
physician or personnel manager, the school principal or superintendent, the hospital nursing staff, other community nursing
services, the welfare worker, and specialists such as the health
educator or nutritionist. For those with major concern for her
program, which would include the nursing supervisor and health
officer when the nurse reports administratively to him, the nurse
will probably want a planning conference.

In preparation for program-planning conferences the nurse
should gather information about health problems of the community, the nursing services rendered in the previous year (or other

planning period), and tentative suggestions for modifications or directions of the nursing program for the coming period. Since joint planning, and not simple approval, is the goal, the nurse should arrange for these conferences before the program has been decided upon, to obtain suggestions and ideas for the coming period. This new information may make the tentative suggestions invalid.

If the planning conference is to be held with persons outside the nurse's own agency she should make clear the limits of her authority to agree to changes that would either require additional budgetary support or would affect her availability for services she is presently carrying. For example, in talking with the nursing supervisor of a hospital outpatient clinic, it may seem that a larger proportion of clinic patients should receive public health nursing follow-up. Once the probable volume of service is estimated, the nurse will need to discuss with those responsible for her total program whether such a change would be possible without detriment to other commitments and responsibilities.

Advance preparation should be sufficient to provide the basic facts and some suggestions for action to be considered; it should be sufficiently unformed to use the help of others in adjusting the program more realistically to the needs of the people served.

SELECTING ACTIVITIES

There are many varieties of activities through which the nurse may realize the objectives of service. These include:
1. Home visits.
2. Office conference, demonstration.
3. Clinic nursing services.
4. Visits to school or industry.
5. Group instruction or group discussion.
6. "Relay" service through preparation of volunteers, nurses in other positions such as in the doctor's office, hospital nurses or nursing students.

The advantages and disadvantages of home visits and other forms of family nurse contact have been discussed in Chapter VI. "Relay" service, in which the public health nurse provides others with the skills or knowledge necessary for them to incorporate public health nursing activities into their own job, has very real advantages. The nurse in the hospital, for example, is in a good position to encourage use of community facilities for care of the well baby, and to explain to the private patient the availability of community nursing or health services which he might need.

In setting up the nursing program, the public health nurse considers the needs of people, and the methods by which these could best be met. She considers the methods of delivery of services in the light of the time cost also, and decides which method is likely to be most effective when the advantage of the method itself is weighed against its cost and probable outcome.

Also weighed is the relationship between reaching a large number of people with a small amount of nursing care as opposed to reaching a smaller number with more intensive supervision. The value of one and two visit cases should be carefully considered. Ten visits made to ten patients may be good if they accomplish the desired result; but if a single visit will *not* accomplish the purpose of the service, all ten visits will have been wasted, since none will profit. It might be better to select five who need the service more and provide two visits each, or select three families to receive three visits each.

It is true that families will vary in the amount of nursing care they need; even when the situation seems the same, one family will gain a good deal from one or two visits, while another will need several more before the desired results can be secured. Education, experience and temperament of family and nurse will cause differences. However, for planning purposes the nurse is concerned with the *average* intensity of needed service, realizing that within this there will be much individual variation.

Within each service the target group should be identified—those within the group for whom the service is first intended. For instance, in acute communicable disease activities those with communicable diseases in which there is great danger to others or danger of complications should be identified for intensive care— those with major illness such as scarlet fever, diphtheria, or poliomyelitis; the very young or older age group with measles; chicken pox in the adult, because of the need to be sure that a medical diagnosis has been secured. "Relay" care might be planned for the parents and teachers in relation to minor communicable disease, using a group approach to inform them of the symptoms and care before the occurrence of actual illness. In some cases, planning to use a resource person who has had training in home nursing and can help to recognize situations that should be referred for professional care to work with small groups may be utilized.

Traditional activities should be reviewed to see whether they are still a valid program entity, or of lesser importance than some new activities. For instance, in one community in which virtually every well child was being seen by the public health nurse there were relatively few prenatal cases under her care, and none of the patients attending the cancer diagnostic clinic and found to need further study were receiving any nursing service or support. Also, it is well to check to see whether some of the things being done by the nurse could be done better by someone else. For example, it has been found that selected non-nurses can teach home nursing quite effectively, and certainly nurse volunteers in a community might also undertake this important activity.[7]

Consideration should also be given to the advantages of a "balanced" program in contrast with a program in which there is an intensive push in one service with others temporarily subordinated. In general, seasonal skewing of services is to be expected— upper respiratory infections swell the general morbidity program in the winter months, school health needs tend to bunch at the beginning of the school year, and if medical examinations are not evenly distributed throughout the year there will be a concentration of service need immediately following them.

Lastly, some activities may be marked for a try-out to see whether there is a new approach that might be more effective, or whether there is really a need for service in a new area. For example, the nurse might talk with physicians and try out a special mothers' class to teach relaxation exercises; or visits might be made to colostomy patients soon after discharge from the hospital to see what could be done by the public health nurse to help with adjustments to home care, with the understanding that referrals might be extended or withdrawn as the hospital and public health nurse evaluate the results of such care.

Estimating Available Time.   As a basis for planning it is also important to know how much nursing time is available. This may be computed on the basis of *effective hours* available, counting as effective hours only those available for direct service. Excluded from this total would be office hours spent in administrative activities, time spent in in-service education activities, travel time, miscellaneous time spent in nonservice activities. Included would be time in clinics, schools or office spent in family conferences and time spent in home calls. These estimates would be based on the daily record if this includes time so distributed, or on a record of time spent for representative weeks during the year. For example, the nurse might record time spent in various activities for a period

7. McGuire, S. H. and R. Freeman, Teaching Effectiveness of Non-nurse Instruction Shown by Tests. *School and Society,* 69: 268–271, April 9, 1949.

of two weeks on three occasions during the year. If this is not possible, it may be possible to make a reasonable estimate on the basis of even a few days' observation.

Unit time costs must also be estimated; for example, a clinic session with appropriate pre- and post-clinic activities, but not including home visits occasioned by clinic findings, may require four hours of nursing time. A home call may require an average of thirty minutes. With this it is possible to estimate the time required for the work included in the program.

When time requirements and the actual effective time available are compared, it is readily apparent whether the program is overly optimistic or not.

Here is an example:

Mary Smith is a county nurse in Payne County, with a population of 3000. She works forty hours a week and fifty weeks a year. Her *effective hours per year* are estimated, on the basis of her records and experience, as follows:

Total hours worked (50 weeks)		2000	
Sick time, 4 days	32 hours		
Holidays, 5 days	40 hours		
In-service education (seminars, etc.), 10 days	80 hours		
Total off-the-job hours		152	
Total hours on the job			1848
Percentage of time spent in travel, office activities other than patient services (based on daily record or special study)	40%		
Percentage of total hours available for patient services	60%		
Effective hours available (60% of 1848 = 1109)			1109

Maternity Service	*Effective Hours Required*	
Birth rate is 21 per 1000		
Total families prenatal and postnatal	63	
Estimated number that would need home visits (primiparas, patients with special problems, etc.)	30	
Average nursing time required for home calls per case, four visits each, 30 minutes per visit	120 min.	
Total time needed for home calls, 3600 minutes or 60 hours		60
Group work—5 sessions, 4 hours per session, 3 groups during year		60
Well baby clinic—2 times a month, 10 months, 2 clinics. Time required per clinic, 4 hours		160
Total time required		280 hours

(Other services computed in similar fashion)

SCHEDULING ACTIVITIES

The method by which activities are scheduled will differ greatly in rural and urban centers. In both it is necessary to plan in a long-range way for the program as a whole. Classes in home care of the sick, school health examinations or special projects will need to be planned well in advance and integrated with the program as a whole.

When much bedside nursing care is included in the program, it may be necessary to make schedules for relatively short periods, since the demand will be fluctuating. In the urban visiting nurse service, daily schedules assume greater importance, and even the weekly schedule will need great flexibility. When there are clinic or class commitments that come at regular intervals, the scheduling for these activities will be for a longer period. Whatever the effective scheduling period, it is important to have a fairly long period scheduled for regularly recurring activities, and a specific immediate work plan for the day, week or month, indicating the specific itinerary.

Scheduling Visits to Schools.   The amount of time to be devoted to school activities will be determined by the responsible administrator in the health or nursing agency and the superintendent of schools. If schools are visited daily it is well to have the visit at the same time of day, to permit most effective use of the time available. The scheduled hours for time spent in the health room or other direct services should not include the total hours assigned for school service, since some time will need to be reserved for committee or health council meetings, or teachers' activities. These may come at a different hour than that regularly scheduled or may occur at irregular intervals.

The nurse should schedule time for special clinics or physical examination periods held in the school, and her schedule should also provide time for the necessary follow-up immediately after the clinic period.

Visits to rural schools should be scheduled well in advance, and usually should be planned for a period of a half day or more. The teacher may then plan for school activities that will enable her to use the nurse's time to good advantage, arranging for conferences with children who have special problems and for conference with parents when that is indicated.

Visits to schools which have new teachers should be scheduled early in the school year, and revisited fairly soon to answer questions that may have arisen and to give the teacher greater confidence. The increasing trend toward consolidation of schools is having the beneficial effect of making fewer schools to be visited, so that visits can be scheduled more frequently. Quarterly visits are highly desirable.

Scheduling Visits to Industrial Plants. When part-time nursing service is provided to an industry the amount of service to be provided will be determined by the administrative officer of the nursing service and the industry.

Visits should be scheduled at regular intervals. As with schools, some time should be reserved for attendance at meetings and for necessary conferences and follow-up work. Wherever possible, visits should be planned so that workers on all shifts have an opportunity to confer with the nurse. In general, not less than two hours of time should be scheduled for a visit.

Scheduling Clinic Time. Hours and days of clinic are usually decided by the administrator and physician providing the medical supervision, although the public health nurse may be asked to suggest suitable times. In planning for nursing time in clinics, time should be allowed for setting up the clinic equipment, and for completing the necessary record and office work following the clinic period. Volunteers may assist with one or both of these activities, with consequent reduction of the nursing time that must be scheduled.

Scheduling Group Activities. This has been discussed more fully in Chapter XII. In scheduling:

1. Choose a time of year that has a minimum of other conflicting demands on time—holiday periods, farm responsibilities (avoid harvesting time, chicken hatching time, etc.), and no special travel hazards or difficulties.
2. The day of week is also important—Mondays and Fridays seem unpopular days in urban areas. In rural communities, days that may coincide with shopping days are usually good.
3. Choose an hour that is suitable. Evening classes may reach men as well as women; late morning or early afternoon hours are less apt to conflict with household or farm chores, or getting children from school; the hour immediately after work may be a good one for industrial workers.

In scheduling, ample time should be allowed for activities before and after the actual meeting session. These may be very important in securing maximum outcomes from the group work.

Scheduling Home Calls. Home calls should be scheduled with consideration for convenience in relation to travel and fitness of time for the service scheduled. Obviously, if insulin is to be administered the time must be adapted to the meal habits of the individual; instruction in bathing the baby will be more acceptable if at the time the bath would ordinarily be given.

Appointments should be made for visits which are not scheduled daily. Noneffective calls will be minimized by good scheduling, choosing a day and time when families are apt to be at home. When visits are made infrequently, a volunteer worker may be asked to phone or send a postcard reminder just prior to the visit.

Sometimes it is possible to make combination calls when several families are near one another and have similar problems. There may be several families in a housing project, for example, who need help with care of measles, or in bathing the baby. Meeting in a group in one of the homes may not only save time, but also allow the patients to learn from one another as well as from the nurse.

Blocks of time for home calls should be scheduled following special clinic activities or physical examination periods at school.

Scheduling in a Rural Service.   The nurse in a rural area will probably need to plan her schedule on a community or zone basis. The public health nurse in a county may have many miles to cover; unless some plan is developed for grouping services and calls on a geographic basis, an exorbitant amount of time may be spent in travel, and the community may feel that it gets little return from the money spent for nursing service. By dividing the territory into zones or subdistricts, each community will receive its allotted share of time and work can be sufficiently concentrated so that its benefits are apparent to the community, and travel time will be held to a minimum.

In planning for such division of the nursing territory, it is desirable that each zone have sufficient population to justify spending at least a day in that community within the scheduling unit (the scheduling unit may be either a week or month). The allocation of time to zones should be such that there is allowance for emergencies, nonservice activities, office work, and for special programs that might develop in one or another of the communities covered. Usually there is provision for some sort of sub-office in each zone, with facilities for taking calls or messages for the nurse. This may be in the school or other public building. Each subdistrict or zone should be visited at a regular time each week or month so that the community members can plan ahead for nursing service and know at what times they may consult with the nurse. Within this framework of zoning, the nurse will plan for her daily activities.

To take an example, in a county that employs one public health nurse there may be three centers of population, the largest one being the county seat in which the nurse's headquarters are located. The county may be divided into three zones of approximately the same area, each including one of the principal towns and surrounding rural territory. A schedule may be devised allowing one day weekly for each of the smaller population zones and two days for the larger one. One day might be allowed for emergencies, special programs or in-service education, and a half day for office or other administrative work. The schedule would then look like this:

> Monday: Zone A (county seat)
> Tuesday: Zone B.
> Wednesday: Open
> Thursday: Zone A
> Friday: Zone C
> Saturday (½ day): Office

FORM AND DISTRIBUTION OF SCHEDULES

The nurse's schedule should be constructed in graphic form whenever possible. It should show 'where' she is, 'when,' in 'what' activity she is engaged and with 'whom' she is visiting. A monthly planning calendar is useful for the nurse in rural areas and will provide general information as to where she can be reached at any given time. In urban services the nurse's daily report form may be written in duplicate, listing each activity on the day's itinerary in order, with one copy left in the nursing office.

The nurse's schedule should be readily available to anyone who may need to reach the nurse or plan to see her. The nurse in a department of health in a rural area will want the health officer or supervising nurse to have her general schedule or itinerary for each month. The nurse in a city agency may leave her schedule of visits in the office where it can be reached easily by the office supervisor or clerk. A schedule of hours of nursing service should be posted in the school or industrial health room when nursing service is on a part-time basis, and copies provided for the school principal, plant personnel director or general manager.

When the public health nurse has much occasion to plan or work with staff members of other agencies, this may require further distribution of her schedule. For example, a public health nurse working in a special program, such as service to cancer patients or a planned parenthood clinic, might want to make her schedule available to the nurses of the health department in order to facilitate planning for consultations or joint visits.

Good scheduling will conserve nursing time and improve the services given to families. Scheduling also promotes sound over-all program planning.

Program planning is an important phase of public health nursing and the nurse should allow adequate time for it. The nursing supervisor and administrator will work with the nurse to get a satisfactory plan, but the nurse herself must use imagination and independence in finding ways to apply the skills of nursing for community betterment.

CHAPTER XVI

Evaluating the
Nursing Program

EVALUATION IS an essential component of planning, and should be "built in" as the plan for service is constructed. The importance of evaluation of the various facets or units of public health nursing has already been stressed as part of the on-going program.

In addition to this concurrent or segmented evaluation, there is need for periodic evaluation of the program as a whole, or for services within the program, as a basis for program planning and service accounting, as well as for the improvement of professional practice.

There is much to be said for the quarterly interval as a time for program evaluation in public health nursing. This usually coincides with the agency budgetary review interval; it is a sufficiently long period to show trends and developments in service, yet short enough to provide for effective re-direction of the program if necessary within the year. Evaluation of program may be required by the agency from each nurse as part of her service, or it may be the responsibility of the supervisory or administrative nursing staff. Responsibility for evaluation will in all cases be a shared responsibility; the nursing supervisor and administrator, the health officer, the school principal or superintendent, the industrial physician, and the general management or personnel director in industry must be concerned with evaluation of nursing service that comes within their sphere of responsibility.

Whatever the pattern, each nurse must initiate and maintain a system of evaluating her own program, using the assistance of others as supplementary to her own value judgment, but not as a substitute for it.

WHAT EVALUATION IS

Program evaluation is a process that is designed to show the relationship between services rendered and the objectives or purposes of the service. It is not synonymous with measurement— measurement may supplement but not replace judgments in deciding what has significance. Mannheim says:

> "Instead of attempting to discover what is most significant with the highest degree of precision possible under the existing circumstances, one tends to be content to attribute importance to what is measurable merely because it tends to be measurable."[1]

Program evaluation is not a record or count of what was done, but of what *difference* the doing made. The number of prenatal visits made is significant only to the degree that the visits caused an increase in the expectant parent's security and confidence, protected the mother from unnecessary danger or discomfort during pregnancy and childbirth, extended the parents' knowledge and improved their attitudes toward parenthood, created new patterns of daily living that might be expected to affect favorably the general health of the family.

Neither quantity nor quality of service alone is adequate in program evaluation; both must be seen as they relate to each other and to the total needs of the group served. For instance, excellent prenatal service that can be provided only to about 10 percent of those who need it may represent a situation in which the quality lowers the level of service to the population as a whole; a larger number of visits of a lower quality might actually produce greater change in the total community health.

Program evaluation cannot be an isolated activity; the nursing program must be evaluated in its relationship to other services within the agency, and other nursing services in the community. The evaluation of well-baby care can be seen only as it relates to the total agency program for mothers and babies, to the hospital pattern of care, and to the services provided by physicians and midwives.

Program evaluation is concerned with human as well as technical achievements; how people feel about the program and the degree to which the program activities produces satisfaction to

1. Karl Mannheim, *Ideaology and Utopia*. New York, Harvest Books, 1936, pp. 51–52.

the family, the nurse and the community may be as significant as the measure of deaths or disabilities prevented. Corley's study of people's testimony regarding the health department is a heartening indication of their expectations and endorsement of the department's activities.[2] The reaction of private physicians, and their understanding of the visiting nurse's program will have real significance in the referral of cases for visiting nursing service, and so affect the degree to which the agency can accomplish its community objective of supplying care for those who need it. Those who receive or use the service should participate in its evaluation whenever possible. Clinic clients, for example, could be very helpful in determining to what extent the clinic is meeting patients' needs.

Program evaluation must be concerned with those *not* served as well as those who were, since public health nursing has the community as well as the individual as a patient. Furthermore, if those *not* served got along just as well as those who were served, the whole basis of evaluating progress may need reconsideration.

Depending upon the policies and customs of the agency, the public health nurse will take varying degrees of responsibility for:
1. Planning for program evaluation.
2. Evaluating the goals or purposes of the nursing service.
3. Collecting data on amounts, quality or results of nursing service.
4. Interpreting and using evaluation findings.

PLANNING FOR PROGRAM EVALUATION

Program evaluation may cover appraisal of:
1. Goals or purposes of the service.
2. Methods of delivering service to the recipients.
3. Service outcomes.

In planning for evaluation, the steps outlined below may provide a useful approach:
1. Write out, with some degree of specificity, the objectives of the service. This has been discussed in Chapter XV, and does not need elaboration here. Be sure they are (a) achievable, (b) important—that they may be expected to make a difference to the people served, (c) consistent with the objectives of the agency, (d) consistent with accepted standards. Fuzzy goals are a primary deterrent to evaluation.
2. Secure evidence of the degree to which objectives are being

2. Catherine Corley, Beyond What Is Required. *Nursing Outlook*, 3: 213–315, April, 1955.

achieved. For example, if the objective is to increase maternal competence, what evidence can be found to show that mothers under care were more able to cope with problems of child care as a result of the service? For example, what indications are there that some were tense and anxious in handling the baby at the initiation of service? Is there any evidence that they are less tense and anxious at the point of dismissal from service? Methods by which such information may be gathered are discussed below.

3. Gather facts about the processes and procedures by which the nurse is trying to realize the objectives of the service. Are interviews the major method? If so, are they essentially directive in character, with the nurse taking responsibility for teaching and advising, or are they essentially nondirective, with the family calling the cues? Are group procedures being used—to what extent, and in what pattern? Which groups are being reached by one or the other methods, and in what intensity?

4. Look for relationships between what was achieved and the methods used. Are the methods working toward or against the achievement of the objectives? For instance, if dependence upon group rather than individual methods results in giving more service to those who need it least, and less service to those with greater need under the present plan of using group work, it would seem to be interfering with the realization of objectives rather than helping, even though the numbers reached may be higher. At this point it may be possible only to obtain a "hunch" as to what effect the particular service afforded is contributing to getting the job done, and the matter may need further study, or separate evaluation of different methods.

Evaluation should inevitably lead to re-planning—trying out new approaches, new methods of case selection, new distribution of services as indicated by the evaluation finding. In re-planning the staff nurse will want to avail herself of consultation with her nursing supervisor, health officer or other consultant, supervisory or administrative personnel.

Evaluation of the program as a whole may be supplemented by evaluation of individual phases of the program; for example, the clinic service may be studied, with the study related to the home visiting services provided, but without a thorough study of home visits per se.

METHODS AND MEASUREMENTS

More precise methods of evaluation and the development of measurements for evaluation are urgently needed.[3] However, there are many approaches which the nurse herself may take to evaluate her program, independently or in coordination with others. Some of the most common methods are discussed here, though it is obvious that comprehensive coverage would not be possible.

Impression of the Nurse or Supervisory Personnel. The impression of the nurse or of appropriate supervisory personnel as to the values of a particular program is frequently used as a basis for evaluation. This measure is one frequently used in medical diagnosis, and may be very useful in evaluation despite its subjective nature. Impression of value is based upon professional knowledge and experience; the nurse's impression that patients are satisfied with the service they received, or that they are more sensitive to their needs, rests on the accumulated though intangible understanding of the meaning of a great many different patterns of physical, social or verbal reactions, and this in turn rests on a multitude of observations the nurse or supervisor has made before. This may be as satisfactory a measure as is feasible for judging the success of home care for psychiatric patients. When bolstered by concurrence of the supervisor and of the responsible medical officer, its value is increased. The use of impression of success as an approach is also safeguarded if there is an outline of questions that might be answered, which relate what the nurse thinks has happened in relation to the objectives of the service. For example, the nurse might ask, in relation to each case carried, and then summarize for the service as a whole, questions like the following:

Was the anxiety of the family reduced in relation to its ability to care for the patient during the course of the nursing service?

Did the family increase in its capacity to accept the patient without constraint, and include him naturally in its activities?

Did the family indicate an understanding of the treatment as a whole—the relationship between drug therapy and the total treatment process?

Was the family-hospital relationship strengthened through the home-care program?

It may not be possible to prove by objective evidence that anxiety was reduced, but the traditionally acute observation of the nurse and the relatedness of her observations will put together

3. Evaluation in Public Health. *Public Health Reports,* 71: 525–529, June, 1956.

facial and bodily expressions, tones of voice, things said and unsaid in a conversation, arrangements made for placement of the patient's bed and his presence at family meals or other occasions into a total impression of increased, unchanged or decreased anxiety in relation to patient care and acceptance of the patient as a person.

Analysis of Statistical Reports. Statistical reports are a valuable source of information for evaluation of a program. From them the nurse may learn to what degree the program is reaching those who need it; for example, she might compare the number of primiparous patients delivered with the number who received nursing care during the prenatal period; or the number of premature babies discharged from local hospitals with the number reported for nursing service.

A study of patients by the census tract in which they reside may give valuable clues to the types of patients reached, since census tracts will differ greatly in the type and extent of health and social problems.[4] If patients are bunched in the localities with a low socioeconomic status the question should be asked as to whether the area does in fact represent the greatest need.

Statistical reports of her own case load will reveal the degree of balance the program has achieved. It may reveal a greatly skewed pattern in favor of certain services that the nurse enjoys carrying, or that represent a strong community interest or demand. For example, school services may have taken a disproportionate amount of time in relation to anticipated service needs; or there may be a very small number of industrial service visits for general health counseling.

Statistics regarding the numbers of patients on home care for tuberculosis and those under the nurse's supervision may reveal deficiencies in service.

Statistics that indicate intensity of care—the number of nursing service units—may reveal over or under nursing patterns in different services.

Statistics regarding the types of service rendered may indicate the balance between personal therapeutic care and teaching or counseling.

It must be remembered that statistics alone do not provide an answer, it is only as they are interpreted in the light of the objec-

4. Rider, Rowland V., Matthew Tayback and Hilda Knobloch, Association between Premature Birth and Socio-Economic Status. *American Journal of Public Health,* 45: 1022–1028, August, 1955.

tives of the service that they gain significance. For example, skewing of time allocation in favor of school nursing may be desirable if the community is shifting from full-time specialized school nurses to generalized nursing service, to ease the adjustment; a decrease in patient load among a group with high needs for prenatal care may be entirely desirable if it coincides with a much-extended teaching program in the hospital.

Record Review. Nursing records may be reviewed for evidence of changes in family health behavior, of patterns of service provided, of family reaction to care, and the approaches or methods used that may have influenced the outcome.

A record analysis plan should be worked out to facilitate collection of relevant material in the light of the objectives of the service. For example, in reviewing clinic records in a well-child service as a basis for evaluation of the service the information might be secured from the record, the types of problem discussed, action taken as a result of clinic visits, and responsibility of the parent as shown by proportion of appointments kept. Figure 19 shows an example of a work sheet that might be used for securing information pertinent to evaluation.

When the number of records is large, a sample of the records may be used. If there is a biostatistician on the staff he will help to indicate what an adequate sample would be; if not, the nurse may review every fourth, fifth or tenth record in the files to secure a number that she feels would be representative of the total clinic case load.

The use of records as an indication of service quality is limited by the great variation in completeness of recording, and by the fact that the record often does not indicate the feelings of the family, or the inter-personal facets of the family-nurse contact. However, records do permit a quick overview of many cases, and may be helpful in providing information not easily obtainable from other sources.

Tests. Paper-and-pencil tests are rarely suitable for evaluation of nursing service. Most of the families cared for are unaccustomed to tests and may even fear them; furthermore the nature of nursing service in many instances does not lend itself to this type of evaluation. Sometimes the use of pre- and post-tests in group instruction, such as instruction in home nursing, may be acceptable to the numbers and a good measure of progress made. Even here, however, evaluating the starting level of knowledge and skill and the degree attained at the end of the class is

Case No.	Date Adm.	Age Adm.	No. Appts.				Feeding		Phys. Care			Prev. Med.		Emotional Reaction			Fam. Rel.		Referral			Comments, incl. Care Other Fam. Members.
			Tot.	Kept	Canc.	Miss.	Sel.	Behav.	Bath	Sleep	Oth.	Imm.	Oth.	TCL	Relax	Sibs.	Hus-W	P-Ch	Med.	Welf.	Oth.	
1	12/5		5	4	0	1	DD (D)	D	(D)							D						
2	8/12		8	2	2	4			(D)													
3	1/18		4	4	0	0	(D)					(D)			D		(D)					Mother tries but very anxious

D = Problems discussed.
D = Action agreed upon.
(D) = Action taken or improvements noted.

Figure 19.   Record analysis work sheet—Well-Child Clinic.

more often based on the nurse's observation of the patient and upon informal conversation, rather than upon a written test. For special studies, tests may prove useful, as in the study of the effectiveness of home nursing instruction by television done by Shimberg and Aird.[5]

Securing Reactions or Opinions from Those Served.   Families, private physicians using the service, hospitals or other agencies referring cases for care, and physicians responsible for medical care of clinic patients will often have valuable ideas regarding the quality and practicality of the service they have received. Reactions may be secured by informal inquiry by the nurse, by the use of some form of questionnaire, or in group discussion.

For example, the nurse in the well-child clinic may ask a small group of mothers to meet with her to discuss how well the nursing service they are receiving meets their needs and those of their friends. Or, at the conclusion of service, the nurse might ask the family members what they would have liked but didn't get from nursing service, or what they felt was most and least helpful as a basis for planning service for other families.

In one visiting nurse service a sample number of physicians who had used the service and an equal number of physicians who had not used the service were visited and asked to indicate what they felt the visiting nurse service should do. If they had used the service they were asked to indicate for what types of problem they had requested service, and what, if any, services they had asked for but could not get. This was very revealing in relation to the degree to which the expectations of the physicians were met.

Process Records.   Process records, a written account of what went on during a family-nurse contact, including what was done, what was said and a description of the evidences of feelings or reactions of all who were involved, may provide a good basis for evaluation.[6] Process recording was discussed in Chapter XI and will not be elaborated here.

Discussion of a process record with other nurses, or with the supervisor, may produce many cues to successful or unsuccessful approaches to nursing service and to inter-personal relationships in the family-nurse contact.

Using Consultants, Individually or in a Team, for Evaluation of Program.   Regularly scheduled evaluation conferences are be-

5. Shimberg, Benjamin and Ellen Aird, Effectivenesss of Television in Teaching Home Nursing. *Nursing Research*, 4: 28–41, June, 1955.

6. Walker, Janet F. and Mary McQuillen, Process Recording in Public Health Nursing. *Public Health Nursing*, 44: 542–547, October, 1952.

coming a more frequent procedure in health departments and voluntary agencies. Sometimes the conference centers around the total service rendered by the agency, sometimes the service of one discipline or department, and sometimes around the work of a single nurse or other professional worker. In a rural health department, for example, the entire staff may meet quarterly to review what has been done. Each service will report what has happened to date, and the staff as a whole will discuss how well this has met the service objectives. The post-clinic conference procedure suggested in Chapter XX is one type of joint evaluation conference.

When consultants are used for evaluation, the nurse's responsibility is to assemble the information needed to show what was done in her service toward meeting the objectives that were set. She may indicate that certain types of visits have increased, and present such information as she can about what was done in these visits and what effect they have had as shown by objective evidence or in her own judgment. She may present evidence about those not reached by the service, or work not done because it was considered to have a lower priority than the selected activities. The group may then discuss the basis of her selection of activities, react to the program outcomes, suggest a new approach or clarify needs that the nurse may have missed. For example, the sanitarian might say that a certain school building is being neglected. The nurse may report that her efforts to get better equipment for the school lunch have been fruitless because there is a movement afoot for a new school building, and the authorities are reluctant to spend anything on the old school. Perhaps a less expensive temporary set-up could be suggested, which would be acceptable to the community, yet provide for safer handling of food.

The same approach might be used in preparing to evaluate the program with a supervising nurse, health educator, or other consultant.

Securing Information on Health Behavior after Service Has Been Given. Direct observation of health behavior may be arranged in many cases if there is good planning. For example, the nurse may plan to visit a home at the time when the baby will be being bathed, or at meal times; she may observe the children's selection of foods at the school cafeteria, or handwashing practices in the washroom. Sometimes evaluation visits may be made to a family after the case has been dismissed to determine what is being done and whether there are instances of change in health behavior.

Case Discussion. Group case discussion and analysis represent another useful evaluation device. Through discussion of a single case, the criteria of excellence in service may be defined, and the nurse may be helped to evaluate some general aspects of her work as well as her performance in this particular situation. For example, in discussing a family in which there is a man with syphilis, the case discussion may revolve around the major objectives of service: to secure early, complete treatment; to locate contacts and get them under care; to protect the individual's personality. In the discussion, there may be much consideration of the relative value of having an individual take responsibility for bringing contacts to the clinic himself, rather than having the health department representative bring them in. Discussion may bring out how one could weigh the professional worker's greater knowledge and skill against the social values inherent in helping one's self and others; or judge the degree of understanding to be sure the infected person is really able to interpret to another the reasons for securing an examination; or sense distress so as to recognize when the infected person may not be able to admit to another that he has exposed her to the disease. Qualitative factors of counseling and interviewing that are applicable to many situations may be brought out with particular clarity in such a case discussion, as would the philosophy and methods of safeguarding a person's good opinion of himself in difficult situations.

These methods are, of course, merely a sampling of the many approaches that may be used in the evaluation of nursing service. Most are within the capacities of the staff nurse to do herself, with guidance from her supervisor. The important thing in using any method of measurement is to remember that measurement is not evaluation, but only a part of it; and to recognize that when only one segment of a program is evaluated it must be seen in its relation to the whole.

INTERPRETING AND USING EVALUATION FINDINGS

There is little value in knowing how well a task was done, unless there is also some understanding of *why* the results occurred, and what might be done to modify them. If the nurse discovers that prenatal patients who are under the care of private physicians are not coming in for care, she needs to know whether it is because the physician does not see the need for it or actually opposes the use of the public health nurse; whether the patients and their families feel that public health nursing is only for the poor, or that health department services are only for the control of communicable diseases and nuisances; whether the services afforded are not adapted to those in the moderate or upper income groups in content, presentation or method of organization. If her success with emotional problems is low, she must know whether it is because she has inadequate information, or because her own emotional needs are so pressing that they interfere with her capacity to help others; or because lack of time has produced a pattern of hurried visits which are not effective for such service.

Tracking down the causes of failure to meet objectives through service may require more time and study. The nurse may have a hunch that her failure to secure much progress in bettering mother-child relations is because of a too directive approach in interviewing. To determine whether this is so, she may need to have someone observe her interviews to see to what extent her practice is really directive, or to make tape recordings and study them herself for this factor. Then she may need to try out a pattern of less directive interviewing with a selected group of patients, and watch as carefully as possible for evidences of its effectiveness. If it seems that her hunch was right, she may then push ahead with the new approach on a more general basis, looking to the next general evaluation period to show what influence this may have on the outcomes.

Discussion with consultant and administrative staff, or with experts in other fields or agencies, may also prove helpful. The health officer might help to decide whether it would be wise to try to reduce the total number of visits, but make each visit more intensive for tuberculosis cases; the social worker in the welfare agency might be very helpful in identifying elements of interviewing that might be critical in influencing others; the maternal and child health consultant might help with specific ways of improving service to premature babies.

Thoughtful evaluation is basic to planning and to the successful accomplishment of public health nursing. The consultant and supervisory staff may provide assistance, but in the final analysis it is the nurse herself who must study her own work in the light of her service objectives.

CHAPTER XVII

Office Management,
Records and Reports

THE PUBLIC health nurse will have varying degrees of administrative responsibility for selection and care of a nursing office or center and for maintaining records and reports of the service. In some agencies the major share of these activities will be the responsibility of the supervisor or nursing administrator.

THE NURSING OFFICE

THE NURSING OFFICE is the nurse's workshop. It serves as a place for planning and appraising work, for conferring with other health workers, patients or families, for receiving calls or messages, and for storing official records and correspondence. Sometimes it doubles as a classroom or clinic, or as a rest room for sick school children or industrial workers.

The nurse in a large agency may have little responsibility for office management, other than to cooperate in keeping the work environment tidy and quiet. In the small agency the nurse may select and equip her own headquarters, office and sub-stations, arrange for clerical assistance, set up office systems for care of correspondence or for management of financial or service records and reports.

Location. The office of the nurse employed by a health department is usually located in a public building. It may be in the health center, the county courthouse or the public school. In the construction of new community hospitals, space is frequently provided for a health center, and the office of the public health nurse may be located there. Sub-stations in health departments may be located in clinic quarters, and the nurse in industry or in school will, of course, have her office in the school or industrial plant.

If the office site has not already been determined, the following criteria for selection may be helpful:

1. The office should be convenient to transportation but not necessarily in the center of town. If patients travel by car, parking space should be available.
2. The office should not be in a church, club or other building that is associated with a particular religious or political group.
3. The office should be convenient to those of related services or agencies when possible. Closeness to hospitals, schools or welfare agencies facilitates planning for conferences and encourages frequent informal contacts that are helpful in building good relationships.

    The industrial health room should be near the employment and personnel offices if possible; the school health room close to the counseling and administrative staff of the school. The county nurse may have her office near that of the health officer, in a school or close to the welfare office.
4. The office should have a separate entrance. Families or patients should not have to go through another room when visiting the nurse's office. Employees who are injured or ill should not go through other workrooms when they go for medical or nursing care.

    If major accidents are a problem, the entrance of the office should be convenient to an automobile driveway.

Basic Facilities.   The office should have certain basic facilities including:

1. Running water.
2. Toilet facilities located in or near the nursing office.
3. Walls clean and in good condition. A light, attractive paint with a dull rather than a gloss finish is preferable to wallpaper.
4. Windows with shades that permit regulation of light.
5. Adequate lighting fixtures and electrical outlets.
6. Adequate ventilation and freedom from unusual noise, odors, dangerous processes or material, or vibration.
7. Floors that are in good condition. Linoleum or composition floors are more easily cleaned than wooden floors.
8. A telephone or telephone service.

When the nursing territory is large, it may be advisable to

establish sub-stations to serve as consultation or service centers or as places to leave messages or calls during the nurse's absence. Sub-stations should be located in places where people are accustomed to go, and that are acceptable to all groups served. They should be near the people to be reached, within a local telephone or single-fare area, if possible. There should be reasonably full telephone coverage, and someone to take calls who is responsible and can be trusted to protect the interests and respect the confidence of families.

Schools, public libraries, clinics, hospitals or other public agencies may provide space for patient consultation on a temporary basis during the days the nurse visits a particular community, or for storage of equipment, supplies or records. The school clerk or librarian may be willing to take calls or messages for the nurse between her visits to the community. Sometimes the chairman or member of the local nursing committee may volunteer to take calls for the nurse, and to keep such interim records and materials as may be needed.

Equipment. Proper office equipment will do much to facilitate the nurse's work.

In states where rural nurses are responsible for office selection and maintenance, the public health nursing unit of the state health department will be able to provide information about equipment that is desirable for the local nursing office. Frequently this is included as part of a manual for public health nursing. The office should provide for:

1. Such diagnostic or testing equipment (vision-testing materials, scales, etc.) as is in current use.
2. Storage for record forms and a locked file for patient records and correspondence, and storage for nursing supplies.
3. Space for office conferences with individuals or families.
4. Instructional equipment for demonstration, audio-visual teaching aids, etc.
5. Basic manuals and reference materials.

Correspondence. In the small nursing office it may be necessary for the public health nurse to set up a system for handling and filing correspondence, bulletins or other official communications.

All correspondence should be professional and business-like. For example, a teacher is asked to make certain preparations prior to the nurse's visit, or is sent information following a school examination session. Such correspondence should be handled as official even though the nurse and teacher are good personal friends and on informal terms. The letters should be typed whenever possible and written on official stationery in suitable professional style. They should be kept as part of the official office correspondence. Informal word-of-mouth agreements should, in most cases, be confirmed in writing to avoid misunderstanding and to forestall forgetting.

Since correspondence forms a part of the official records of the agency, it should be stored in such a way as to keep it safe and accessible. A metal file case with a lock is desirable. If the file drawer of the nurse's desk is used for such correspondence, the desk should be provided with a lock to protect correspondence of a confidential nature.

Bulletins, directives and other official communications should be filed where they are easily found and accessible, usually by subject. Correspondence and bulletins should be filed promptly to avoid loss or misuse.

Use of Clerical Assistants.   The public health nurse on a large staff will work with paid clerical personnel. This clerical staff may be supervised by an office manager or administrative assistant, and the nurse's responsibility is usually limited to understanding and cooperating in the procedures that require both professional and clerical service. In a small branch office or substation where a single clerk or volunteer or part-time personnel may be used, the public health nurse may have greater responsibility for directing and supervising the work.

Selection of clerical staff or volunteer is important. Such workers should be responsible and not prone to gossip, able to work with confidential material without betraying the trust of families or of the agency. They should be friendly and interested in helping people, since the office assistant or clerk may be the person the patient or family meets first in the agency. If the clerk or office assistant is responsible for taking requests for nursing service, she will also need good judgment since it will be necessary to decide under what conditions a situation is sufficiently important to warrant calling it to the attention of the nurse at once, and when calls may wait for the nurse's regular visit to the office or community.

CASE RECORDS

Individual or family health records are a valuable administrative and family guidance tool. To the degree that records are selective in content, comprehensive, accurate and organized for effective use, they will contribute to the total care of the family, as well as provide a dependable account of the patient's condition and of treatments or other services rendered. They provide the basis for relating nursing service to that of other workers or agencies.

Form and Content. Record forms and general content are usually determined by the administrative staff of the agency. On the basis of experience of many agencies, state health departments or national professional agencies or agencies such as the National League for Nursing, the Public Health Service or the Children's Bureau may suggest record forms or supply standard forms for use in local agencies.[1] The public health staff nurse may, however, make valuable suggestions regarding content or format based upon her own use of the forms provided.

Records may be constructed on an individual or family basis. There may be separate record forms for each type of health situation or service, such as a tuberculosis record, an infant health supervision record or a maternity record, or a single record may be used for an integrated statement of total health needs. Sometimes the health record is combined with a personnel record or a school-guidance record. In some agencies a record that provides for machine tabulation may be used, either in addition to or in place of other record forms. In this type of record a code is used to designate the necessary information regarding the situation and the care provided. Much experimentation is underway to determine the best ways of using machine tabulation for nursing services, and this will undoubtedly bring many changes in case recording.

Whether a single, integrated health record is used for the entire family, or a group of records is assembled in a family folder or envelope, or as part of another form, the total record should contain essential information as listed below:

1. Identifying information.
2. Significant health history and present health status.
3. Family factors that affect care.
4. A statement of health needs.
5. A statement of plans for health care.
6. A statement of nursing services rendered.

1. The Department of Public Health Nursing, National League for Nursing has a Record Loan folder that may be borrowed for study.

7. A statement of changes in the situation and results of service.

Certain items may be specifically indicated in particular instances. For example, under health history and present health status the industrial record might provide for history of dermatosis or allergy, and for work-capacity rating; the tuberculosis record, for names and addresses of contacts and results of diagnostic tests; the infant supervision record, for a report of medical findings.

The amount and type of *identifying information* will vary somewhat from one service to another. Names, age and sex of family members (including maiden name of mother); address and telephone number, including travel directions in rural areas, floor and apartment numbers in urban communities; location within the service unit, for example, the grade in school, the department or section in industry; in the hospital or clinic, the clinic or health service number is commonly required. Color, citizenship and insurance status including policy or social security numbers may be required both for identification and for determining eligibility for certain types of care.

In most instances, all necessary identification data are indicated on the record form, and the public health nurse has only to see that all items are completed. When the record form does not include information regularly used (such as name of the county in which the family resides, or type of housing), a rubber stamp may be secured and the item added to the form. This avoids having to remember to collect the information each time, and makes it easier to secure a complete record.

History of past illness, pregnancies and accidents and of health practices provides a basis for appraisal of the present situation. In the history of pregnancy or disease it is important to know whether recovery was prompt and uneventful. Possible precursors of disease should also be noted when relevant: use of unpasteurized milk, exposure to communicable disease, dietary deficiencies, and so forth. In certain communicable diseases such as typhoid fever an exhaustive study of possible disease-related activities will be necessary. A record of contacts is especially important in tuberculosis, syphilis and gonorrhea.

Present health status includes medical diagnosis (if there is disease or impairment), general condition as reflected in physical examination or inspection, and health practices when they are significant. If there is frank illness, the medical diagnosis should be recorded in detail and the condition of the patient should be described carefully, including general appearance, any observable or reported symptoms, the temperature, and pulse and respiration rates. The medical diagnosis should be secured directly from the physician, hospital or clinic rather than from the family, in order to avoid error. The physician may be asked to write his diagnosis and orders on the nursing record that is left in the home, or the nurse may telephone or see the physician and request the diagnosis at the time she talks with him about the patient's care.

When there is no disease or impairment, the present health status may be the nurse's statement of the general health condition as shown in physical examination findings, reports of other health services, or her own observation. General vitality, emotional stability and maturity, freedom from minor health conditions and unusual fatigue should be noted. Present health practices should be considered, and when significant should be noted on the record. For example, if a young man habitually gets only five or six hours of sleep, or a young woman uses her lunch hour to shop because she never eats lunch, these facts are significant even though there may be no evidence that they are producing any physical reaction.

Family factors that affect care include the facilities, attitudes and experiences of the family that will make a difference in planning to meet health needs. The adequacy of the home as a place to care for a sick person, or as a place where children can practice desirable health habits; family income as it affects purchasing power in terms of food, shelter and medical care; educational background as it provides a basis for present health teaching or ability to solve problems independently are examples of family factors that are important to know and record.

Attitudes of the family toward this illness and toward illness in general, as well as its attitude toward the community agencies that provide health care are also important. There will be families who "don't believe in doctoring" and those who call the city ambulance at every sneeze; those who refuse surgery because they "know cancer is hopeless" and those who take an intelligent interest in their disease and the possibility of cure; those who welcome the representative of the health department as someone who can help, and those who give a false address so they "won't be hounded." Each needs to have plans for health care adjusted to meet its particular need.

Attitudes of the family members toward one another may also be significant. For example, in one family there may be a strongly paternalistic pattern. Children may be taught to obey, to be quiet and polite, never to question the decision of their elders. In another family the group may be closely knit, interdependent, with parents and children sharing responsibilities and fun. In still another family, its members may seem to be residing in the same house by accident, each going his own way, with few common bonds or interests. Obviously, health problems must be met quite differently in each of these family groups.

The *statement of health needs* should include needs for nursing care, for health instruction guidance or emotional support, and for referral to other health or related social or educational agencies.

The *statement of plans* for health care should include the physician's orders and directions for care as well as the family's plan for action. Physician's orders should be secured directly from him, either in writing or by telephone or personal conference. Dates on which orders were given should be indicated, as well as the date on which they were discontinued. When the doctor advises that routine care be given or standing orders followed, the nurse should be certain that these statements are adequately defined. If the agency does not have printed standing orders or routines for care, the nurse should indicate to the doctor her understanding of what would be included in such care, and be certain that it has his approval.

The family's plan for care should be clearly and concisely stated. The nurse may note modifications or extensions of this plan that may be made at a later time. Services planned or to be rendered by another agency should also be indicated when they are pertinent.

The statement of *nursing services rendered* to the family should include treatments or nursing care given by the nurse; demonstration or supervision of nursing care given by the family or other worker; instruction, guidance or other supportive measures offered; and referral to other agencies or individuals. The record of nursing care or treatments given should be free from expressions or abbreviations that are not commonly used. When instruction or guidance is recorded it should be specific enough to serve as a basis for future visits. "Advised about prenatal care" means nothing. "Discussed the importance and content of prenatal physical examination, assured patient that hospital records are confidential" indicates the scope and direction of the instruction. When referrals are noted they should be specific also. In a large city, "referred to prenatal clinic" is not very helpful; "referred to St. Jude's Hospital prenatal clinic, Thursday afternoon" enables the nurse to follow through intelligently on the next visit to the family. When several different nurses are involved or if visits are infrequent, a more complete description is necessary than when all care is given by a single nurse within a relatively short span of time.

The statement of *changes in the situation and results of service* should include a description of the patient's condition and re-action to treatment, and the results of nursing guidance and in-struction. In acute illness the nurse's observation of the patient is particularly valuable, since the frequency of the physician's visits is not great, and the physician is apt to depend upon the nurse's report. Treatments given and the patient's reaction to them should be fully described. Evidence of changes in health behavior or increased skill in caring for sick members of the family should be noted. Use of community health facilities and the family's reaction to their use are also important indices of progress.

The *summary note* should provide a statement of the situation at the time the case is closed, and a brief evaluation of the nursing service provided to the family. If the family is to stay under the supervision of some other health agency that infor-mation should be noted. If the situation has not been satis-factorily resolved at the time of dismissal the reason should be indicated if it is known. For example, if a family is dismissed from care with no noticeable improvement in health practices, the nurse may indicate that the family resists all assistance and instruction, and that further service would probably be wasted. If a child with impaired vision has not secured glasses, the reason may be that the family did not have the money for glasses, or that there was no community agency that would provide them.

As has been previously mentioned, additional or slightly dif-ferent information may be required for records in specific situa-tions. By studying the uses to which the records will be put, the public health nurse should be able to recognize the need for additional or modified record content.

This description of necessary record content has not been or-ganized to conform to any particular record format. Identifying data may be recorded on the face of the record, on a family folder or envelope; the statement of needs and plans for care may be recorded on the face of the record, on a family folder or envelope; the statement of needs and plans for care may be segregated with the medical diagnosis or may appear as part of the nurse's narrative notes; planning and progress may be recorded in the narrative notes or placed on a summary sheet or designated column on the record. Whatever the record format, the public health nurse should secure and put in writing the information that is essential for family nursing care and health guidance.

Securing Record Information. The method by which the nurse gathers record information will make a great difference in the type and quality of the information obtained. It is important to secure the understanding and cooperation of the family in obtaining the necessary facts; to exercise sufficient imagination to uncover significant information that might otherwise not be mentioned; and to devise methods for checking the accuracy of the data.

Interpreting the purpose and confidential nature of health records will help to assure a free response to questions. The individual or family should understand that records are used to make nursing service more effective, and that they may provide an account of health conditions and treatment that will be important in future medical care. Families may also appreciate knowing that the information they provide, when combined with that from hundreds of other families, may serve as the basis for increasing medical knowledge or for promoting more adequate community facilities for care.

It is also important to emphasize that the *information secured is confidential* in nature, and will not be available to anyone but professional health workers. The family should know if others do have access to the record (such as teachers, personnel directors, social case workers), or if no information is released without the consent of the family.

Requesting only essential information will help to avoid resistance to supplying necessary record data. Sometimes agency policy demands that the nurse collect certain items of information for every case, and she is not free to adapt record content in accordance with need. She may, however, interpret to supervisory and administrative staff some of the problems associated with collecting information that is seldom if ever used, and present evidence of the fact that the information is not necessary. For example, questions about family income may be resented if not needed to determine eligibility for care. For those who are not requesting subsidized care it may be sufficient to note that the income is adequate, or to note the occupation of the wage earner, without specifying the exact amount of income.

An *easy, conversational approach* helps to secure information. Such an informal approach serves the further purpose of providing an occasion for counseling or for investigation of health needs that have not been reported or discussed before. For example, in recording the ages of the children in the family, one nurse may simply ask the question and record the answers. She finds out the ages of the children and nothing more. Another nurse, when mother says "Johnny's six" may note the fact, but add, "That's certainly an interesting age!" or "Then he's in school. Does he like it?" The second nurse may find that Johnny's mother is worried; the mother might say, "It may be interesting, but Johnny's so fresh I don't know what to do with him"; or "He likes school all right but I get worried because he seems to get so excited about it; I can't seem to calm him down after school." The nurse has built a feeling of mutual interest, has secured fuller information and has an opportunity for counseling if it is needed.

Indirect questioning is rarely desirable. Examples of this approach might be securing information about the family income by asking a general question such as "Do steam fitters get a very good salary these days?" or determining a woman's age by getting the date she was married and her age at that time. Such circuitous questioning is apt to give the family the feeling that they are being "pumped" for information.

Probing for relevant facts may require special skill. For example, in completing an epidemiologic record, the nurse should be familiar with the ways in which the disease may be spread, and be prepared to follow up every possible lead. In typhoid fever investigations, when food may be suspected as a source of infection, the nurse's questions must be focussed so as to secure the fullest possible information about all food eaten by the family. She will ask questions about food eaten at home and where it was purchased, about meals taken in restaurants, or food brought to the home by neighbors or friends. She will ask who prepared the food, and double check for foods that are high on the suspect list. When recording food intake she will check information by supplementary questions such as "Did you have any snacks between meals?", or "Did you have coffee or anything at any of your neighbor's homes?". In a similar manner, the industrial nurse will direct questions so as to secure information about reactions to irritating substances that are used in the particular section where the man works, or check on all possible contributing causes such as improper handwashing or home repair activities that may be factors in determining the cause of a dermatosis. The nurse must have a broad knowledge of the health conditions common to the group she serves, and sufficient imagination to obtain all of the relevant facts.

Rephrasing questions may be necessary when accuracy is particularly important. For example, in determining the date of onset of a communicable disease, the family may report that the child became ill three days ago. The question may be asked in another way to check the information by saying "Then Johnny was in school on Tuesday." The answer to the second question may reveal that Johnny wasn't well enough to go to school on Tuesday, and that the onset of the disease was four rather than three days prior to the visit.

Writing the Record.　　Information should be recorded at the time and place most likely to insure accuracy and completeness. Some record information may be secured and recorded prior to the visit. It may be possible to ascertain the physician's diagnosis and orders for care, the report of hospital or clinic treatments, physical examination findings and recommendations, or a summary of previous contacts with the nursing service.

In general, it is desirable to record identifying information and such facts as are necessary to determine eligibility for certain types of care or are required for planning on the first visit. Properly prepared, families will accept the need for providing necessary information at this time. Of course, if the family is greatly upset and the household disorganized, as it might be if the nursing visit coincided with removal of the patient to the hospital, it might be necessary to postpone recording. Prompt completion of records, however, provides a basis for planning future nursing visits. It also minimizes the danger of failing to secure necessary data; it is easy to forget to collect information in later visits.

The report of each family-nurse contact should be written during or immediately following the visit, to insure accuracy. When the visit is made in the patient's home, recording may be done there or in the nurse's office, depending upon the type of information to be recorded. When direct patient care is being provided or treatments are being given, information is usually best recorded in the home at the same time the report is being written for the physician. Instructional or guidance information, on the other hand, may sometimes be more easily recorded in the nurse's office where there are fewer distractions, and when there is time to consider wording and organization of the record content more carefully. Some agencies, because of their method of cost accounting or for other reasons, may require that records be written in the home. When such regulations exist they will, of course, determine the way in which recording will be done.

Securing Information from Other Agencies. Information from physicians, teachers, social workers, hospitals and other individuals or agencies concerned with the family's health may be incorporated in the health record. Such information should be collected with discrimination, requesting only that material that might be expected to contribute to the care of the family.

When asking another agency for information, the nurse should explain her interest in the family, and indicate what nursing service is being given. A written request should be used if the information requires that the other agency review and abstract their records. When information is requested by telephone, the nurse should try to select a convenient time to call.

It is seldom necessary to collect information about families from other than agency or professional sources. When information is secured from relatives, neighbors or employers great care should be exercised to protect the patient and family, and to avoid any implication of "snooping."

Methods of Recording. However valid and pertinent record content may be, it cannot serve its purpose if the information is not clear and readily located.

Wording is important. An overlengthy record makes it difficult to locate essential information and to establish the relative importance of the various elements in the situation. By conscious attention to the wording of record notes, and use of the dictionary or thesaurus to select the most descriptive word, the nurse can improve her ability to write in a comprehensive yet succinct manner. Such care in the choice of words will also produce a record that is not subject to misinterpretation. For example, to describe a young mother as "immature" is bound to result in many different interpretations of the situation. More accurate description is necessary if misinterpretation is to be avoided.

Abbreviations should be used with care. Some nurses develop their own system of abbreviation that cannot be understood by others. Abbreviations may also grow up in a particular hospital or agency and be meaningless to anyone outside that particular situation.

Information of primary importance in guiding care should be so placed or specially indicated that it can be located quickly. Such information may be placed in a specially designated place on the record (as the surname, that almost invariably appears in the upper corner of the record to facilitate filing), or it may be marked by the use of a different colored ink, underlining, or a marginal notation.

It is particularly important that health needs and plans for care be clearly stated and readily located. Without some provision for marking this information there is danger of fragmentary planning and inadequate follow through on problems.

Reports to Other Agencies.   When other agencies are providing care to the family, reports of nursing visits should be made to them as necessary. In some instances, reports should be sent following each visit or contact by the nurse. The physician, for example, will probably want to be informed of the condition of his patient, the nursing care given and progress made following each visit. This report may be left in the home if the physician is calling regularly. In cases of acute and chronic illness the home nurse should be encouraged to keep a record of care as well, to supplement the information provided by the public health nurse.

When the physician is not visiting the home, reports should be mailed promptly. Emergency matters may be reported by telephone, but in general it is better to send the report in writing as it can then be easily incorporated with the medical record.

In some instances it is sufficient to send periodic reports. For example, the nurse may report to the industrial health service when the first visit is made to an employee who is ill at home, giving a report of his condition and the plan for care. It may not be necessary to report further until the patient is ready for convalescent care, or is to be discharged from the nursing service.

When there is no specific form that defines the content of reports to other agencies, the public health nurse should be certain that the following information is included: (1) the date service was instituted, (2) the plan for care, (3) service given and results of care, (4) referral to other agency, (5) information that has a special bearing on the service of the cooperating agency, such as the student's reaction to missing classes, the effect of employee's condition on work capacity, and so on, and (6) termination date and plans for follow-up. The degree to which the report considers these matters in detail will depend upon the situation and the uses to which the cooperating agency will put the report.

Safeguarding Confidentiality of Case Records. Health records are usually considered confidential, and information is not released from them except under policies of the agency. These policies usually provide for release of information to designated agencies or individuals, such as case work agencies, hospital personnel, and physicians responsible for the care of the patient. Release of information from health records to other sources should be only with the consent of the family.

When health information is included in general records—such as the cumulative school record or the personnel record of the industrial worker—its content is determined by the purposes of the over-all record. For example, the school record may include a notation regarding vision-test results, or may indicate that the child has rheumatic fever and requires some adaptation of his school schedule. However, the more extensive and confidential nursing interviews, consultation regarding family emotional or social problems might not be included in such a general record except to refer to the fact that the case is being carried by the appropriate health service.

ADMINISTRATIVE RECORDS

In addition to case records, records are needed for service planning and accounting. Usually administrative recording procedures will be defined by the agency; if not, the state division of public health nursing will be prepared to make suggestions, or the procedures suggested by the National League for Nursing may serve as a basis for planning.[2]

Requests for nursing service provide valuable information for case planning and service evaluation. They should indicate the reason for request for care, the referral agent and the medical supervisor. Minimum information secured on this form should include complete identification information (including name, address, directions for locating home such as apartment number or

2. National League for Nursing, *Statistical Reporting and Costs in Public Health Nursing.* New York, The League, 1953.

route when not on named or numbered streets, and telephone number); name of medical attendant and directions for reaching him for orders or other information, and whether or not a report of service is requested. In some instances it is possible to secure medical orders, or social information relating to care that will influence service planning, which may be noted by the person taking the call for care. This information may be incorporated in a standard form used on a community-wide basis to facilitate

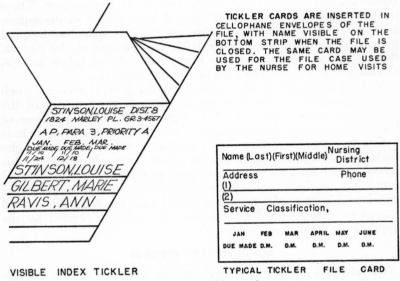

TICKLER CARDS ARE INSERTED IN CELLOPHANE ENVELOPES OF THE FILE, WITH NAME VISIBLE ON THE BOTTOM STRIP WHEN THE FILE IS CLOSED. THE SAME CARD MAY BE USED FOR THE FILE CASE USED BY THE NURSE FOR HOME VISITS

STINSON,LOUISE DIST. 8
1824 MARLEY PL. GR.3-4567
A P, PARA 3 ,PRIORITY A
JAN.   FEB. MAR
DUE MADE DUE MADE DUE MADE
11/24   11/10 12/18
STINSON,LOUISE
GILBERT,MARIE
RAVIS , ANN

Name (Last)(First)(Middle)	Nursing District				
Address				Phone	
(1)					
(2)					
Service Classification,					
JAN	FEB	MAR	APRIL	MAY	JUNE
DUE MADE D.M.	D.M.	D.M.	D.M.	D.M.	

VISIBLE   INDEX   TICKLER   TYPICAL TICKLER   FILE   CARD

Figure 20.   Tickler cards.

continuity of care between hospitals or other sources of medical care and community nursing services.

A tickler file is essential if the case load is at all large. The purpose of a tickler file is to provide a reminder of service needed at a particular time—patients due to attend clinic for physical examination or for home visiting, or for reminder notices of various sorts. This may be in the form of index cards filed chronologically, entries on a dated sheet, or a visible index file or book. Figure 20 shows typical tickler forms.

This reminder form should contain the minimum information for scheduling service or follow-up—the case record itself is the real planning basis for service. When more information than is necessary is put on the tickler card or sheet, copying time is high, and the record will still give too little information for total case planning. Usually it is sufficient to include identifying information, the time the next visit is due, and the type of service provided. If the tickler file is kept in a different place from the case records (as when the school health record is in the school and the tickler file in the nurse's office at another address), it may be necessary to include somewhat more information to facilitate case selection.

Cards of a different color, or identifying stickers or tabs, may be used to differentiate types of service. For example, records of maternal and child health cases may be put on white cards, of communicable disease follow-up cases on blue ones; or in a tuberculosis tickler file a different colored card or tab may be used for active, inactive and contact cases. Such differentiation should not be used unless it is warranted by the use to which the cards are put, since it means a more complicated problem of ordering and storing and a slightly longer time requirement for maintaining the file.

Sometimes the nurse carrying a small case load may file her case records chronologically, and in this instance it is not necessary to maintain a tickler. The nurse who carries a heavy bedside care program and provides intensive service to a small number of patients may find this method entirely satisfactory.

An alpha file will be needed as a means of locating case records. This is an alphabetical index of all cases for which records have been made. The alpha card usually contains only name and address, dates service was given, and, in some cases, an indication as to where the record may be located. The alpha file serves as a sort of summary indicating the dates on which the case was opened or closed to nursing service. When inactive records are not easily accessible or when some records are stored in other buildings, additional summary information may be included. Cards 3 by 5 inches in size are usually most suitable for the alpha file.

FINANCIAL REPORTS

The staff nurse is rarely responsible for complete budgets or financial reports, but there are some financial records she must keep. These include records of fees received, petty-cash expenditures and travel or maintenance expenditures. Each agency will have definite policies and procedures for such accounting, and the nurse should be thoroughly acquainted with them.

When fees are collected or contributions received, receipts should always be given, indicating the person paying and receiving, the amount and the service for which the fee was paid or the purpose for which the contribution was made. Receipts should be in duplicate, one for the donor and one for the agency record. Cash collected should be deposited daily with the designated person or in accordance with established procedure.

Petty-cash expenditures should be recorded, and receipts for all expenditures appended. A petty-cash book should be maintained and balanced monthly. The nurse working alone should be clear as to the limits of her authority in relation to expenditures for incidental needs.

Travel vouchers will be required in many agencies, and there will be definite regulations regarding reimbursement. When car expenses are reimbursed on a mileage basis, the voucher should indicate distance traveled between assignments or during each day. This should be recorded daily to avoid error; some daily report sheets include this mileage item. When the car is agency owned, the nurse should carefully record all car expenditures and mileage, and secure receipts for all charges not billed directly to the agency.

When maintenance or other expense items are to be vouchered, the nurse should find out what receipts are required, and should familiarize herself with the conditions under which reimbursement is made.

Vouchers should be submitted promptly in accordance with agency regulations.

SERVICE REPORTS

Service reports are essential for program planning and evaluation, and to provide for service accounting. They will include statistical reports of services rendered and narrative reports.

Statistical Reports.   Statistical reports may be compiled directly from the nurse's case records by a clerical worker, from a daily report sheet, or from individual service records for each case or service unit. Records may be designed to allow machine tabulation.

Daily report forms provide a record of the nurse's work. They report time on duty and all activities undertaken within that time—office, clinic, home visiting, in-service education and any other service or nonservice activity. Time may be recorded for each visit or activity, but more frequently only total time spent in each type of service is recorded except for specified sample periods. The daily report form suggested by the National League for Nursing is shown in Figure 21.

Agencies will differ in what is considered a service unit; in some instances it will be a nursing "incident"—a particular health situation requiring nursing service. Thus, within a year an individual with a long-term illness may have several units of care for the same condition. In some instances the family rather than the individual is the unit of service, regardless of the number of problems that may be represented, or the number of individuals served during a single visit. The National League for Nursing recommends that a visit to an individual be counted as one regardless of the number of conditions present, and that when care is given to more than one person in the family the visit to each individual be counted.[3] For accounting purposes, all patients may be discharged at the end of the accounting year, readmitting the active ones en masse for the new year, or patients may be carried over to the new year, indicating the first visit in the new reporting period.

Visits will be classified in accordance with an agency plan. Telephone contacts are not generally counted but may be included in some instances, as well as office or school conferences, visits to families, and visits to others on behalf of the family. The National League for Nursing has suggested a classification scheme.[4]

Individual service unit statistical reports are being used more frequently, since they permit machine tabulation and greater flexibility in study of records for planning purposes. Figure 22 gives an example of this type of report. Compilation and tabulation of statistics may be done by clerical workers directly to cards for machine tabulation.

In some instances, as in schools and industrial establishments, more than one compilation of statistics may be needed, since the school or industry may want to analyze the data for different purposes than does the health agency providing the service.

There is an increasing trend toward having compilation of statistics done in a central office, rather than by the individual

3. National League for Nursing, *Statistical Reporting and Costs in Public Health Nursing.* New York, The League, 1953, p. 4.
4. Ibid., pp. 2–9.

NURSE'S DAILY REPORT

On Duty_____A. M.   Off Duty_____P. M.

		Hrs.	Mins.	Type of (✓) Visit		
Total Time						
Lunch Time Off						
Other Time Off Duty						
Total Working Time						

Clinics, Classes and Group Conferences (Specify)	Ses- sions	Attend- ance			Therapeutic Nursing	All Other (Exc. Cols. 2 & 4)	Not Home and Not Found
		New	Rev.				
School, Industry, Other Activity (Specify) _____							

Patient (Name and Address)	Column 1	2	3	4

Home Visits	(All Codes with A. Fv. R)			
Office Visits	(All Codes with A . Fv . R)			
Cases Admitted	(All Codes with A. Fv. A . Fv)			
Cases Discharged	(All Codes with D)			

Code: A—Case Admission   Fv—First Visit in Current
                                              Year to Carried Case

Mead & Wheeler Co., Chicago, Ill.
   Exclusive Publishers

Nurse_____

District_____

Date_____

Visits Classified by Service Program (Code)

Maternity			Health Guidance								Communicable								All Other							
			Infant								TB		Other													
			Under 1 Yr.																							
Antepartal	Postpartal		Premature	Neonatal—Other than Premature	Other Infant	1–4 Years	5–14 Years	15–19 Years	20 Years and Over								Cancer	Cardiac	Diabetes	Other Dis. and Conditions					
5	6	7	8	9	10	11	12	13	14	15	16	17	18	19	20	21	22	23	24	25	26	27	28			
																								Total (Add Across)		
																								Total (Add Across)		
																								Total (Add Across)		
																								Total (Add Across)		

R—Revisit   D—Case Discharged   Indicate Office Visit
by Circling Code Letter
(December 1952) Form NLN64

Figure 21. Daily report form. (From *Statistical Reporting and Costs in Public Health Nursing*. National League for Nursing, 1953. Reprinted with permission.)

nurse. When compilation of statistics of services rendered must be done by the nurse, the form of the daily report should be such that it is easy to maintain cumulative totals.

The nurse should be aware of the possible uses of statistical data, and may want to collect information not required by the agency or included on the report form as a basis for her own program evaluation. For example, the month of pregnancy in which the first nursing visit was made, and the number of well-

(1) No._____ CT_____	(18) CLASSIFICATION OF SERVICE	DAILY RECORD DEPARTMENT OF PUBLIC HEALTH

```
(1) No._____ CT_____        (18) CLASSIFICATION      DAILY RECORD DEPART-
        Birth                               OF SERVICE          MENT OF PUBLIC HEALTH
                                        00 Infant.......  ____
(10) Date: Mo.__Day____Yr.____         10 Preschool....  ____   Name_____
                                       20 School.....    ____       Last      First     Middle
_____    30 Venereal Dis.  ____   Address_____
(13)  Male: W__N__ Other (Sp.)_        40 Ac.Com.Dis.(Sp.)____   Name of                 School
      Female: W__N__ Other (Sp.)_                               father____
                                       57 Contract....   ____   Single          Future
(14) New to Dept._____          58 Suspect.....   ____   visit only____   visit indicated____
     Old to Dept. New to Service___    59 Carrier......  ____
                  Readm. to Serv.__       TBC. (Check Stage)     TYPE OF          TYPE OF
                  Old to Service___    61 Minimal.....   ____    ACTIVITY         DISPOSITION
                                       62 Moderate....   ____       (22)             (24)
(15) First visit Subsequent            63 Far Adv.....   ____   1 Culture____    1 Ret. visit____
     this year____ visit this yr.____  67 Unknown....    ____   4 Sputum____     2 Disch(rel)____
                                       68 Suspect....    ____   7 Investigate____    Refer to:
(16) Place of visit:                   69 Contact....    ____   8 Quarantine___  3 Priv. M.D.____
     Field:     Not      Note             Other (p.)             9 Demo.bedside  4 Hosp. In-P____
     At home__ home__ left____                                    nursing____.   5 Hosp. Out-P___
     Other (Sp.)                       70 Other Disease (Sp.)   10 Hlth. supv.__ 6 Sanatorium____
     Office:                                                      Other (Sp.)    7 Nurs. Agen.___
     Cl-Conf:____ D.P.H.____           90 Defect (Sp.)____                          Other (Sp.)

(17) Type of Medical Supervision          Other Service (Sp.)
     Priv. M.D.____  Vet.____
     D.P.H.____     Unknown____                                 (26) Date____19__  (34) Insp.____
     Hosp. O-P.___  Other (Sp.)                                 (30) Nurse____     (35) School____
     TBC League__                                               (32) M.D.____      (38)_____
```

Figure 22.   Report form for home visits. (From *Records and Reports of Local Health Departments*, Public Health Monograph #15. Washington, D.C., U.S. Government Printing Office, 1953, p. 42.)

baby conferences which include guidance on emotional problems of the family, may be important items for evaluation.

Monthly and annual statistics are compiled from the daily record sheet or from the individual service unit reports. These include information required by the agency itself and by other groups such as state or federal agencies, sponsoring or coordinating groups such as the community chest or council, and by contracting agencies such as industrial firms or voluntary agencies that pay for service.

When the nurse is responsible for compilation, she usually maintains cumulative totals of services provided on a monthly basis, totalling monthly reports for the annual one. Monthly reports may be kept in a loose-leaf notebook, and the data entered each month in columns headed "total this month," "total to date this year." In this way the nurse has a quick source of reference of the service accomplishments at any particular time during the year. It may also be helpful for comparison to have a third column headed "total to date last year."

Narrative Reports of Service. Narrative reports of service may be required on a monthly, quarterly or annual basis. In large agencies this report may be compiled on a group basis by the supervising nurse or administrator. However, there is real benefit in such reporting by each nurse, since it provides an excellent opportunity to review accomplishments and problems, and serves as a base for planning and for securing consultation from the supervisor. In general, a monthly report serves little purpose, since the degree of change within the service is not great in such a short period. Annual reports are the minimum, since planning and budgeting periods for the agency are apt to be on an annual basis. Quarterly reports are highly desirable as they provide for check points within the year, and for re-direction of efforts when the program appears to have diverged from its objectives.

The narrative report—and in particular the annual narrative report—needs to be related to the statistical report. Sometimes the statistical report items need to be interpreted or evaluated, or may be expressed in different terms for clarification of their significance. For example, charts or graphs may express the meaning of trends in service more clearly than do the figures or tables; a case example may explain why increased time cost per visit reflects better care.

The annual statistical report should also be related to reports of previous years, to indicate the trends in service. For example, there may be a marked change in the distribution of service among the various types of case—an increase in the number of industrial employees who received general health counseling services; or in the method of delivering the service—a greater or lesser proportion of home visits as compared to office or school consultations or clinic visits.

The annual report should show:
1. Major accomplishments of the year, indicating qualitative as well as quantitative achievements.
2. Trends in service needs and activities.
3. Relation of service rendered to estimated needs for such services, and to the stated objectives of the service.
4. Problems and unmet needs.

5. Plans for change.

In writing the annual report, attention should be given to its interpretative value as well as to its content. The following suggestions may be helpful:

1. Collect information and illustrative materials for the annual report during the year. Keep notes in a folder for ready reference.

2. Choose a style that will suit the audience to be reached. The administrator will be reviewing many such reports. He will want a succinct summarization, with a clear and readily located summarization of progress and problems. Reports for the general public or for advisory committees will be more interesting if they include illustrative case materials. Statistics in reports for the lay public should be quickly comprehended—"last year each family received an average of three visits; this year they received four." A simple graph may mean more than a table of the total visits made.

3. Organize the report so that essential material is readily located. Sometimes different colored sheets are used for sections of the report; or a summary sheet may appear at the beginning, with more detailed reports following so that the parts of the service are related to the whole.

4. Give recognition to other agencies, divisions or persons who assisted with the program during the year. Sometimes it is helpful to translate volunteer services into professional time equivalents.

5. Place this year's activities in relation to what has gone before and what is to come during the next report period.

6. Use volunteers to help to write the report when possible.

Records and reports make a valuable contribution to the management of the nursing job. They provide the information necessary for appraisal; they show highlights and gaps in service; they focus attention on the service as a whole. Properly used, they provide a good and economical channel of communication among workers in the agency and between agencies in the community and between the agency and the public. The staff nurse can make a real contribution to total agency management by providing record and report material that is selective, pertinent, and significant; she can also make valuable suggestions based on her field experience, regarding record content and utilization.

CHAPTER XVIII

Working with Committees and Citizen Groups

THE PARTICIPATION of interested citizens, organized into committees or boards, has been traditional in the work of voluntary public health nursing agencies. More recently, it has come to be a recognized adjunct of official public health nursing services as well. Wise use of the general public in furthering the work of public health roots the work deeply in the structure of the community. This in turn provides a channel for relating public health nursing services to the community in such a way that the efforts of the services are directed toward the most important of the community's problems. In time of trouble—such as "economy drives" —it provides a group of informed and concerned citizens who are able to interpret the need for service to the public.

TYPES OF COMMITTEE

There are several types of citizen committees, each serving a particular purpose. They may be:

1. Policy-making, administrative, responsibility-bearing groups, such as the Boards of Directors of Visiting Nurse Associations.
2. Advisory committees, which serve as a bridge of communication and understanding between the agency and the public.

3. Technical committees, which advise in special technical areas, such as the medical advisory committee of a visiting nurse service, or a special committee on rehabilitation.

4. Action committees, which are set up to do a specified job.

It is important that both staff and committee members be clear about the purpose for which the committee exists, and the extent to which its authority is executive, or merely consultative. An advisory committee which construes its responsibility as administrative may attempt to control aspects of the program in a way that is not only disturbing, but may also be harmful to the community.

Administrative or Policy-Making Groups. The board of directors of a voluntary agency is the type of administrative and policy-making group most commonly found in public health nursing. The functions of a board of directors are:

1. To determine the general policies under which the agency will work.

2. To raise the necessary funds and to take responsibility for the expenditures of the agency, and for approving its budget.

3. To approve the program and activities of the agency, and make certain that they are consistent with the policies established.

4. To authorize necessary contractual agreements.[1]

While much responsibility may be delegated to the director of nursing service, the final responsibility for the work of the agency remains with the board. The board is accountable to the public for spending the funds of the agency for the purposes for which they were intended, and for the general direction and efficiency of the operation.

In addition, the board of directors serves as a unit and through its individual members acts as a sounding board for public opinion and as a channel of communication between the agency and the public.

Advisory Committees. Citizens' committees may serve as advisers to either voluntary or official public health nursing services. An advisory committee may and usually does make *recommendations* regarding policy and program, but does not have the authority to actually put them into effect. The authority and responsibility for planning and implementing the program rest with the designated administrative officer—the health officer or nurse director. The advisory group, however, serves a valuable purpose in

1. Wensley, Edith, *The Community and Public Health Nursing.* New York, Macmillan Co., 1950.

presenting the point of view of the general public and of allied professional groups in relation to community needs and methods of meeting them through nursing services. Sometimes the committee may provide guidance in particular phases of the program —for example, one member of the committee may be a newspaper man who could advise on matters relating to the public information aspects of the work; another may be an educator who could advise on problems of relationships with the schools or of setting up family educational programs. As informed and conscientious consumers of nursing service the committee members review and render judgments on the program as a whole, advise on general trends and on nontechnical matters of administration; they interpret the program to the general public through personal influence and through organized public relations and public information programs.

Technical Committees. Technical committees may serve on a continuing basis or for a temporary period as needed. A medical advisory or medical consultant committee may serve continuously to review and advise on agency policy as it affects medical practice and medical relationships. It may recommend policy regarding the treatments that may be given by the nurse in the patients' homes, or on the procedures to be used. It has a particularly important role in deciding under what conditions new drugs or treatments may be administered with safety. A rehabilitation committee, on the other hand, might be set up to establish or revise policies and procedures used by the agency in this field, and be disbanded when the job has been finished. While the technical committee is usually labeled as "advisory" or "consultant," it actually carries somewhat more authority than does the general advisory committee because of the expertness of its members.

Action Committees. Action committees are set up to carry through a special assignment, and usually carry performance as well as advisory or judgmental responsibilities. For example, a committee may be set up to assist with the work of a mobile clinic; or to help with medical examinations or with vision or hearing tests in the school; or to organize a home nursing class. These committees usually work under the direction of the nurse or other professional worker to plan, organize and help to implement the special activity with which they are concerned. Subcommittees of boards of directors or of advisory committees may serve in the capacity of an action committee.

An agency often has more than one type of committee functioning. Whatever the pattern, each committee should know its purpose, its authority limits, and its channels of communication with the agency and the public.

SELECTION OF COMMITTEE MEMBERS

Volunteers or paid consultants who participate as committee or board members should be selected with great care. The qualities of the individual members and the composition of the group as a whole will have much to do with the quality of the committee's decisions and actions, and its influence upon agency program and public impact.

Members selected for boards or committees that have administrative or policy-making functions should be representative of the community as a whole. Individuals from different political, religious, racial, economic and vocational groups should be included as far as possible. Representation from the medical and nursing professions, from the health department and from related health and welfare agencies or from special interest groups may be very helpful. Both men and women should be included. The tendency to select members only from the professional and economically privileged class should be avoided; representatives of labor or of residents from housing developments, for example, may be most helpful.

Sometimes members are chosen by having representative agencies or organizations appoint official representatives. The Medical Association, Parent-Teacher Association, or Health Department may be asked to name members to a committee or board. This procedure may be useful in securing medical and nursing representation, using the local professional groups as the selecting mechanism. However, it is usually preferable to select individuals known to have particular interests or capacities, being sure to have broad representation among those so selected. This usually produces a more vital group. The committee should include some members with experience and competence in handling financial matters.

The committee or board should be small enough to function effectively as a group. If it is impossible to keep the board small and at the same time secure adequate representation of the various interests in the community, organization into working committees may help to counteract the difficulty of a cumbersome deliberative body. It may be possible to secure wide representation and still keep a small working group through rotation of membership. For example, the clergy might be represented by a priest for one term, by a minister or rabbi the next. Twenty or thirty comprise a manageable group for a board; committees that are not responsible for multiple functions or for broad responsibilities might well be limited to eight or ten.

Members should be selected for leadership and deliberative qualities. Every community has certain natural leaders, who have status within their own group and who have the capacity to influence the behavior of others. Such leadership is important in board and committee members who carry policy responsibilities, since they are expected to represent the views of the group they represent, and in turn to interpret the agency's program and needs to the community. They must be able to think carefully about the problems and needs of the community and of the agency, and about the relationship between the two. They must be able to participate actively in making sound decisions that may have far-reaching implications.

Selection of *advisory* committee members should be in terms of special competence in the area of advisement. If the committee is to serve primarily as an interpretative body, broad representation from different community groups is of great importance. Individuals should be included who are expert in communication, such as journalists or editors, as well as representatives of such membership groups as Kiwanis and Rotary Clubs, church or social organizations, veterans' organizations, professional groups and parent-teacher associations.

If the purpose of the advisory group is primarily to relate the agency program to that of other community health activities, representation on an organization-representative basis may be desirable. For example a "liaison" committee might be composed of representatives of the health department, the voluntary public health nursing agency, industrial or commercial nursing services, school health services and other agencies whose work impinges on that of the public health nursing service.

An advisory committee may be larger in size than an administrative or policy committee if the purpose is primarily interpretative. This permits broader representation, and the personal involvement of a larger number of people. Decision making and detailed planning may be done by an executive committee elected by the larger committee.

If the primary purpose of the committee is to offer technical advice, members should be selected for the technical competence they possess in relation to the total activity. For example, a medical advisory committee might well be composed entirely of physicians. It should, however, include physicians in private practice as well as in public health and hospital services, and if the work of the agency includes much bedside care it may be necessary to include specialists in the area of special concern of the agency, for example, in heart disease. A committee to give guidance to a rehabilitation program might include physicians, nurses, physical therapists, educators and vocation rehabilitation workers. Such a committee could give advice concerning organization of the rehabilitation program, approve procedures to be carried out, and indicate desirable qualifications or training for the staff in this field. It could also advise on the relation of this particular agency program to total community planning for rehabilitation.

Sometimes an existing organization or committee may agree to serve as a technical advisory committee. For example, a small local medical society may agree to serve as a medical advisory committee to the local visiting nurse or county nurse; and existing committee of the nurses' association may serve as a liaison between the agency and nursing as a whole—as when the committee on personnel practices of the nurses' association advises in relation to salary scales; or an industrial health subcommittee of the local health council may serve as an advisory committee on part-time service to industrial workers.

Selection of members for an action committee proceeds on a somewhat different basis. Here the responsibility of the committee requires members who have time to devote to the activity, who have the necessary training or are willing to get it, and who are acceptable to the community and able to work well together. For example, if the activity involves patient transportation, it is important to select someone with a car, with suitable insurance coverage and who is able to get along well with members of the committee and with the patients whom he will transport. No great capacity for deliberative thought is required, but sensitivity to people and their needs would be a prerequisite. Usually an action committee requires people with varied interests and backgrounds. Because the work of an action committee is not as clearly prescribed as that of some of the others, and because it involves a larger measure of implementation, the chairman assumes particular importance. He must be able to push forward the work of the committee to a successful conclusion, to organize and to work with others on the committee with unusual skill. The person who "gets things done" is a good chairman for an action committee.

In all committees that carry on work over a long period of time, rotation of membership is important. In this way the number of people directly involved with the work of the agency is increased, and fresh ideas are encouraged.

The chairman is a key person in any committee, not only for his own wisdom and help, but also because he will have a great deal of influence on the enthusiasm and contribution of other members. In selecting a chairman it is well to look for someone with a real interest in the community problem with which the agency is concerned, and preferably someone who is already familiar with the agency. Prior board membership is very helpful. Equally important, the chairman should be one who has shown himself through other civic activities as one who is good at following a task through to its conclusion. Willingness to work with others without domination of them is also important in a chairman.

ORGANIZATION OF A BOARD OF DIRECTORS

Committees or boards having policy-making or administrative responsibilities should function under by-laws that define duties, responsibilities and authority of the board itself, and of its authorized standing committees; the number and functions of officers; and the regulations governing voting, meetings, financial accounting, election of officers and members and the conditions under which they serve.[2]

Officers should include at least a president or chairman, vice president, secretary and treasurer. With officers as with members, rotation of membership is desirable to prevent development of an "ingrown" board. Officers should be chosen for their knowledge of the agency, preferably after serving for a time on the board; for their acceptability to the group; and for their special competence in leadership or in the recording or financial management skills needed by the secretary and treasurer.

Meetings should be held frequently enough to keep the board actively concerned with the affairs of the agency and currently informed of its progress. If the board is large, it may meet as infrequently as once a year, but in that case an executive committee with power to act should meet regularly at more frequent intervals. Once a month is not too frequent for such a meeting.

Where possible, meetings should be on a regularly scheduled

2. Suggested form for by-laws may be secured from the Department of Public Health Nursing, National League for Nursing, 2 Park Avenue, New York, N.Y.

rather than on an "on call" basis, to promote fuller attendance and continuing interest. Meetings should be conducted in accordance with accepted parliamentary procedure even though they may be quite informal in spirit.[3]

Subcommittees should be formed as needed on a standing or temporary basis. It is not necessary that all subcommittee members be members of the board, but it is usually desirable for the chairmen of subcommittees to be board members. No subcommittee should be formed, even though it is authorized in the by-laws, unless there is a job for it to do. A paper organization that does not keep members busy dissipates interest.

Delegation of work to members of the board or committee should be thoughtfully and aggressively undertaken. In general, the committee member who has a specific job to do has greater and more continuing interest in the total agency work. Every member of the board or committee should be reached with specific assignments, both to distribute the work and to maintain the active participation of the entire group.

Minutes should be recorded by the secretary at all meetings, and a record should be kept of other official activities of the board. These minutes should be considered a permanent record, and kept in the nursing office or agency file rather than in the homes of the officers of the board. Dates of meetings, attendance, a record of all action taken and recommendations made should be included in the official minutes.

Any correspondence carried on by board or committee members should be considered official agency correspondence and handled as such.

ORGANIZATION OF ADVISORY, TECHNICAL OR ACTION COMMITTEES

Advisory, technical or action committees do not have the same need for formal organization as does the administrative or policy-making board. However, there should always be provision for a responsible chairman; for an orderly method of arriving at and recording the recommendations of the committee; and for involvement of every committee member. Recommendations should be kept as a part of the permanent records of the agency.

Meetings of advisory committees may be held regularly, with the frequency determined by the functions of the committee. Quarterly meetings are often proposed as a minimum to keep a

3. Roberts, *Rules of Order, Revised,* is considered a standard text for parliamentary procedure.

general advisory committee in touch with the agency's total program. However, meetings may be scheduled monthly, if the problems are many or the program is being intensively reviewed. Sometimes irregular schedules are desirable. For instance, a health advisory committee in a school may meet twice a month during the last two months of school, to lay the groundwork for next year's program, or to discuss recommending parent participation in school inspections and physical examinations. During the balance of the year it may meet only at bi-monthy periods.

Sometimes an advisory committee may be in the nature of an *ad hoc* committee. For example, a health officer or visiting nurse association may call a citizens' conference to obtain the views of a representative group on a particular problem or proposed activity. This conference may meet only once or for a few times, to consider this special problem, and be disbanded as soon as this has been done.

Technical committees are usually made up of busy professional and business people. Meetings of such groups should be called only when there are real problems to be discussed or procedures to be reviewed.

Action committee meetings must by their nature be irregularly spaced, and no single pattern of meetings can be suggested for them.

TRAINING

Training of board and committee members is the responsibility of the board itself and of the staff of the agency. Thorough training is essential if the board as a whole is to make sound decisions, accept full responsibility without overstepping proper authority or exceeding its sphere of competence, and have the vision and sense of direction so necessary for effective leadership. The following are basic:

1. A thorough indoctrination in the functions, purposes and scope of the work of the agency in relation to over-all community provisions for health care. In this connection, observation of the services of the agency in action is particularly helpful in giving a feeling for the work being done.
2. Thorough instruction as to the authority and responsibility of the board or committee.
3. An understanding of the ways in which decisions are made within the board or committee. This should include an

interpretation of the relative autonomy of committees, responsibility of the professional staff or others in technical matters; limitations set by legal provisions or by community habit.

4. Budgetary and personnel limitations.

The board or committee should be given current information on the general progress and activities of the agency. Frequent reports should be submitted by the professional staff, and the committee should be kept informed of projected or on-going special programs or activities. Such service reports should be written in full or in abstract form so that they may be filed with the board or committee records. Sometimes it is useful to have informal reports of activities or case reports in addition to the formal service report. These informal presentations may be very effective in transmitting the flavor of the service, and its human aspects. These would not, of course, become part of the permanent records of the committee.

Members should have full and accurate information on all matters to be considered. Sometimes this information is gathered by standing or special committees; it is often provided by the nursing or other technical staff. For example, if salary changes are to be discussed, the committee should have salary schedules of comparable agencies in the same or similar communities, and recommendations of professional associations regarding salary ranges when they are available. If the prenatal clinic organization is being discussed the committee members should know the prenatal case load, the type of medical supervision patients receive, the present facilities for prenatal care, location of cases in relation to existing or planned clinic locations, possible costs of materials, facilities or personnel. Such information should be compiled in concise and easily readable form. The committee should be provided with facts rather than opinions of the staff. The materials should represent data basic to the deliberations of the committee, and not a proposed course of action presented for unquestioning approval.

INCREASING THE USE OF COMMITTEES

The staff nurse in an urban community may have little opportunity to work directly with the policy-making or advisory committees of her agency. The rural nurse, on the other hand, must often organize, train and work with advisory and action committees which function in local communities and in counties or other political jurisdictions. Often she will be able to see new ways in which citizens organized into committees or action groups can extend the work of the nurse, or can help to keep the nursing program close to the needs and feelings of the public. Through the application of good techniques of group discussion and problem solving in groups, the nurse can contribute to the effectiveness of committees and boards, either through her own functioning as a member of the group, or by helping prepare committee members for effective group action.

CHAPTER XIX

Working with
Volunteers, Auxiliaries
and Students

W$_{\text{ITH}}$ INCREASING frequency, public health agencies are using the services of volunteers, practical nurses and aides for the furtherance of public health programs. Volunteers, who have been a traditional part of the voluntary agency and in rural nursing services, are taking an important place in urban health departments as well. The use of practical nurses has increased so that on April 1, 1955, 205 practical nurses were reported to be employed in public health agencies.[1] To a lesser extent, and in unknown numbers, public health agencies are finding a place for nurses' aides, especially in clinics.

VOLUNTEER WORKERS

Volunteer workers serving without pay have played an important part in the development of public health nursing in America. They have served in two ways—as policy makers, advisors and fund raisers; and as "doing" volunteers who participate in the daily activities of community nursing. It is with the latter group that the staff nurse is most likely to be concerned.

Purpose of Volunteer Assistance. The purpose of volunteer assistance is to extend and supplement the work of the paid pro-

1. *Facts About Nursing*, 1955–56 Edition. New York, American Nurses' Association, 1956, p. 145.

fessional and ancillary staff. Volunteer services should not as a rule be used for continuing basic functions that ought to be or could be provided by paid workers, since they may lead the community to delay or avoid taking necessary action to provide basic health services for its citizens. For example, the nursing supervision of selected prenatal patients is a basic part of the community nursing service, and should be assured by adequate budgetary support and by the inclusion of this service in the regular work load of the professional staff. However, if volunteer workers are used it might be possible to extend the service to reach some expectant mothers whose needs are not as great as those in the "must see" group, or to provide for more intensive service or additional niceties within the service. Instead of form notices, personal notes may be used for invitations to parent classes; hospitality activities such as serving simple refreshments or using a volunteer receptionist may ease the class member's adjustment to the class group; additional opportunities for class or group experience that might not otherwise be available in nutrition, parent-child relationships or accident prevention may be afforded.

Selection of Volunteer Workers. Volunteer assistants should be selected from all kinds of groups. The banker may be an excellent amateur carpenter; the housewife may assist with care of small children while their mother sees the doctor; the retired nurse may teach a home nursing class; high school children might visit homebound patients; the psychiatric patient in the hospital might make posters for the well-baby clinic; the secretary on her day off might shampoo and set the hair of an arthritic patient.

Sometimes there are organized community sources of volunteer service. The Junior League, The American National Red Cross, various veterans' organizations or religious groups may maintain regular training programs for volunteers who may be assigned to community agencies. Girl and Boy Scouts, 4-H Clubs or special interest groups in schools such as Future Nurses' Clubs or Young Homemakers' Clubs may urge their members to provide community volunteer services or carry certain activities as a group. Some communities have a centralized volunteer bureau that recruits, trains, and assigns volunteers to community agencies on request.

When the agency recruits its own volunteers, helpers should be selected who are capable of doing the job that is needed, and might be expected to be responsible in carrying out the assigned work. There will be an almost unlimited number of activities that may be undertaken by volunteers—assisting the physician in a clinic; making a rack to hold health information pamphlets; preparing supplies for use in the nurse's bag or in clinics; assisting with office procedures such as telephone service, filing or typing; preparing publicity releases; maintaining an office library. This means that with thought the nurse will find work that needs to be done and that will suit the capabilities and interests of almost any type of person who would like to help. Volunteer services reach maximum usefulness when many sources are tapped.

Placement.   Volunteers should be fitted to the job. It is important that they are assigned to work which they feel uses their full skill and ability. For example, a group of high school boys or a handicapped older woman might like very much to prepare unsterilized supplies for the clinic, which involves work of a simple repetitive nature. A young and enthusiastic college graduate, on the other hand, might be irked by such a task, but might enjoy analyzing nursing records and making graphs of the service trends, writing publicity materials, handling or preparing sterilized supplies, or assisting the doctor in the treatment room. Moving volunteers to more and more responsibility as they gain experience and skill also helps to maintain their interest, and provides for full use of volunteer time.

When professional services are to be given by volunteer workers, as when nurse-volunteers are used in blood collection centers or to make follow-up visits after a community chest x-ray program, only those who are fully qualified to carry the responsibilities should be assigned. For example, a nurse who has been inactive for many years and out of touch with modern nursing practice could not make visits to patients needing further study following x-ray, unless she could secure some additional preparation. Even the volunteer with good background preparation will probably need special briefing. When direct patient care is to be given, the responsible administrator should give his approval, and ascertain any liability the agency may be assuming.

Organization of Volunteer Services.   Volunteers may be recruited, trained and assigned by another agency, such as the volunteer bureau. Sometimes these agencies have comprehensive regulations under which their volunteers serve, as is the case with the nurses' aides or Gray Ladies of the Red Cross. When such services are used the nurse should, either herself or through her administrator, determine the conditions under which the sponsoring agency will undertake to provide such service, and the extent and nature of the service to be provided. When necessary, agreements should be made, defining the respective responsibilities of the sponsoring and receiving agencies, and the conditions under which the volunteers will be used. These agreements need not be formal documents—a simple exchange of correspondence may be adequate. However, some written statement of the cooperative arrangement should be made to avoid misunderstanding.

When volunteers are recruited and trained by the agency in which they serve, they may work directly under the supervision of the nurse who may serve as the coordinator of the services afforded. If the group is large, one volunteer worker may be asked to serve as director or coordinator of the volunteer services, arranging with the nurse or with the board of the agency for general management of the program.

Special work units may also have a leader or chairman. For example, a group of school children might undertake to make certain supplies for the nurse's bag, perhaps to fold the paper squares used for a clean work surface in the home. One of the group may be elected as a leader, to take responsibility for allotting the work; arranging the work schedules; teaching new recruits the proper methods of handwashing, the method of folding, and the technique of keeping the materials clean during folding and storing. The chairman of the publicity committee may supervise and direct the work of volunteers who write, speak, or give radio or dramatic performances for the agency, arranging, of course, for necessary clearance of all materials used with appropriate staff members.

The use of volunteers to direct and supervise the work of other volunteers has many advantages. It not only saves nursing time, but also provides recognition and responsibility for a volunteer of unusual ability. A volunteer director who is herself a volunteer understands the problems of others rendering a similar service. An organized volunteer service also makes it easier to find and use substitutes when a regular volunteer must be absent.

Training.   Volunteer assistants need careful training if they are to make their best contribution to the agency. Such training should include the following:

1. Introduction to the agency. This includes a clear interpretation of the philosophy, objectives and program of the agency, its organization and management, and its place in the total fabric of community health services. The volunteer worker wants and needs to know how the organization came into

being, what it is trying to do, what sources are used for its support, how it runs and what kind of activities it carries on. In addition, he needs to get the "feel" of the service. For example, volunteers who are helping set up clinic supplies and equipment and in the reception of patients will see more sense in what they are doing if they have an opportunity to visit patients in their homes with the nurse, or to see how the physician works with the supplies they prepare.

2. Specific job training. This includes the special skills or techniques used in the work, the demands for the work, the amount of service needed, seasonal, hourly and daily variations in need, and ethical considerations. For example, the volunteer assisting the school nurse during a health examination clinic might be assigned to securing the record from the file, entering the student's height and weight, and bringing the record to the nurse or physician. She will need training in the use of the file, in ways of checking to be sure the right record has been secured, in techniques of weighing and measuring school children, and in methods of recording information on the record. Important ethical considerations include scrupulous courtesy in working with patients, safeguarding the confidential nature of record information, and leaving advisement of student or parent to professional workers, even though she may feel competent to advise. She will need to know the approximate speed with which she must work to keep a steady flow of patients to nurse or physician, and at what times and for approximately what duration her services will be needed.

3. Continuing supervision of work. Except when the volunteer is functioning in an area outside of nursing (such as carpentry or specialized instruction by a professional worker), the volunteer assistant will need the support and assurance that comes from supervision by the nurse. Immediately after the training period it is helpful to talk with the volunteers or to observe them at work to be sure that they know what to do and how to do it. Subsequent observation, review and discussion of the work offer an opportunity to suggest ways of enriching or extending what the volunteer is doing.

Inefficiency should not be expected nor should it be overlooked because the worker is not paid. It is better to find a new volunteer than to have the service disrupted by one who is inefficient and so interfering with the work's progress.

Furthermore, when regular service of good quality is expected, the volunteer can feel that what he or she is doing is of importance, and is apt to take more pride in the performance.

Some supervision—that which has to do with the mechanics of assignment or of non-nursing tasks—may be delegated to other volunteers. However, the over-all responsibility must rest with the public health nurse herself.

Job Descriptions.   A clearly outlined job description will help the volunteer to function with greater confidence. A step-by-step description of each task, kept available for volunteer helpers, simplifies the task of supervision, and makes it easier to introduce a new worker to the job. The importance of regular attendance, of reporting for the job at the time agreed upon, should be emphasized in the job description.

Starting a Volunteer Program.   Occasionally the public health nurse is in a position where no volunteer assistants have been used, and she may wish to take the initiative in establishing such a program. In this case, the following steps are suggested:

1. Develop a clear statement of the reasons why such a program is needed.
2. Secure necessary administrative clearances. Approval of the health officer, nursing supervisor or director, or board of directors or nursing committee may be necessary before instituting a volunteer program. If volunteers are to be used for direct patient care, the administrator will want to clear any legal aspects of such service.
3. Outline the specific functions to be carried by volunteers.
4. Canvass prospective participants. If possible, look early for someone who can help with the organization of the program, and provide leadership for other volunteers who may be recruited.
5. Write out specific job descriptions and schedules. If there is a volunteer who may develop into a leader in volunteer services this person may help with this.
6. Interpret the program to anyone who may be affected by volunteer assistance. Physicians working on a part-time basis in clinics, and patients who may have communications from volunteer workers should be informed about the plans as they are being made.

Holding Volunteers.   Once recruited and trained, the volunteer worker's interest in the program must be maintained at a high level, so that the agency may be assured of continuing participation and a good quality of performance. The following suggestions may be helpful in maintaining continuity and quality in volunteer service:

1. Every volunteer worker should have a specific job to do.
2. The extent and limits of the job should be clearly understood.
3. The worker should be identified with the agency. A smock, uniform, arm band or other insignia may identify the volunteer as a regular member of the agency. Inviting the volunteer to staff meetings that would be of interest to him, or to social functions of the staff help to make him feel a part of the organization. Sharing reports or stories of accomplishments or of program developments also contributes to his sense of belonging.
4. A plan should be made for recognition of service. This may be done by:
   a. Reporting on volunteer activities at board or staff meetings, or in agency publications, or in the local newspaper.
   b. Use of service pins or insignia. Some agencies provide pins, bars or other recognition symbols for specified periods of service.
   c. Providing for advancement to positions of greater responsibility within the volunteer service.
   d. Reporting on the value of volunteer service in terms of nursing time saved, dollar equivalents of services provided by volunteers, or statements of additional nursing services that were made possible because of the volunteer activities.

Interpretative Functions.   Every volunteer is a potential emissary for the agency. Volunteers may serve as speakers during fund drives, or as a part of the general public information program of the agency. They may interpret the service to their own special interest groups, or in incidental social contacts among their friends. The enthusiasm and concern of volunteer workers is a valuable asset; it should be fostered by good training programs that will keep the volunteer accurately informed of agency policies, needs, and programs, and also by a whole-hearted acceptance of the volunteer as an important and respected member of the health team.

PRACTICAL NURSES AND AIDES

Many of the principles and procedures that are effective in working with volunteers are equally effective with paid auxiliary nursing personnel. The practical nurse member of the staff will usually be employed by the administrator and the nurse will not be involved with her selection. Since most agencies employing practical nurses require licensure, the initial training of the practical nurse will have been completed before her employment. When licensure for practical nurses is in force, only licensed practical nurses should be employed because of the fact that they must often work without immediate supervision. All but three jurisdictions in the United States provide for such licensure.[2] When working with the practical nurse, the public health nurse may be in the position of team leader, and have responsibility for over-all management of family care.

The agency should have a list of specifically designated activities which the practical nurse may undertake. If there is no such designation of activities, the nurse should take steps to clarify the activities the practical nurse may undertake with the nursing supervisor and the appropriate administrative officer. It is particularly important to have clear authorization in relation to giving medications, and especially medications that are given by hypodermic injection. There are wide variations in the amount of responsibility the practical nurse takes in different agencies.

The practical nurse and the aide also need to have an orientation to the over-all purposes and program of the agency, and the place of their own work in relation to the whole. Specific job-training will be needed to acquaint the auxiliary worker with the particular procedures and regulations of the agency, even though she comes with good pre-employment preparation for the job. When the practical nurse or clinic aide deals primarily with equipment and relatively routine procedures, initial briefing, a clear job sheet and occasional supervision is usually adequate.

In long-term patient care, however, when public health and practical nurse work in an integrated way with much interchange of specific activities, there is no such clear delineation of duties. For example, the public health nurse may give insulin to a patient during a period of rebellion against the disease, or with a person who appears not to understand his dietary restrictions; the practical nurse may give the same treatment at a later time when the patient has adjusted to his disease and when there is less need for counseling and emotional support during the nursing contact.

When responsibilities are shared with auxiliary workers it is necessary to:

2. *Facts About Nursing*, 1955–56 Edition. New York, American Nurses' Association, 1956, p. 155.

1. Keep the total management of the family nursing care the responsibility of the professional worker.
2. Have a clear understanding of the family nursing care plan. The practical nurse or aide must understand what the public health nurse is doing and why, and the over-all purposes of the total nursing service, else the practical nursing responsibility is not clear.
3. Be sure that the practical nurse or aide understands the conditions that would require consultation with or referral back to the professional nurse. For example, if a man with a cardiac impairment reports that he is not sleeping well, or if he shows a slight but consistent increase in pulse rate, or says he "feels nauseated at the idea of food," the practical nurse should be able to recognize these symptoms as an indication that a professional nursing visit is needed. If the mother of a preschool child who is being readied for a medical examination seems exasperated or tense with him, or the woman with a hip-and-leg cast complains of cold toes the aide should recognize the need to report such things to the nurse. Joint case-planning is an essential element in the use of auxiliary workers.
4. Give status to the auxiliary worker on the team. It is easy to build up family confidence in the practical nurse or aide; to show one's own confidence in her work by commenting on things done especially well; by talking things over with her and asking advice; by sharing with her educational materials or opportunities that may be available.
5. In observing the work of the practical nurse's aide, or in making suggestions for improvement of her work, the same helping approach that would be used with families should be employed. When changes need to be made, make clear that you both share the same objective—to provide better family health care—and recognize her concern as well as your own. If a different procedure is suggested, be sure to give the reason why, and explain that it is the situation and not you personally that requires the change.
6. Discuss the nursing care of families frequently and informally, especially if the public health nurse's visits are infrequent. Having a specific time each week to review cases and to plan for care makes for effective use of time. However, it should be clear that cases can be discussed at any time. Problems should not wait for a scheduled conference if they

are worrisome or important, or even if they are just of nag-
ging concern to the practical nurse or aide.

Working with volunteers and with paid auxiliary workers requires the exercise of sound leadership. The public health nurse
does not turn over her responsibility for family care—the case
management responsibility must stay with her. All members of
the team work together to do the job, with the public health nurse
maintaining over-all responsibility, while at the same time giving
full recognition to the importance of volunteer and auxiliary staff
in bringing better nursing care to the families served.

STUDENT PROGRAMS

The public health nurse will have many opportunities to participate in the basic professional education of nurses and of related
professional workers. She may:

1. Arrange for field or clinic observations.
2. Work in a coaching relationship with nursing students assigned for a period of clinical practice in public health
   nursing.
3. Participate in family care courses by attending case discussions, or by conferring with individual students about
   families.
4. Teach in formal classes or seminars.

Through all of these approaches, the nurse brings to the student
a live contact with community nursing—an opportunity to get the
feel of such service as well as to obtain facts about it.

Whatever the type of experience provided, it is important to
remember that the student will see only part of the total program
—he will see the service only at a given point in time. The field
nurse has the responsibility for being sure that the student relates
his actual observation or experience to the total nursing or health
program, and to the direction of changes occurring in the service
on a long-term basis. For example, the nurse may indicate that
the school nursing service which the student observes represents
a compromise between a previous type of program which was felt
to be ineffective but was much liked by the school administrator,
and what will probably be a different pattern in the future when
it is more acceptable.

The nurse should learn, whenever it is possible to do so, what
information the student has already had about public health nursing or about public health services in general, and whether there
are special aspects of the service that the sending agency feels
are particularly important to this particular student.

Arranging Field Observations.   The "day in the field with a public health nurse" can be a very profitable experience for the medical or nursing student, or it can be a complete waste of time. Unless carefully planned, such a brief contact may produce serious misconceptions of function and service. One medical student, for example, after a day with the visiting nurse explained to a fellow student that the visiting nurse did the work that involved the "laying on of hands," while the health department did the teaching and preventive work. He had visited with an excellent nurse, who included a great deal of teaching and preventive work in her contacts with families. However, the selection of families to be observed was such that what the student actually saw was personal care of the patient. If he had had an explanation of what had already been done in the family, or what was projected, he might have seen the service whole. Through record reading followed by discussion, or through conversation before and after the visit, the student might have been given a much clearer concept and deeper appreciation of the work of the voluntary agency. For example, the nurse might have said, "Mrs. Smith is quite cheerful about her disability now, but at first she had a very hard time accepting it. She had to have a great deal of attention and we made many more visits than would have been warranted by her physical condition alone; this gave her and her husband also a chance to blow off steam and voice their bitterness about this affliction, and to realize that we were really standing by and wanting to help. Usually with patients getting along this well the practical nurse gives most of the care, but today I had hoped to start Mrs. Smith thinking about doing something for someone else. She has enough control in her hands now so she can write letters, and I thought she might like to write to some of our new patients who need cheering. Her writing may look a bit shaky, but she would probably get a great deal of satisfaction from such an activity. But when she seemed so upset at the news that she and her family will have to move to a new apartment, I realized it was not a good time to bring up this idea. She was too upset even to talk about her moving problems. I'll revisit in a few days, and try to help her with the problems of moving, and after the family is settled again I'll suggest the friendly writing." In this way a sense of the whole plan would have been conveyed, and the concept of helping as contrasted to simply giving treatments would have been emphasized. Through informal discussion the student should learn what has gone before and what is planned for the future; the family's share in decision making and in providing nursing care; and the relationship between the nursing care and that given by other professional workers, such as the physician, social worker, or physical therapist. If the service provided on the observed visit to the family is atypical, it is particularly important to explain how and why this differs from usual care, and the basis upon which modifications in the pattern of care are made.

Observation of a clinic session may also present only a partial view of family service. The student must see the clinic service as it is related to other family service provided through home visits, office conferences, group work, or other methods. The tendency of the student to focus attention on the operation of the clinic must be balanced by an interpretation of the place of the clinic service in the total pattern of family care. This approach is facilitated if the student becomes identified with a patient or two. He can then observe the clinic procedure through the patient's eyes. He should also be helped to see this service as it relates to other community services provided to the patients he is observing especially, and to services being rendered to family members who are not enrolled in this particular clinic. The medical or social work student might follow a patient as he goes through the clinic. Through record reading and conference he might learn what home follow-up has been provided or planned, what other members of the family have had care, or are now under care. For non-nurses especially, it is important that the teaching facet of clinic care be interpreted clearly.

Sometimes services afforded in clinics for some of the population are duplicated in part for patients under private medical care. For example, the medical or social work student should know if the group conferences or individual counseling services provided to clinic patients who meet certain eligibility requirements are also available to the patients who are under the care of private physicians.

Coaching. In some situations, especially in rural areas, nursing students are assigned to work with a field nurse for a period of clinical practice. Usually the selection of the field practice agency and a framework of policy agreement and general planning will have been effected between the appropriate administrative officers of the school and of the agency or the state or unit health department. However, the field nurse will have great influence in the selection of activities for the student. Even more important, the field nurse will affect the student's concept of public health nursing as a whole, and her concept of public health as a component in all nursing activities.

Families selected for student care should be typical rather than problem cases. Usually students find it easier to manage cases in which the problems are well defined, and such cases should make up the bulk of the early case load. Later in the student's experience, handling more subtle problems will be more profitable. For example, it is relatively easy for the nursing student to provide care to the expectant mother who has a common complication, such as an elevation of blood pressure. This type of service parallels that the nurse has given in the hospital. However, the expectant mother who comes from an economically secure home, and is having a second baby that is welcome, and who is without any physical problems associated with the pregnancy requires the kind of nursing assistance with which the nurse may be less familiar. She will need help in preparing the sibling for the new baby, and anticipatory guidance in relation to the differences that may be expected in siblings, in methods of avoiding fatigue, or in training baby sitters or grandparents. In these areas the student is apt to have had much less experience, and she will need to build some competence and assurance before she can manage them easily.

In general, it is better for the student to give intensive care to a small number of families than to have a scattered experience which covers many different types of illness or health condition, but which permits little consecutive care for the families served. Public health nursing procedures are quickly learned, and may in fact have been taught in the classroom. But the process of providing comprehensive family care, and relating this to the health care of the community as a whole is less easily mastered. This experience in depth is an essential part of public health nursing practice.

Ample time must be allowed for conference and discussion. This provides an opportunity for exploring service potentials in relation to a particular family, for reviewing the care given as it affects family health behavior, and for relating the service given in this instance to the general program. For example, the student caring for a cardiac patient needs to savor the full depth of service to *families* in which there are cardiac patients. She needs to see that the care of cardiac patients cannot follow a set pattern, that each patient will differ in needs and in the type of care he should have, depending upon family as well as patient characteristics.

Through conference and discussion the student can also be helped to see the service as a whole, and the trends and developments that are anticipated. She should see the degree to which the period of her observation and practice is typical of the year-round program. If she is present in the early fall when school activities predominate, she should have an opportunity to discuss the ways in which the various services are balanced during the year, and the way in which the service plans are developed. Almost always there will be some aspects of the program that are incomplete or otherwise unsatisfactory. The student can learn much from discussion of plans that are not being carried out, or activities that are not running smoothly. Through such discussion, the problems and principles that underlie program planning, the basis on which compromises are effected, and some of the human elements that interfere with accomplishment of objectives can be clarified.

It is important to know the educational program from which the student comes, so her experience can be related back to her work in the classroom. The field nurse may confer with the instructional staff of the school, secure copies of class outlines, or talk with students about the content of their classwork and how it relates to what they are seeing and doing in the field. Some schools arrange for regular meetings of faculty and field staff to whom students are assigned, to promote integration of classroom and field experience.

The field nurse will get much assistance from her supervisor or from nursing consultants from the unit or state office. The school may also provide faculty members to work directly in the field, who will assist the staff nurse in the student program. Usually there is at least one opportunity during the student's experience for a three-way conference with the staff nurse, the student and the educational director or supervising nurse who is responsible for the over-all student program.

To summarize, in arranging for clinical field experience when the staff nurse acts as a preceptor it is important to:

1. Provide "experience in depth," through thorough exploration of the services given, their potential effect on family

health behavior, and their relation to the objectives of the total public health program of the community.

2. Relate the field experience to the theoretical instruction the student has had.

3. Discuss and evaluate deviations from the ideal in the program in which the student is participating, and the reasons why the deviations exist.

PARTICIPATION IN FAMILY-CARE COURSES

An increasing number of professional schools—especially medical schools—are offering courses in family care. In these courses the student "follows" a family during the entire period of his student preparation, at first observing and gradually providing an increasing amount of professional service as his skills and knowledge develop. A similar experience, but of shorter duration, may be offered when students participate in home care programs of various types. The students, usually in the last year of their program, act as family practitioners under the guidance of the faculty of the school.

The public health nurse may participate in family care courses by:

1. Attending and participating in case presentations and discussions, bringing to the seminar her knowledge of the family and its problems.

2. Planning or conferring with medical or other professional students about the care of a family that is included in her case load.

3. Serving as one member of a multi-disciplinary panel in presenting a case for discussion.

The public health nurse has special information and competences that are important in the student's understanding of the meaning and depth of family health care. She should be prepared to assist in appropriate ways in family-care courses, when families under her general supervision are also used as teaching cases.

FORMAL TEACHING

Occasionally the public health nurse will be asked to participate in formal classroom instruction in schools of nursing, medicine or social work, either through presenting one or more lectures or discussion periods or by teaching an entire course in public health nursing.

The public health nurse can bring a great deal to courses in public health or preventive medicine; her close contact with the community and the "live" nature of her teaching material cannot be duplicated by those who are not in a direct service situation. Teaching at one or two sessions in a course may be mutually beneficial to student and field nurse, bringing the student closer to immediate public health nursing problems, and giving the field nurse an opportunity to organize her thinking and renew her faith in public health nursing as a means to improve community health.

In presenting material through a lecture or discussion period the nurse should:

1. Find out what is covered in the course as a whole, and how this session fits into the total plan.
2. Select vital, specific problems to discuss which exemplify the principles the student should identify and remember.
3. Protect families from identification and the agency from criticism while discussing problems.

Requests for more extensive classroom teaching should be considered very carefully, and accepted only after consultation with appropriate supervisory and administrative officers. Such requests should be granted only when:

1. It is clear that the job could not be done better by a member of the faculty of the school, thus providing more opportunity for integration of public health with other aspects of the curriculum.
2. The field nurse has the necessary breadth of experience and preparation to undertake the job.
3. The time necessary for teaching—and, even more important, for the preparation for teaching—can be taken without sacrificing essential public health nursing services.

Regardless of the degree to which schools provide their own field supervisory staff, or the agency functions through an educational director or director of student programs, the practicing nurse is bound to have an important influence on students working with or near her. Faith in one's job and its importance, enthusiasm, and a thoughtful concern for patients, for their families and for the community are catching. Even when the staff nurse has no direct responsibility for students, she should appreciate the force of her incidental communication with students, and direct that force toward the improvement of the students' understanding of public health nursing practice.

SUGGESTED READINGS

Part III

Program Planning and Coordination

Adams, Mary C., Case Selection and Planning. *Public Health Nursing*, 44: 140–141, March, 1952.

American Public Health Association, *Guide to a Community Health Study, 1955.* New York, American Public Health Association, 1955.

A Study of Selected Home Care Programs, *Public Health Monograph No. 35.* Washington, D.C., U.S. Government Printing Office, 1955.

Baumgartner, Leona, Maternal and Child Health Services. *Public Health Reports*, 68: 397–404, April, 1953.

Bergsma, Daniel, A Method of Recording Public Health Programs. *American Journal of Public Health*, 46: 72–74, January, 1956.

Department of Public Health Nursing, National League for Nursing, *Nursing Activities of Public Health Nursing Agencies.* New York, The League, 1955.

Department of Public Health Nursing, National League for Nursing, *Communication between Nursing Services.* New York, The League, 1957.

Erskine, W. L., A Health Program for Migrant Workers. *Nursing Outlook*, 3: 333–335, June, 1955.

Farrisey, Ruth M., Continuity of Nursing Care and Referral Systems. *American Journal of Public Health*, 44: 449–454, April, 1954.

Ferguson, Marian, W. G. Hollister and Florence Ullman, What Does the Consumer Want? *Nursing Outlook*, 2: 571–574, November, 1954.

Foster, G. M., Guidelines to Community Development Programs. *Public Health Reports*, 70: 19–22, January, 1955.

Hubbard, Ruth and Matilda Sheuer, Organization of Referral Programs. *Nursing Outlook*, 4: 18–19, January, 1956.

Identification of Social Components in Health Department Programs. *American Journal of Public Health*, 44: 125, January, 1954.

Kirkwood, S. B., Complete Maternity Care. *American Journal of Public Health*, 46: 1547–1549, December, 1956.

Knutson, Andie, Human Behavior Factors in Program Planning. *Public Health Reports*, 70: 1129–1134, November, 1955.

Kotinsky, Ruth, An Approach to Interprofessional Understanding. *Children*, 1: 203–206, November-December, 1954.

Kurlander, A. B., and B. Carroll, Case Finding through Multiple Screening. *Public Health Reports*, 68: 1035–1042, November, 1953.

Leader's Digest. Chicago, Adult Education Association of U.S.A., 1954. pp. 63–69, "Program planning."

McKeever, Nell and M. Derryberry, What Does the Changing Practice of Public Health Mean to Health Education in Program and Practice? *American Journal of Public Health*, 46: 54–60, January, 1956.

Minkoff, A. B., A Community Based Home Care Program. *Nursing Outlook*, 2: 516–518, October, 1955.

Nathan, M. R., Some Steps in the Process of Program Planning. *American Journal of Public Health*, 46: 68–71, January, 1956.

Rives, Ruth, The Staff Nurse Develops Her Own Priorities. *Nursing Outlook*, 1: 266–268, May, 1953.

Sheahan, Marion, The Public Health Nurse's Contribution to the Annual Planning of a Public Health Program. *American Journal of Public Health*, 37: 1586–1588, December, 1947.

Vaughan, M. S., Priorities for Public Health Nursing Visits. *Public Health Nursing*, 43: 17–20, January, 1951.

Yankauer, A., K. Gross and S. Romeo, An Evaluation of Prenatal Care and Its Relationship to Social Class and Social Disorganization. *American Journal of Public Health*, 43: 1001–1010, August, 1953.

Young, R. F., A Scientific Approach to Fetal Wastage in Halifax County, North Carolina. *Public Health Reports*, 71: 1065–1068, November, 1956.

PROGRAM EVALUATION

Beasley, Florence, and William C. Rhodes, An Evaluation of Public Health Nursing Services for Families of the Mentally Ill. *Nursing Outlook*, 4: 444–447, August, 1956.

Corley, Catherine, Beyond What Is Required. *Nursing Outlook*, 3: 213–215, April, 1955.

Corley, Catherine, Study of the Results of Public Health Nursing Procedures As Judged by Infant Welfare Records. *Nursing Research*, 3: 92, October, 1954.

Densen, Paul M., and Janice Mickey, Evaluation As a Basis for Progress. *Nursing Outlook*, 2: 383–385, July, 1954.

Dunlap, Mary, The Tape Recorder As an Aid to Education. *Nursing Outlook*, 3: 338–340, June, 1955.

Evaluation in Public Health (Conference Report). *Public Health Reports*, 71: 525–529, June, 1956.

Hilleboe, H., Public Health in a Changing World. *American Journal of Public Health*, 45: 1522–1523, December, 1955.

Knutson, Andie, Evaluating Program Progress. *Public Health Reports*, 70: 305–310, March, 1955.

Knutson, Andie and Benjamin Shimberg, Evaluation of a Health Education Program. *American Journal of Public Health*, 45:21–27, January, 1955.

Leader's Digest. Chicago, Adult Education Association of the U.S.A., 1954, Chapter 7, "Evaluating progress."

McGuire, J. H., and R. Freeman, Teaching Effectiveness of Non-nurse Instruction Shown by Tests. *School and Society*, 69: 268–271, April 9, 1949.

National Organization for Public Health Nursing, Desirable Organization of Public Health Nursing for Family Service. *Public Health Nursing*, 38: 387–388, August, 1946.

Prock, Valencia, Analysis of the Health Services Given by a Voluntary and an Official Agency. *Nursing Research*, 4: 4–23, June, 1955.

Shetland, Margaret, *Family Health Service*. New York, Community Service Society, 1943.

Shimberg, Benjamin, and Ellen Aird, Effectiveness of Television in Teaching Home Nursing. *Nursing Research,* 4: 28–41, June, 1955.

Walker, Janet and Mary McQuillen, Process Recording in Public Health Nursing. *Public Health Nursing,* 44: 542–547, October, 1952.

Wallace, Helen, and others, Use of a Review Committee in the Evaluation of a Program for Handicapped Children. *American Journal of Public Health,* 45: 751–758, June, 1955.

RECORDS AND REPORTS

Dahlin, Bernice and Helen Hotchner, The New Family Record. *Public Health Nursing,* 44: 142–145, March, 1952.

Densen, Paul, Administrative Use of Records. *American Journal of Public Health,* 39: 1025–1026, August, 1949.

Dickerson, L. A., Coordinating Medical and Nursing Records. *Public Health Reports,* 68: 1205–1239, December, 1953.

Fulton, W. J., Records—the Seeing Eye of Industrial Medicine. *Industrial Medicine,* 13: 1, 36, 154–155, 1944.

Gallagher, Constance D. and J. R. Gallagher, A Tab System for Use in the Follow up of Health Examinations. *American Journal of Public Health,* 42: 969–971, August, 1952.

Hazard, W. G., Putting Absence Records to Use. *American Journal of Public Health,* 41: 1087–1095, September, 1951.

Jones, Mary E., Nursing Activities in Erie County Department of Health and Their Reporting. *American Journal of Public Health,* 45: 324–327, March, 1955.

Kenney, Alpha K., Simplifying Local Service Records. *Public Health Reports,* 68: 1200–1205, December, 1953.

McCabe, Anne and Dorothy Clark, Family Record. *Public Health Nursing,* 43: 624–627, November, 1951.

The Narrative Record—a Nursing Tool. *Public Health Nursing,* 43: 620–623, November, 1951.

National League for Nursing, *Statistical Reporting and Costs in Public Health Nursing.* New York, The League, 1953.

Records and Reports in Local Health Departments, *Public Health Monograph No. 15.* Washington, D.C., U.S. Government Printing Office, 1953.

Swanson, Marie, *School Nursing in the Community Program.* New York, Macmillan Co., 1953, Chapter 14, "The nurse's part in school recording."

Tolleris, B. K., *Annual Reports: How to Plan and Write Them.* New York, National Publicity Council, 1946.

Webster, Robert G., Public Health Operating Statistics. *Public Health Reports,* 68: 467–473, May 1953.

Weisner, M., The Industrial Nurses' Annual Report. *American Journal of Nursing,* 55: 697, June, 1955.

COMMITTEES AND BOARDS

Adult Leadership, 3: 13–24, November, 1954. A series of articles comprising a "Workshop on the Volunteer."

Blumenthal, L. H., *How to Work with Your Board and Committees*. New York, Association Press, 1954.

Carp, Bernard, *Your Annual Meeting*. National Publicity Council for Health and Welfare Services, 1955.

Fauber, J. C., G. Laue and others, Building Committees That Work. *Adult Leadership*, 2: 11–19, September, 1953.

Koos, E. L., New Concepts in Community Organization. *American Journal of Public Health*, 43: 466–469, April, 1953.

Round Table on Health Councils. New York, National Health Council, 1956.

Seering, Esther, Our Board Works with the Health Department. *Nursing Outlook*, 3: 206–207, April, 1955.

Sorenson, Roy, *How to Be a Board or Committee Member*. New York, Association Press, 1956.

Strauss, Bert and Frances Strauss, *New Ways to Better Meetings*. New York, Viking Press, 1951.

Two Sample Manuals for V.N.A. Board and Committee Members. *League Exchange No. 14*. New York, National League for Nursing, 1956.

Wensley, Edith, *The Community and Public Health Nursing*. New York, Macmillan Co., 1950.

VOLUNTEERS, AUXILIARIES, STUDENTS

Belin, Constance, The Citizen's Contribution to Nursing. *Nursing Outlook*, 4: 25–28, January, 1956.

Bell, Marjorie, The Staff Nurse As Senior Adviser. *Public Health Nursing*, 44: 286–289, May, 1952.

Dawson, Jessie, The Public Health Assistant in a Health Department Program. *Public Health Nursing*, 44: 443–444, August, 1952.

Field Training of Public Health Personnel. *American Journal of Public Health*, 45: 1351–1355, October, 1955.

Joint Committee on Practical Nurses and Auxiliary Workers in Nursing Services, *Practical Nurses in Nursing Services*. New York, American Nurses' Association, 1951.

Lott, Merle K., Volunteer Aides in a County Health Department. *Nursing Outlook*, 2: 622–624, December, 1954.

Menkin, Paula, Supervising the Volunteer. *Adult Leadership*, 4: 19–20, October, 1955.

Olson, Apollonia, Rural Affiliations with a New Look, *American Journal of Nursing*, 51: 621–624, October, 1951.

Phillips, Elizabeth, The Role of the Practical Nurse in Public Health Nursing Services. *American Journal of Public Health*, 42: 717–722, June, 1952.

Thomson, Ann, Field Instruction in Public Health Nursing. *Nursing Outlook*, 2: 597–598, November, 1954.

Services in Clinics, Schools and in Occupational Health Programs

CHAPTER XX

Public Health
Nursing in Clinics

Most public health agencies carry some clinic activities in which the public health nurse participates. Certain group procedures such as medical examinations in school and industry are also conducted on a clinic basis.

Clinics may be open on a continuing basis, or scheduled for only a single session or series. The clinic may be organized by the agency in which the public health nurse is employed, or sponsored by some other agency. For example, clinics in which a county nurse participates may be established under the auspices of the local or state health department, hospital or other community agency. They may be set up in permanent headquarters or may function on a mobile basis. Sometimes groups of physicians may establish a "pay clinic" that operates as a private venture.

Most states have legislation controlling the establishment of clinics or dispensaries, as well as laws that control any agency that seeks support from public contributions. Fees may be collected for clinic service under policies established by the agency board of directors with advice from the medical advisory committee, or by the appropriate administrative officer. Clinics set up under the auspices of tax-supported agencies rarely collect fees from patients.

In the large, well-organized clinic the public health nurse's responsibility may be limited to following established procedures and maintaining supplies and equipment. She may make suggestions, but determination of procedures and materials used may be prescribed by experts in the field of planning medical facilities or by staff or executive committees. In the small clinic the nurse may have to find clinic quarters, secure and set up equipment, and assume responsibility for over-all management.

The public health nurse may be called upon to advise or assist in clinic services in the following ways:

1. Determining need for clinics.
2. Assisting with preclinic organization activities, such as notification of patients or promotional activities.
3. Arranging for housing and equipment.
4. Securing necessary clearances and setting up routines for patient management.
5. Organizing an instructional program.
6. Organizing and supervising services of subsidiary workers and volunteers.
7. Planning record systems and follow-up procedures, such as notification of patients, referral and reporting to other agencies, and arranging supplementary home care.

SUGGESTING NEED FOR CLINIC FACILITIES

The public health nurse, especially in rural areas, may assist in determining the need for establishment or continuance of clinics. Since clinics involve medical care, no recommendation or request for such service should be made without consultation with the medical advisory committee or medical director of the agency, or, in the absence of these, with the local medical society.

Clinics should not be proposed if existing facilities for care are or could be made adequate. Special clinic facilities (such as orthopedic or mental hygiene clinics) may be necessary if specialist services are not available in the community of nearby hospitals, or if such service is not available to those unable to pay the usual fees for care. It is important to know approximately how many individuals might be expected to avail themselves of the service offered.

HOUSING AND EQUIPMENT

Selection of a Clinic Site.   The public health nurse may be asked to find suitable quarters for either a continuing or special clinic. If there is a well-organized nursing committee, its members might undertake the search for facilities, or a special subcommittee might be appointed to work on this particular project.

The following criteria should be considered in selecting a clinic site:

1. Convenience to transportation. In rural areas the clinic should be easily accessible by automobile or bus and have adequate space for parking cars. If the clinic is in a center that makes it possible to combine the clinic visit with shopping, school consultation or some other activity, it is even more satisfactory. In urban areas the clinic should be easily reached by main line trolley or bus, and when possible within a single fare zone.

2. The clinic building should not be one that is associated with any particular religious or political group. Unless the community has virtually one religious faith, clinics should not be held in churches or denominational meeting places. (An exception is a first-aid or treatment clinic set up during a disaster or other emergency when such considerations can be temporarily ignored.) Political meeting places should also be avoided as clinic sites.

3. The clinic should be in a familiar place, if possible. People in a particular community may be used to meeting in the settlement house auditorium, in the rural school house or in the 4-H Clubhouse, and it is easy for them to identify that location.

4. The clinic site should provide for the special needs of the clinic patients. Well-baby clinics should have space to park baby carriages; prenatal clinics should not require the patient to walk up several flights of stairs; syphilis treatment clinics should not be isolated from other services so that the patient's diagnosis is made apparent to others.

5. Handwashing and toilet facilities should be available as well as provision for sterilization of equipment if necessary. A one-burner gas plate or solid alcohol stove might be adequate for some clinics; others would require plumbing outlets for sterilizers.

6. Heating and ventilation should be adequate. Open heating units such as gas burners should be avoided because they present an accident hazard, especially when small children may be expected to attend the clinic.

7. Waiting space should provide adequate seating facilities.

8. Space should be adequate to provide privacy for patient interviews with the physician and the nurse, either in separate rooms or by the use of screens.

9. The rooms should be easily cleaned. Floors should be covered with some hard-surfaced material such as linoleum or asphalt tile, and walls should be painted rather than papered.

Securing and Organizing Clinic Equipment. In large urban clinics the nurse will have relatively little responsibility for selecting or purchasing equipment. Her concern will be in arranging and caring for equipment and in assuring maintenance of supplies. In rural clinics the nurse may be responsible for securing all equipment and supplies by purchase or loan, or for supplementing the equipment and supplies provided by a mobile clinic.

In the purchase of equipment and supplies for clinics, the following points shoul be kept in mind:

1. If the clinic is a permanent one, equipment should be efficient. Improvised equipment should be scrutinized carefully to be sure it is not actually wasteful of time. For example, poor equipment for filing records, occasioned by attempting to use cast-off filing equipment, may cause much loss of time on the part of the patient or the clinic clerical staff.

2. Equipment that must be transported should be light in weight and packable. Experimentation will develop methods of packing that make for compactness, protection of breakable or chip-prone equipment, and rapid unpacking and arrangement of materials. If sets of equipment are frequently used, they may be set up in advance and packed in well-labeled cartons or specially constructed boxes.

3. When equipment is borrowed there should be a clear understanding about the costs and methods of transportation, service charges and the date on which equipment must be returned.

4. Supplies should be purchased locally when it is possible to do so. Some items may be purchased by the agency or provided through the state department of health. For supplies not centrally purchased, it is good public relations to procure them locally since it identifies the agency more closely with the community.

5. Storage for supplies should be adequate, and, when the clinic space is used by other groups, supply closets should be kept locked.

6. Record and report forms should permit comparison with other services. Most state departments of health have recom-

mended forms for use in various nursing services, or forms may be purchased from the National League for Nursing.

PLANNING WITH OTHER CLINIC PERSONNEL

Planning conferences with other clinic personnel are essential for good management. The post-clinic session, in which all workers meet to discuss the clinic, the problems presented by patients and the need for follow-up service, is becoming more and more common. If this is not possible, occasional informal discussion periods might be arranged with the physician and any other professional workers involved to evaluate and plan for family care through the clinic and related services.

CLINIC MANAGEMENT

Securing Necessary Clearances. When treatments are to be given to minors, it is necessary to secure written consent for the treatment or diagnostic procedure from the child's parents. Parental approval should be secured for such measures as immunization, x-ray examinations, tuberculin tests, and blood tests for syphilis. If diagnostic findings or statements regarding services rendered are to be released to other agencies, physicians or individuals, the patient may need to give his consent for release of this information. (Many states have legislation forbidding release of such information to anyone but the patient.) In some instances it is desirable to have the consent of private physicians for their patients to use special diagnostic facilities; for example, a private physician may be asked to indicate his approval for having his patient attend the state-sponsored orthopedic clinic for posture appraisal, or a multiphasic diagnostic clinic. If minors are to be transported to the clinic in private cars, parents' consent and release of responsibility in case of accident should be secured.

Routing and Handling of Patients. The nurse must plan to avoid confusion by orderly handling of patients.

1. Receive and register each patient and secure his record for referral to the physician or nurse. At this step a certain amount of screening may be done, and obviously disqualified applicants referred for consultation with a professional worker. At this point, too, much can be done to reassure the incoming patient and to make him feel welcome and secure.
2. Route patient through dressing, examination or treatment,

conference, redressing and appointment stations. A one-way flow of traffic, when possible, avoids confusion. Adequate waiting space must be provided at each station in the process to avoid having patients mill around in the clinic and add to the confusion.

3. Arrange appointments. An appointment system may be used or patients may be given a number, or the receptionist may list names or place case records in the order of registration so the patients may be called in turn as their records are taken to the physician or to the conference desk or room. A receptionist (who may also register the patient), and a hostess, both of whom may be volunteers, help to keep patients properly directed and to make them feel welcome.

4. Record findings, services or instruction. The nurse usually records her work during or immediately following her service to or consultation with the patient. The physician's findings and recommendations may be written on the patient's record by him or by a recorder who sits beside his desk and takes notes as he dictates them. This recorder may be a volunteer worker or a medical or nursing field student who uses this method to obtain an over-all view of the type of medical services provided.

ORGANIZING AN INSTRUCTIONAL PROGRAM

Clinic attendance should be a learning experience for every patient. Patient instruction may be general and incidental, such as is provided by posters, pictures, exhibits, charts, fliers or leaflets placed in the waiting room. It may be more formalized group instruction as is given when a demonstration or discussion class is given during the first half hour of a prenatal clinic, or a motion picture is shown to patients in a syphilis clinic prior to or following their conference with the physician. Individual teaching interviews may be arranged for each patient or for selected patients to interpret the doctor's recommendations or to supplement his instruction. For example, following an eye examination, the patient may be scheduled for an interview with the nurse who discusses the doctor's findings and recommendations, demonstrates or explains treatments if necessary, answers questions or provides general health instruction if such is needed. Usually the instructional program in a clinic will use more than one of these methods.

It is the nurse's responsibility to plan with other professional personnel of the clinic for the type of instruction that will be provided, and for the methods that will be used. For example, in a preschool health clinic there may be a nursing interview with each parent to discuss the child's particular problems and needs. In addition to this a variety of exhibits may be planned on food selection, homemade toys, clothing that permits freedom of activity and is easy for the child to manage, or books of interest to the very young child. Motion pictures on growth and development may be secured and showed prior to or following the clinic session. Parents' clubs or discussion groups may be formed to supplement clinic instruction. Leaflets or pamphlets on child care may be distributed, or parents may be given direction for securing such materials. Posters, graphs or charts may be used to emphasize some particular aspect of care.

Whatever method is used, each should be part of a planned program of instruction, not a haphazard addition. Posters, for example, should be varied and changed frequently to meet the seasonal and regional differences in patient interest, instead of the dispirited display of old pictures that is too often found. Exhibits should use materials familiar to the group attending the clinic; a display using mayonnaise jars as containers for baby bath supplies should not be used if the people attending the clinic do not use mayonnaise. Food displays should be made of items actually liked and frequently purchased by the group. Individual conferences should not be limited to interpreting findings and recommendations of this particular clinic visit, but should be planned to meet individual and family needs in exactly the same way they would in counseling in the home.

CLINIC ORGANIZATIONAL ACTIVITIES

Depending on the size and type of clinic or agency, the public health nurse will assume varying degrees of responsibility for organization. In large agencies, community organization experts, health educators or management assistants may carry the greater responsibility, while in small rural services the nurse may have much responsibility for organization. For example, in setting up a physical examination session in a public school, the public health nurse may take full responsibility, in coordination with the instructional or guidance staff of the school and the medical supervisor. In a large city tuberculosis clinic, promotional activities and procedures for notification of patients may be developed by specialists or office staff entirely, with the public health nurse's role limited to offering suggestions on procedure.

Checking and Confirming Arrangements.   When clinics are not held continuously it is necessary to check and confirm arrangements carefully before the session is scheduled. This may be done by the public health nurse herself, by an administrative officer, or, if arrangements are being made by a committee, by the committee chairman, but the public health nurse should see that it is done. All arrangements should be confirmed in writing. In preparing for a school examination session, for example, the school superintendent or principal should have a letter confirming the date and general arrangements with copies for such classroom teachers or other instructional staff as are affected by the activity; the physician should have a letter giving the time and place of the examination; all helpers should be similarly informed.

A check list of the steps that should be taken and materials to be assembled may be prepared for the person or group responsible for general arrangements. The nurse herself may prepare and use this guide or send it to the local person or committee responsible.

General Publicity or Promotional Activities.   For noncontinuous clinics the nurse may be asked to organize or to help with publicity or promotional activities. Working with the health educator when one is available, she may suggest methods of publicity, explain the purposes of and need for the particular service, or approve publicity materials prepared by nonprofessional volunteer or paid workers. For example, if a mental hygiene clinic is coming to a small community, the nurse might work with a special promotion or publicity committee. She might suggest the value of short talks or announcements of the clinic, help to prepare an outline or fact sheet for speakers to use, suggest facts that might be suitable for incorporation in newspaper items, or suggest that notices of the clinic be posted in gathering places such as stores, clubs, or churches. Members of the committee could then follow through with the necessary action. Plans for promotion and publicity must be started well in advance of the clinic. Planning groups should be organized several months in advance and general publicity started at least a month before the clinic is to be held.

Plan for Clinic Attendance.   Patients should be notified of the time and place of the clinic; if an appointment system is used the importance of promptness should be stressed. If special information or permission slips are needed, this information should be provided in advance to assure that patients will come properly prepared. An appointment card may be given at one clinic for the next session, invitations may be distributed to entire groups of school children or employees, or individual invitations may be sent to a particular clinic. It may be important to know how many plan to attend the clinic. A double postcard may be used for the invitation so that the patients may use the return part of the card to indicate whether or not they plan to attend. Sometimes if the number invited is not too large or if clinic attendance is particularly important to the community, volunteer workers may telephone or call on families a few days in advance to check whether they plan to come to the clinic.

Some system must be devised to check those who do not keep appointments or respond to the invitation. The tickler file may be used for this. If the invitation or appointment has gone to persons already enrolled in the clinic, records of those expected to attend the clinic may be drawn from the file in advance. Then as the records of those attending the clinic are withdrawn and transmitted to the physician or nurse, those remaining constitute the delinquent or nonattendant group.

Sometimes a list of those invited may be prepared, with columns to check those who indicated they would attend and those who actually reported to the clinic. It may be necessary to plan for facilitating clinic attendance by securing volunteer assistance for transportation of patients (Red Cross Motor Service or neighborhood car pools may help here); arranging for care of children during times parents are to be at the clinic; arranging for special parking privileges for those attending the clinic, and so forth.

Training Clinic Assistants. Clinic assistants will need to be prepared for the service they will give. In some instances this will necessitate direct instruction by the nurse in advance of the clinic; for example, teachers may be taught to administer vision tests on one of the nurse's visits to the school prior to a physical examination period, or a group of helpers may be briefed just before the opening of a community orthopedic clinic. On other occasions the nurse may be able only to refresh the assistants' memories on previous duties, or send written instructions or guides. Sometimes it is possible to use volunteer professional nurses of the community to instruct clinic assistants.

FOLLOW-UP PROCEDURES

Follow-up procedures must be planned if clinic attendance is to be maintained, and continuous and comprehensive service assured for every patient. Clinic patients who do not report for appointments must be contacted, and individual counseling and instruction arranged to meet problems discovered during the clinic visit.

Checking Missed Clinic Appointments.   Some system should be devised for investigation of reasons for failure to keep clinic appointments. In some instances a letter or card to each patient who did not report, reminding him that the appointment was not kept and suggesting a new date, may be sent immediately after the clinic session. In other instances it may be better to wait a week or so, leaving with the patient the responsibility for informing the clinic of the reason he didn't come, and letting him take the initiative in making a new appointment. Some workers feel that too prompt a check-up makes the patient feel that he is being "hounded." In cases where clinic treatment is essential for the protection of others, an immediate home visit may be indicated.

Checking Action Taken.   It is important that plans be made to provide whatever supplementary service to patients may be needed to assure that the recommendations made at the clinic are carried through satisfactorily. For example, in a physical examination clinic in an industrial plant, Mr. X. may be told he should secure an examination by an oculist. The public health nurse must devise some method of ascertaining whether this advice has been followed and what corrective measures are instituted so that supplementary guidance may be given if necessary. Various methods may be used for this. Sometimes the worker is asked to report back to the health service by postcard, telephone or personal visit. A tickler file or follow-up flags or signals on the case record may be used to check whether a report has been received that recommendations have been carried out.

Supplementary Counseling.   A certain proportion of patients seen in clinic will need additional help in the form of home visits or subsequent conferences. These should, if possible, be scheduled at the time of the clinic.

Referral and Reporting to Other Agencies.   Reports of clinic service may be sent to private physicians, to other clinics or to health or social agencies. Appropriate forms for such reporting may need to be developed to conserve time of the clinic staff and to get information out promptly.

Definite reporting procedures should be established, defining to whom reports may be sent, who shall write them, whether they must be checked by nurse or physician before sending, and whether the patient's approval must be secured before the information is released.

Referral to other agencies will be facilitated if the necessary information is kept in the clinic or brought with other clinic materials. If a community resource file or book is available the patient may be referred directly and exactly to the other agency, thus reducing the need for subsequent office work or home calls.

SURVEY OR DIAGNOSTIC CLINICS

Special problems arise with survey or diagnostic clinics that are arranged for a single session or at widely spaced and irregular intervals. Tuberculosis diagnostic clinics, multiple blood-testing clinics for diagnosis of diabetes, syphilis and other diseases revealed by blood tests, and the recently developed multiphasic mobile diagnostic clinic create problems of management that do not arise with continuing clinics.

Advance Plannning. Advance planning for "spot" clinics should be begun at least three months before the clinic is scheduled,[1] and an intensive public information program should be instituted during the month prior to the clinic. A citizen committee for preliminary planning and action and to assist with follow-up is imperative. Such a committee should have representation from the local health department, nursing organization and important civic groups or civic-minded individuals. If there is a local health council the committee may be organized under its sponsorship; it may be under the auspices of the health department, or it may be set up as an independent body. Sometimes an already organized committee, such as a tuberculosis subcommittee of the health council or a health advisory committee of the health department of parent-teacher association may be the logical group to take on such a responsibility. It should be organized at least three months before the clinic is to be held to:

1. Assist with necessary interpretation of the program through talks, newspaper articles, interviews with leaders in the community, and similar activities.
2. Assist with physical set-up for the clinic.
3. Provide volunteer assistance in making preliminary contacts with patients and sending out invitations, screening records to find those who should be invited, making home or group contacts to explain the service.
4. Provide volunteer assistance in manning the clinic.

1. National Tuberculosis Association, *Chest X-ray Service in Action*. New York, National Tuberculosis Association, 1948.

5. Provide necessary volunteer assistance or assist in recruiting paid staff for follow-up procedures.
6. Set up necessary training courses for volunteers who will assist with the various aspects of the program.
7. Assist in reaching special groups that may be served as a unit. Industrial plants, schools, professional or fraternal organizations may agree to participate as a group. For example, a tuberculosis x-ray unit may be set up in an industrial plant or department store and employees released long enough to attend; a Rotary Club may agree to have a mobile blood collection unit service all of their group at one of their regular meetings, or the schools might release students from classes for an orthopedic diagnostic clinic.

Adjustment of the Work Load. Diagnostic or survey clinics are often of a rather specialized nature and organized like a campaign. During the period when the clinic is held and a short time before and after it, selection of patients to be visited and activities to be scheduled by the nurse will need considerable adjustment. For example, in a community tuberculosis x-ray program, approximately 3.4 percent of those who have an x-ray may be expected to need some further study.[2] Notices, letters, home and office conferences and telephone calls will be required to inform the patient of the findings, to interpret the need to him and to provide necessary guidance to those whose examination reveals some abnormality. While the proportion of patients who will need further care will vary with the type of clinic, it may be expected to be sufficiently large to distort the nurse's usual case load. The effectiveness of such follow-up procedures is greatly enhanced if they are provided very soon after the examination of the patient. The need for intensive nursing care in a particular field as a result of intensive diagnostic or treatment service may be met by:

1. Rearranging other responsibilities so as to clear the decks for this particular activity. Other programs may be held at a minimum level for a short period of time to permit intensive service in the areas being studied or examined.
2. Arranging in advance for some responsibilities ordinarily carried by the nurse to be carried by selected non-nurse volunteers for a short time. Such duties should be carefully

2. Roemmick, William, F. J. Weber, F. J. Hill and Lucille Amos, Preliminary Reporting in a Community-Wide Chest X-ray in Minneapolis, Minnesota. *Public Health Reports,* 63: 1285–1298, October 1, 1948. Similar results were found in other community surveys.

chosen and suitable volunteers mobilized and trained to assist. Volunteer nurses' aides, women who have had home nursing courses, or men who have served as corpsmen in the Navy might provide especially valuable service with a minimum amount of additional training.

3. Arranging for the use of an auxiliary staff of paid or volunteer professional nurses. In many communities there are inactive nurses who may be available for special peak activities. The local nursing association or nurses' registry may be able to suggest names. The American Red Cross chapter may maintain a roster of nurses who have agreed to help meet unusual community needs, usually on a volunteer basis. Nurses enlisted for such special services must have training or orientation to the program, and the responsibilities of the various groups or agencies that are participating in the program should be clearly understood. Also, instruction will be needed in the methods of the diagnostic or survey programs, as well as review of current concepts of the health conditions being studied, or of treatment methods and significant concurrent effects of the condition. It may also be necessary to give instruction in interviewing techniques.

Clinics offer a real opportunity for sound and comprehensive health guidance. Proper planning and efficient administration will enable the nurse to give her full time to nursing activities, delegating nonprofessional duties to volunteer or subsidiary personnel. She can promote full use of available medical time through proper management of patients and equipment, and enhance the value of medical services through a strong and soundly conceived program for patient instruction.

CHAPTER XXI

Public Health
Nursing in School and in
Occupational Health Programs

Pᴜʙʟɪᴄ ʜᴇᴀʟᴛʜ nursing provided in schools and that given in industrial establishments are similar in that the service is supplied by an agency organized for a purpose other than health care—health services are supplemental rather than central objectives. Both are characterized by multiple channels of responsibility for public health nursing—school nursing is the responsibility of school as well as health authorities, and industrial nursing is the responsibility of health and general management groups. Both require careful planning with health services offered by other community agencies to assure coordinated family care; both include nonmedical personnel on the health team. The services afforded are also similar. Although the age group involved creates differences in content, both are concerned with health appraisal; with the special types of problems created by the environment; with control of environmental factors of significance in accident control and general health care; with general health education and counseling growing out of specific problems in the environment, but encompassing the broad objectives of comprehensive care; and both utilize the activities of other professional groups, such as teachers and foremen, to further the health program.

The priorities assigned to activities and case selection will be influenced by the primary objectives of the agency as a whole, as well as by the objectives of the health service. For example, in industry it is important that priority be given to activities which tend to keep the worker on the job, since his absence slows down production of others as well as interrupting his own; in school, health services that promote good citizenship or living skills may have priority because of their contribution to the school's objective of producing better citizens.

In this chapter some of the special problems of school and industrial nursing will be discussed, but counseling and teaching procedures and principles of planning will not be considered as differing from those used in general public health nursing.

PUBLIC HEALTH NURSING IN SCHOOLS

Practice of public health nursing in schools involves the same procedures and processes as in other fields—there is the same need to help to develop the individual, to sense needs and adjust services to emotional as well as physical conditions, to consult with rather than to advise. Administrative and service relationships are based on the same principles; planning requires essentially the same steps. The difference lies in the locale and the environment rather than in the service itself.

Studying the School Community. Health is only one of the school's many objectives, and nursing only one facet of the health program. Unless the nurse has a concept of the whole, her efforts may miss maximum productivity. The nurse in the school has the same obligation to know her community—in this case the school community—as does the general public health nurse for the community as a whole. She needs to know how the school is organized to do its work—the relationship between the classroom teacher and the specialists; the regulations or laws under which the school functions, especially those relating to health requirements or exclusion from school. She needs to understand the philosophy on which the educational program is based—the concept of the school's responsibility for living skills as well as for academic content areas; the patterns of student responsibility that have been developed. She should be familiar with the agreements between the school and the health department relating to the health services provided for school children and faculty. Regulations regarding exclusion from school will be worked out jointly by the departments of health and education.

The degree to which the school is "community oriented" will influence the types of nursing service provided; if the school is used by the community as a regular meeting place and the school staff participates actively in community affairs, a broad approach is possible. The role played by the Parent-Teacher Association will make a difference in parent education plans and in volunteer recruitment.

The pattern of communication between teacher and administrative staff, and the degree of autonomy teachers have, will influence the methods of nurse-teacher planning and action.

The financing of the school system is also of interest, since it determines the degree of flexibility in use of funds, and the possibility of increasing budgetary appropriations for additional services.

The preparation of faculty in health care and education is also of significance in planning the nursing program. The degree of responsibility that faculty members can assume will hinge upon their knowledge of content as well as upon their attitude toward health promotion as a function of the school. If they feel it is a nuisance, or the nurse's responsibility and not their own, it is difficult to delegate responsibility for health inspection or pupil observation. The nurse's program will have to be adjusted to teacher expectations.

The pattern of use of school facilities is also important. Behavior in and use of the school cafeteria and the playground, and after-school use of school facilities will influence the safety program; availability of library resources may affect methods of health counseling; adult education facilities may open new channels of improving school health through adult education in health.

Relationships with Administrative and Instructional Personnel. The nurse in the school has a three-way responsibility—to the school administration for the over-all administration of the program in its relation to the total school program; to the school physician or medical adviser for nursing care which is part of the plan for medical supervision of pupils; to the nursing supervisor or community health agency for the professional nursing aspects of the work and the qualitative aspects of nursing practice.[1]

The public health nurse will want to arrange for periodic conferences with the appropriate administrative officer of the schools in which she works. This may be the county superintendent and the individual principals in a rural setting, or the principal in the urban community. These conferences provide an opportunity to

1. Department of Public Health Nursing, National League for Nursing, *School Nursing Services*. New York, The League, 1956, p. 57.

reach agreements regarding the scheduling of services, the content of the nursing program, and clearances that are required or desirable. Arrangements for teacher conferences in relation to schedules, classroom activities, plans for medical or dental examinations in the school, and methods of notifying parents of defects found are examples of things that require such clearance.

Regularly scheduled nurse-teacher conferences are also important. These provide an opportunity to discuss the health of the pupils under the teacher's surveillance, for exchange of information, and for consultation by the nurse in matters relating to health care. Such conferences may be scheduled monthly in urban schools; in rural schools, three or four times a year may be manageable and the conference may be combined with the nurse's observation of the children in school. Parent conferences may also be scheduled in the school on the same day.

The nurse in the high school will need to plan with the health teacher, the physical education teacher, the counselor or student adviser, and the home-room teacher.

In addition to scheduled or informal consultative conferences, the nurse will participate in the work of the instructional staff through active membership on school committees or councils, and through participation in parent-teacher meetings. She may be a member of the health committee of the school, or of the curriculum committee; in the rural district she may be a member of a county-wide school-community health committee or school health committee. In many schools there will be a school health council, with membership from the general teaching staff, administrative group, teachers in special health areas, health service personnel and, in some cases, student body. If the school nursing service is provided by the community health agency, the nurse may serve as representative of that agency on the health council, asking the responsible medical administrator to be present only as necessary. If school nursing is under the administrative direction of the Board of Education, a representative of the health department may also be a member of this council. The nurse should be an active participant not only in presenting information or suggested action, but also in recognizing the potential contribution of others, encouraging them to participate, and providing them with necessary factual material.

Health Appraisal Procedures.   Health appraisal of the school child is a joint responsibility of the school health service staff, the teacher, parents and family medical adviser. The nurse's share in this activity will vary depending upon the preparation and interest of the instructional staff, availability of private medical facilities, habits of the community in relation to use of preventive medical services, and the amount of time the nurse has available for school work. In communities that are accustomed to using community facilities for preventive medical services, the nurse's part may be one of supplementation and referral. When few of the group take advantage of available sources for preventive medical care, the nurse will place more stress on briefing teachers on the problem and teaching possibilities in this field, on "build-up" activities prior to the school health examination including work with individual families, on follow-up activities after the examination.

The *growth record,* maintained for each pupil on a monthly or quarterly basis, provides one index of development and health. It may be kept by the teacher or, in high schools, by the pupil himself. With younger children the routine weighing and measuring may be undertaken by a volunteer (the Parent-Teacher Association usually includes mothers with special interest in health work who may be recruited for this activity). The public health nurse's participation in weighing and measuring should be limited to those occasions on which she is using this activity as a channel for health education, or for building a satisfactory relationship with school staff and pupils.

Teacher observation of pupils should be a continuous process, and is the most potent means for detecting departures from normal health. The public health nurse should work with the teacher to enhance this observation, which is usually done on an informal basis. When special disease conditions are anticipated (as when there is an increased incidence of communicable disease), the nurse may provide special focussed instruction to teachers; for example, she may discuss the symptoms of measles and procedures for isolation and exclusion from school.

The teacher should be alerted to general symptoms of importance in judging student health—evidences of visual or hearing impairment; fatigue or listlessness; behavior such as withdrawal from the group, or belligerence, that may indicate emotional stress. The cumulative health record provides a guide for observation (Fig. 23). If the teacher is working in a rural environment she should know how to take the child's temperature and recognize other symptoms of illness and should be cognizant of procedures for isolation, since she must make judgments about sending the child home.

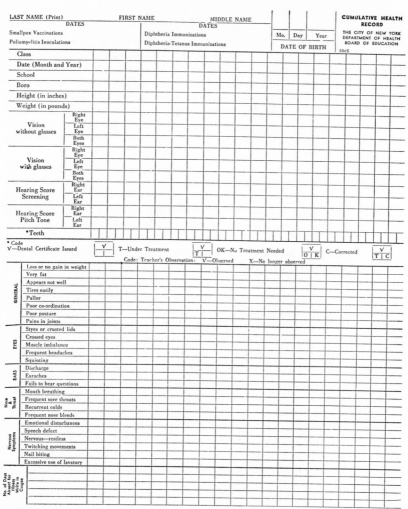

Figure 23. Cumulative Health Record, City of New York Department of Health and Board of Education. The reverse side provides space for narrative notes of nurse, teacher and physician.

During the teacher-nurse conference, when the status of all pupils is discussed, there is an opportunity to stress the observational procedures that may be followed, and to increase the teacher's sensitivity to deviations from normal behavior. This may also be a subject for discussion at teachers' meetings, before the beginning of the school year or during the year.

Vision and Hearing Screening Tests.   Vision and hearing tests may be required by law for students at specified intervals. Hearing tests may be given by a technician, or the nurse may be asked to administer them. The public health nurse should be familiar with the use of an audiometer; if she is not, arrangements should be made for her to observe a technician, and to secure the literature available about the use of the machine. The American Hearing Society sets standards for hearing tests. The pure-tone audiometer has been shown to be effective, economical and reliable, and testing hearing with it is considered the method of choice.[2] The nurse should be familiar with the problems that arise in hearing tests, and the indications for re-check, such as the presence of an upper respiratory infection at the time of the test. About 5 percent of the student group might be expected to have some hearing impairment.

There are several vision screening tests in use; perhaps most commonly used are the Snellen Chart and the Massachusetts Vision Test. The former is a simple test, in which children read a simple chart at a specified distance, testing each eye separately and then both eyes together. It measures visual acuity only. The Massachusetts Vision Test uses specially designed spectacles to test visual acuity and parallelism between visual lines. A study of the comparative effectiveness of vision testing methods done in 1948–49[3] showed that such tests are useful for rough screening only. The National Association for the Prevention of Blindness or the State Department of Health will provide information on testing procedures and their use.

In the testing of hearing and vision, it must be remembered that the observation of the teacher may be as significant as the tests themselves. The teacher who is alert to children who have a strained look as they listen or who seem inattentive without

2. Swanson, Marie, *School Nursing in the Community Program*. New York, Macmillan Co., 1953, p. 188.

3. Crane, Marion and others, Screening School Children for Visual Defects. *Children's Bureau Publication 345*. Washington, D.C., Government Printing Office, 1954.

reason, or who rub their eyes frequently or hold their heads at an awkward or unusual angle, or seem unduly sensitive to light will be able to reveal many problems even before the screening test gives evidence of impairment. Both vision and hearing tests should be made, if possible, during the first year of school.

In preparing for such screening tests, teachers, helpers and the children to be tested must be prepared for the test, know why it is given and understand their part in the process. Agreement should be reached as to the criteria that will dictate referral for medical follow-up, so the nurse is not placed in the position of referring a large number who do not need medical care, or of failing to send those who should have it. There will be some variations in these criteria, especially in the marginal areas of deviation, depending upon the community facilities for follow-up and the attitude of the medical group about it.

Other Screening Procedures. In rural areas the public health nurse will participate in a general screening observation of the children in small schools. She may observe and talk with each child or with the class as a whole, will discuss each child with the teacher, and will observe those students who seem to have a problem.

Dental screening is rarely useful unless it includes examination with a mirror and explorer, since by simple inspection only obvious cavities will be located, and failure to see cavities may lead to a false sense of security. For this reason, dental screening is usually done by the dental hygienist.

Special screening surveys for tuberculosis or cardiac impairment may also be made, as well as for ringworm, speech or postural defects.

The Medical Examination. Medical examinations may be required at stated intervals for all school children. These examinations will vary a great deal in frequency and comprehensiveness, depending upon the community philosophy and facilities and the availability of medical personnel with special interest in this field. There seems some indication that such examinations are not always useful as a case-finding device,[4] since the great majority of defects can be located with simpler screening procedures. However, they serve as a means of parent and child education and should be considered as an educational opportunity. There is a trend toward increasing the quality of medical examination by

4. Yankauer, Alfred, A Study of Periodic School Medical Examinations. *American Journal of Public Health*, 46: 1553–1562, December, 1956.

decreasing the frequency, or by being more selective in the group examined.

The nurse will have much responsibility for setting up the plans for medical examinations, and organizing the school for carrying them out. She will work through the schedules for such examinations with the principal of the school, so that the examinations do not interfere with other important school activities; she will arrange for the necessary facilities and supplies, recruit and train helpers (including teachers, students, community volunteers), and set up the necessary record and report systems. In addition, she will have to plan her own program so as to be available for the necessary follow-up; there is little value in a medical consultation unless there is some way of following through to see that the findings and recommendations are used to promote the health of the child and his family. Probably most important of all, the nurse can encourage parents to understand and participate in this activity.

It may be necessary to secure certain permissions from parents —for example, to remove clothing for examination, or to give diagnostic tests. Plans must be made for clearance with the local medical society (usually this is done by the school medical adviser), and to secure its agreement to and understanding of what is to be done, and to establish the procedure by which patients will be referred to the private medical practitioner or clinic for follow-up. A woman—one of the parents or another volunteer worker—should be present when girls are examined.

In general the nurse should avoid getting herself tied up in assisting the physician or in routine activities such as routing patients, forwarding records or doing routine tests during the examination period. She should be free to work with students, teachers and parents.

If parents accompany the child at the time of examination, follow-up seems to be greatly facilitated.[5] However, the effectiveness of such a plan will depend upon the availability of consultation by the nurse or other professional worker at the time of the examination.

Methods of notifying parents of conditions found, when the parent is not present at the examination, must be carefully worked out so that they are administratively and psychologically sound. A "required notice of defects found" may need to be accompanied by a warm personal note inviting parents to talk with the nurse, or

5. Nyswander, Dorothy, *Solving School Health Problems*. New York, The Commonwealth Fund, 1942.

explaining just how to follow through. Wording of reports should be considered in the light of the parents' interpretation of them, as well as of their scientific accuracy. And, of course, the follow-up system and the school health records should be organized to give adequate control; it should be possible to know which students have not taken action about a problem, what progress has been made, and what pupils need further follow-up or care.

Students should be prepared for the examination; they should know what to expect and how they can help. Older children should be aware of the purposes of the examination and its relation to general preventive medical service in family health care.

The same principles that apply to management of clinics will, of course, apply to the management of examinations of school groups.

When reliance is placed on facilities outside the school for periodic health examination, the public health nurse still has a responsibility for seeing that this experience is an educational one for the students, working with the appropriate medical officer to see that the type of examination given meets the school's needs, and arranging for the necessary nursing or related follow-up services.

Absence Records.   The study of absences and their causes is also a valuable method of analyzing the health of school children. The child who has frequent absences due to colds may need general health supervisory assistance; the child who is absent because he has not appropriate clothing may be brought back to the school by making necessary referral to a social welfare agency, or sometimes by counseling of family and student as to the relative importance of "keeping up with the Jones" and of taking full advantage of one's educational opportunity; the child who stays home because he is not doing well in classes and feels lost and frustrated may need consultation with the educational adviser in the school, and perhaps some adjustment of the school schedule. The expressed cause of absence is not, of course, always the true one. In some cases, careful study of the frequency and patterns of absence will help to reveal the true causes.

Emergency Care.   First aid supplies should be immediately available, and the nurse should recommend what supplies will be kept, where they will be kept, and how they will be used. She should also see that they are replenished as necessary.

First aid can be provided adequately only when there are several people in the school setting equipped to handle emergencies. The physical education instructor in the secondary school will

almost certainly have such preparation. In other cases, the nurse
may have to suggest that interested school personnel take the
necessary courses to fit them for emergency care in the nurse's
absence. Emergency care should provide a channel for education
in safety.

Emergency care should be provided under definite understanding as to the procedures that will be followed and the limits of
such care. Sometimes the emergency procedures are outlined and
approved by the medical supervisor or the medical association of
the community; the American Red Cross Textbook on First Aid
may be accepted as the recommended procedure.

Provision should be made for care of emergency illness, and for
isolation of those with suspected communicable disease until such
time as they can be returned to their homes. Some kind of cot
should be available in the health room or, in the small school, for
the accommodation of those who need additional rest during the
day, or a short period of rest when they are ill.

Environmental Control.   In an urban setting the nurse's responsibility for environmental control will be limited; she works
with the school custodian and administrator and may make suggestions for decreasing safety hazards in the school or playground.
She also may suggest educational procedures and scheduling for
decreasing stress. Stress due, for example, to inadequate time
between classes when classrooms are not close together, or when
halls are too narrow for easy flow of traffic, may affect both pupils
and teachers; poor scheduling may produce peak loads, delay and
hurried eating in the school cafeteria.

In schools offering vocational training, the nurse should be familiar with the materials and equipment used, and work with the
shop teacher on special health problems growing out of the shop
situation. For example, the use of solutions in leather work may
produce a dermatitis unless careful handwashing procedures are
instituted. The nurse can be helpful in selection of the handwashing method and of a soap or detergent that will minimize the risk
of skin irritation, or may consult with the shop teacher about procedures that may be used to decrease contact with the irritating
substance. Safety in use of equipment is also essential, and the
nurse may make helpful suggestions about this.

Reduction of exposure to infection is an important factor in
reducing illness in schools. Helping to develop an attitude of
responsibility on the part of students and faculty for staying out
of the school environment when they have a cold, and providing

counseling that will encourage teachers to use facilities for routine chest x-ray (when this is not required by law) are examples of ways in which the nurse may reduce the hazard of infection. The education of the teacher in procedures for screening children for symptoms of illness will also promote more prompt recognition of communicable disease and reduce the exposure to other pupils.

In the rural setting, the nurse's responsibility for environmental hygiene will be broader. Working with the sanitarian or the public health engineer, who may make joint visits to the school with her, the nurse will be concerned with the water supply; with the handling of hot-lunch equipment and food used in preparation of the school lunch or food brought by individual students; with toilet and handwashing facilities; or sometimes with suggestions for improvised equipment, facilities for seating, lighting, and the control of fire hazards.

Services to the Child with Special Needs and Incidental Nursing Care. Nursing service to the child with special needs and to his family will require the same planning and counseling skills as in other services. In the school, however, there is greater need to help in the adjustment of the school educational and recreational program to meet the child's particular needs, while at the same time avoiding isolating him from other students. The child with epilepsy, for example, needs special care in relation to rest and avoidance of stress; he may need emergency care when he has attacks. It is important that the teacher and other pupils in his group understand his needs, stay calm in face of seizures, and accept him without stress on his difference.

Although emergency care has been a traditional responsibility of nursing services in schools, provision of incidental direct nursing services of other types such as supervision of orthopedic exercises, has been less generally accepted.

It is important to balance the responsibility of the family for the health care of its members against the great desirability of having children remain with their classmates during the school day so they can engage in the usual school activities without interruption. For example, if the school child who is diabetic can have his lunch in the school cafeteria, provided there is some supervision of his selection of foods, he has an opportunity for significant social contacts with his fellow students. If he must go home for lunch, his difference is accented and his identity with his group may be reduced.

Referral to other sources of nursing care may be necessary if the school nurse is not herself carrying a generalized program. Children who need intensive home supervision may be referred to the health department nurse or to the visiting nurse service. Arrangements will need to be made for exchange of information and coordination of services offered through the school and through the other community agencies. Regularly scheduled case-review conferences are helpful.

Preschool Activities.   The school program must extend backward to the preschool period for maximum effectiveness. Preparation for school might include an orientation in which the prospective student comes to the school to get used to the surroundings in advance of registration. Parent-teacher associations and other community groups may help to publicize the need for a comprehensive preschool examination, and the medical society may also lend its support and guidance to such a program. In rural areas or when the school medical adviser is available only on an occasional basis, the nurse may need to make these contacts with the medical group.

Ideally, the preschool health supervision program should be a continuous one, with no need for acceleration just prior to admission to school. However, in most communities the proportion of preschool children under continuing medical supervision is not large, and special efforts are necessary to secure a health appraisal before school admission. The school health program may contribute to preschool health in an incidental way through education of the school child or parent counseling.

Counseling Students and Parents.   The nurse will need a program of general health counseling of students and their parents directed toward maintaining the health of the school-age child. The processes and procedures do not vary from those used in general public health nursing practice and are discussed in Chapter X. Because the children are in a group, and much of the program is addressed to the group as a whole, it is particularly important to emphasize and strengthen the responsibility of the family for its own health care, and to relate school health services to total family health needs.

Much counseling can be done in the school. In rural schools particularly, it is economical in respect to time to have parents come to the school during the nurse's visit. However, as discussed in a previous chapter, there are certain advantages to the home visit that make it an indispensable part of the total service. When a child has special problems, appraisal of the home situation and enlisting the help of the family group are necessary to meet the child's needs—the school cannot function alone.

Some problems of students may be handled through scheduled group or educational activities, or in group sessions such as parent-teacher meetings. If a large number of high school students are having little or no breakfast, for example, a committee of faculty and students may act as a subcommittee of the school health council to work on this particular problem. The importance of a good breakfast may be stressed in physical education and health education classes; it may become the subject of a PTA meeting; the Future Nurses' Club or the Future Homemakers' Club may take on the project of preparing informational materials and posters, or may develop a school-assembly program centering around this problem. Problems of importance to the entire school community need the full-scale treatment that is only possible when all faculty members who are involved with the problem or who have competence in the subject matter work with the students themselves to effect a change in behavior.

To supplement work in these general problems, individual counseling must be planned around those needs which are peculiar to the individual or family. Such a counseling program should be carefully planned and developed, so the intensity of service is sufficient to meet the need. A single counseling contact, or contacts so widely spaced that there is no sense of continuity, may produce little or no result.

The nurse may need to increase her knowledge of growth and development as a means of strengthening her counseling service with parents and teachers and her understanding of the children she serves. Other areas of special need growing out of the characteristics and needs of the age group served include control of communicable disease, accident prevention, and for the junior and senior high school group a knowledge of the particular problems of adjustment faced by the adolescent.

Selecting and Scheduling Activities. The problem of scheduling for school nursing services becomes particularly important when the nurse is serving more than one school, or when she is carrying school nursing as part of a generalized public health nursing program.

When the nurse is in a school on a full-time basis, her problems of scheduling revolve around setting times for health-room activities or office conferences with teachers, parents and pupils; scheduling special activities such as medical examinations or screening procedures of various types; and arranging for conferences with teachers and administrators.

There is need for some concentration of teacher-nurse conferences either before the formal opening of school or during the first few weeks of school, particularly for new teachers who will require orientation to the school health program and their part in it. Conferences with teachers on a continuing basis should be arranged so as to create minimum disruption of teaching responsibilities. Scheduling sufficiently far in advance allows the teacher to plan for using the time of the nurse's presence as a resource for special class activities, and for involving the class in the program, and to arrange her teaching schedule to accommodate to the nursing visit. The administrator should approve the general plan for scheduling teacher conferences.

Conferences with administrators should be arranged just prior to natural planning periods; for example, it is frequently the custom to discuss school programs for the following school year in the late spring. This would be a natural time to talk about plans for the school health program for the coming year. The school physician, other health education personnel and the nurse might well choose this time for a conference. Conferences about problems which are common in the school and of concern to the administrator, or of particular immediate significance, should, of course, be discussed as soon as they become apparent.

The hours at which the nurse is in the health room should be scheduled at a regular time as far as possible—at the same hours daily or the same days each week—and the schedule posted.

The nurse who serves the school on a part-time basis has even more need for a definite schedule. If a large number of small rural schools are to be served, the schedule usually needs to be set up on an annual basis. Schools in which there are new teachers, or where there are known problems (as in schools where there has been a great influx of population in the community), should be visited early in the year. This provides an opportunity to interpret the service, and to help the new teacher in the problems of screening, health instruction and environmental control. It may be possible to plan this as a joint visit with the public health engineer or sanitarian who can at the same time advise about environmental sanitation problems. If there is a health educator functioning in the school health program she may plan a visit with the nurse, to get the program started; or, in some cases, when visits must be infrequent, the health education supervisor may prefer to schedule her visits between those of the nurse to provide more frequent support for the teachers. In this instance, both scheduling and content of consultation will need careful coordination.

The nurse in a generalized program, carrying a large number of rural schools, will probably have to skew her program during the early fall months in favor of school activities to accommodate to these needs.

The content of activities in the school program must be subjected to close scrutiny, to select those activities which are most productive in relation to the time available. Student loads will vary widely; a full-time nurse may have anywhere from 300 to 5000 children under her supervision. Swanson suggests alternative activities for nurses who have ample time, moderate time and restricted time available for school health work.[6] A recent Children's Bureau publication also lists priorities for the school health program as a whole.[7] Emphasis is placed on the child's opportunity for experiences that will help him to learn to live healthfully in his world, on relating the school health program and its needs to community development, on problems of high incidence such as dental caries and of mental health.

When school visits are widely spaced the teachers' meeting and the initial conference with the new teachers will help to define the kinds of help the nurse might be expected to provide. Prior to the visit an informal note or telephone conference may help the teacher to plan. The teaching schedule should, if possible, be arranged so the teacher has time to discuss with the nurse the general condition of each student (this means arranging tests or "busy work" for the student); for requesting parents of children who have special problems to come to the school to see the nurse; to assemble the particular problems she may want to discuss and perhaps ask the nurse in advance of the visit for materials or suggestions about special areas of interest or teaching units.

The nurse in the school plays an important part in health promotion and protection. She can also make a very real contribution to planning and to the general educational program.

6. Swanson, Marie, *School Nursing in the Community Program.* New York, Macmillan Co., 1953, pp. 130–141.

7. *Better Health for School Age Children.* Washington, D.C., Children's Bureau, Department of Health, Education and Welfare, 1952.

PUBLIC HEALTH NURSING IN OCCUPATIONAL HEALTH PROGRAMS

The purposes of an occupational health program are indicated in the definition propounded by the World Health Organization Committee on Occupational Health:

> "Occupational health should aim at the promotion and maintenance of the highest degree of physical, mental and social well-being of workers in all occupations; the prevention among workers of departures from health caused by their working conditions; the protection among workers in their employment from risks resulting from factors adverse to health; the placing and maintenance of the worker in an occupational environment adapted to his physiological and psychological equipment."[8]

Industrial and commercial establishments and labor organizations have shown an increasing interest in health programs for workers. This interest undoubtedly arises from the fact that both industry and worker pay a high price for the estimated four to five million man days lost annually. About three-fourths of these lost days are due to common and often preventable illness, and it is likely that in-plant health programs might reduce these lost days by one-third to one-half.[9] Because of her close relationship to workers and the fact that she is usually seen by both worker and management as a "middle" person, the nurse is in a strategic position to forward the program. In 1952 there were 11,096 nurses employed in industry.[10] The American Nurses' Association, Industrial Nurses' Section, and the American Association of Industrial Nurses have outlined the functions and responsibilities of nurses in industry.[11, 12]

Studying the Industrial Community.　　Employee health programs, and nursing within those programs, must be seen in re-

8. Committee on Occupational Health, World Health Organization, Second Report. *World Health Organization Technical Report Series No. 66.* New York, Columbia University Press, 1953.

9. Health Maintenance for Greater Efficiency, *Small Business Management Series No 16.* Washington, D.C., Government Printing Office, 1954.

10. American Nurses' Association, *Facts About Nursing,* 1955–56 Edition. New York, The Association, 1956, p. 45.

11. *Functions, Standards and Qualifications for an Industrial Nurse in a One Nurse Service in Industry or Commerce.* New York, The Association, 1956.

12. *Duties and Responsibilities of the Professional Nurse in an Industrial Medical Service.* New York, The Association, 1955. Or in *American Association of Industrial Nurses Journal,* 2: 13–14, June, 1955.

lation to the major goals and operating philosophy of industry. A major objective in industry is to secure maximum production. To a somewhat diminishing degree, industry is concerned also with maximum profits; this objective is influenced by an increasing sense of obligation on the part of industry toward its social responsibility, and for the achievement of maximum wages.[13, 14] Good relations with the public and employee are considered essential for effective industrial management and the industrial health program may make a very real contribution to both.

The industrial community in which the nurse works needs the same careful study that would be accorded the general community. It is important to know what kind of people work in the plant—what proportion are women; the age distribution; the proportion in different types of work, such as "white-collar" employment, skilled or unskilled labor, professional workers such as research or technical consultant personnel. It is important to know the processes involved in production, and their special hazards. The nurse should plan early to observe the processes in production to obtain an understanding of how the product is made, and what kinds of activities are required of workers in various positions.

She needs to know, too, how workers and management relate to one another—what procedures exist for communication between groups, how people are organized into functional units, and the kinds of responsibility assumed by those at different levels. For instance, in one industry, managers and owner may have a very easy, informal relationship in which problems can be discussed without too much concern about lines of authority or delegation charts. In another, there may be a tight top control, in which virtually all decisions are made by the top-management group. In another, there may be a carefully organized system of joint committees and representatives of worker groups who consider and advise on most problems of significance.

It is important, too, to know under what laws or regulations the industry operates. Requirements such as those relating to the employment of women, compensation for accidents, inspection and standards for safety equipment will vary from state

13. Mayo, Elton, *The Social Problems of an Industrial Civilization.* Boston, Harvard University Graduate School of Business Administration, 1955.

14. Smith, H. C., *Psychology and Industrial Behavior.* New York, McGraw-Hill Book Co., 1955, p. 9–14.

to state. Agreements with local or state health departments or with insurance carriers are also important; recording and reporting may be much influenced by these agreements. Compensation laws in particular are significant in the nurse's work; the way the nurse records in history taking or in writing the accident record may be important in establishing compensation status. Her ability to explain and interpret them will influence employer-employee relations. If a copy of the laws is not available on the job, it may be secured from the state department of labor.

Relationship with Administrative and Production Personnel. In the large plant with a well-organized health service and a full-time medical director, the relationships with management will channel through the medical director. In the plant without such direction, where part-time or panel physicians are used, the nurse may be responsible for keeping the management group informed of needs and plans in relation to employee health service.

Whether through the channel of the medical director or directly, the nurse will be concerned with maintaining interpretative and planning relationships with the staff in personnel management and in general management; with private physicians responsible for the care of individual employees; and with community health agencies which provide services for employees and their families, or promulgate regulations that apply to the industry, such as reporting certain communicable diseases or excluding workers from certain occupations when stated diseases are present.

When there is an organized health committee in the plant the nurse may be a member of the committee or serve as a consultant to it. The use of health committees is gaining increasing acceptance in industry, and the use of safety committees is well established.

The pattern of medical direction should be clearly outlined. Standing orders that govern emergency care of employees should be written and clearly understood. Procedures for referral of employees for medical care should likewise be thoroughly discussed and outlined, since they will involve the responsibility of the plant for its own health services, absence from the job and, in some instances, compensation benefits.

It is important to plan for safeguarding the confidence of workers in relation to health records by indicating clearly the conditions under which information from the record may be given to foremen, management, or personnel officers.

In general, it is important wherever possible for the nurse to avoid being aligned with either the management or labor force. A neutral position is very helpful in promoting the health program, and in making nursing service effective.

Health Appraisal Procedures. Health appraisal procedures in industry include pre-employment and periodic health examinations; inspectional or checking procedures for evidence of illness associated with a particular occupational hazard; screening procedures for illness associated with the occupation or with illness common to the working adults. The type of appraisal procedure will vary with the sex and age distribution of workers and with the processes used in the plant. Absence and health records also provide valuable information on the collective health status of employees.

A pre-employment examination may be conducted in the industrial plant by the plant medical staff, or may be required but performed by private physicians or group medical clinics outside the plant. The nurse will participate in in-plant examinations much as she would in any clinic, arranging for appointments, physical set-up and for conferences with those examined.

When the examination is done away from the plant, the nurse may review the record for completeness, and secure additional information from the physician or clinic as necessary. She can do much to interpret to the worker the purposes of this examination, explaining that it is not to bar him from employment, but to permit safe and satisfactory placement that will protect him and the organization. She may also explain that the personnel department or management group classifies positions in relation to their physical demands, and that this plus the physical examination record help with placement.

In some industries, periodic physical examinations are required of all employees, and are made either in the plant or by a private physician or industrial clinic. If this is not the case, the nurse may urge all employees to take advantage of opportunities for preventive medical care, and urge those in especially vulnerable groups to arrange for their own health examinations. Those in the late middle years, for example, might be urged to have more frequent examinations because of the need for early detection of chronic disease.

When examinations are not required of all employees, there may be a plan to provide examination for those in high priority groups—those with known physical defects, with a higher than average accident history, or those whose work exposes them to dangerous processes or materials. The nurse can be helpful in estimating the number of people that can be accommodated within the personnel and facilities limitations of the situation, or in suggesting groups that might be included in such a plan.

As in the school situation, a medical examination without provision for adequate follow-up is of limited value. Scheduled conferences with workers who have problems revealed by the medical examination, referral to community sources for assistance, and a system of follow-up that shows which of the conditions found is actually under treatment are all needed.

Sometimes the cumulative reports of medical examinations reveal an unusual incidence of illness or disability in particular sections of the plant. The nurse should be alert to such indices of possible trouble, as they may demonstrate need for environmental or managerial measures to produce a more healthful environment.

Screening Tests. Screening tests may include vision and hearing tests; diagnostic surveys such as chest x-ray, diabetic or cancer detection tests; or tests to detect unfavorable reactions to industrial processes or materials. For example, there may be a special search for dermatoses, or periodic x-rays when silicosis is a potential hazard, or for early indications of lead poisoning.

Absence Records. Absence records may provide a valuable clue to individual or group health problems. The *pattern* of absence is significant. The person absent for forty days for major surgery presents quite a different picture from the person absent forty days without surgery when his record of average duration of absence has been less than two days. The worker whose record is dotted with short absences due to colds, minor gastric upsets or dysmenorrhea may need special help with general hygienic practices, or may reveal emotional problems associated with the job situation which are amenable to managerial control. Unusually high absence rates in a department or section of the plant may also be important. Excessive absenteeism may be related to poor physical conditions such as excessive drafts, or poor housekeeping that is conducive to accidents, or poor morale among the workers which is producing some degree of stress.

Emergency and Incidental Care of Illness. First-aid care may be provided by the medical and nursing staff directly, or in smaller plants by specially trained personnel who take the responsibility for first-aid care. In general there is a trend toward using the health office for first aid, since it promotes more accurate recording of accidents, and may be a safer place for care. However, when nursing service does not cover all shifts, or is available only on a part-time basis, or when the various departments or sections of the plant are widely scattered, this is not possible. In the latter case, the nurse is usually responsible for maintaining first-aid kits at strategic points throughout the plant, and for working with the management group to be sure there is someone trained in first aid available at all times to give the necessary care.

The procedures to be used in first aid should be agreed upon by the medical director or advisor, and followed in the training of first-aid personnel.

First-aid care should be used as a method of safety training; in each instance the possibility of avoiding future injury should be discussed. Reporting of accidents—even very minor accidents—is especially important in industry, since compensation claims may be involved.

There is much variation in the degree to which incidental care is provided for minor illness in the industrial plant. Since it is important to keep the worker on the job with minimum interruption, it may be advantageous to have the girl with dysmenorrhea lie down for a short while rather than go home for the day, or for certain treatments such as heat treatments or small dressings to be done in the plant rather than have the worker absent while he goes to a clinic or physician's office. When the patient is under private medical care, it is particularly important to clear with the physician the care that might be provided for his patient by the nurse in the plant and secure his approval.

Often there is a tendency for the health room to be a place where the worker can get an aspirin or other medication for minor ills, given in accordance with standing orders authorized by the medical supervisor. The dispensing of pills should be minimized. The worker with a headache or dysmenorrhea should be helped to get at the cause of the disturbance, rather than given relief of the symptoms; the worker with frequent intestinal upsets should be helped to find and correct the dietary or emotional causes as well as to stop the immediate distress.

Environmental Control. Control of the environment is especially important in relation to the prevention of accidents. It is estimated that approximately 2,000,000 disabling injuries occur annually in industry, and cost a minimum of two billion dollars.[15] Environmental control plus worker education could undoubtedly greatly reduce this burden.

In large plants, control of environmental hazards will be the responsibility of the plant engineer or a safety engineer, and the nurse's job will be to understand the basis of such rules or regulations as may be made and to help make them effective. In the smaller plant the nurse's responsibility will be greater. There may be a safety committee which takes much responsibility, but the nurse must be concerned with seeing that safety devices are really used, and help employees to understand the need for them. There is little benefit from a guard that is removed by the worker because it "gets in the way."

Good housekeeping is also a factor in accident control; wet, slippery floors, equipment not put away or placed so it may be stumbled over, and masks or safety goggles kept in poor repair are all accident hazards. Supervision of lighting, ventilation or seating of workers may also be problems in the small plant.

The nurse should work closely with the safety engineer and designated safety and first-aid workers in the plant on matters of environmental sanitation. When the plant does not employ such personnel, the state health department or the insurance carrier may provide consultant services. If there are regular safety committee meetings it is easy to exchange information. If not, the nurse may need to find ways of keeping in touch with the work of safety engineers and allied personnel.

Services to Those with Special Needs. The nurse may be called upon to provide counseling or other assistance to workers with special problems. Women represent a growing component in the labor force and may present special health maintenance problems. The proportion of women in the total labor force rose from 14 percent in 1900 to 28 percent in 1947.[16] Problems arising from conflicting demands of the job and of the home, from pregnancy, or from disorders of menstruation or menopause may require counseling, special care or referral.

The older worker, too, may present special problems. In addition to physical problems associated with aging itself or with chronic disease or disability, there are the emotional and social

15. Smith, H. C., *Psychology of Industrial Behavior*. New York, McGraw-Hill Book Co., 1955, p. 76.

16. Klem and others, *Industrial Health and Medical Programs*. Washington, D.C., Government Printing Office, 1950, p. 22.

problems attendant upon job adjustments and retirement that may seriously affect total health. Accident proneness may also increase with age in some situations.

There is increasing interest in employment of the handicapped, since they have been shown to be a valuable addition to the labor force. This group may also place special demands upon the nurse in industry, especially if there is need for continuing treatment or supervision during working hours.

Counseling with Employees and Their Families.[17]   Counseling with employees and their families is an important phase of industrial nursing and an integral part of any nursing service. The accident-prone employee may be the employee with poor vision or poor general health; he may be the worker who is anxious about his work or worried about his family; he may be the worker who has not grown up to his years and his responsibilities and shows it by adolescent "horsing around" which leads to accidents. Through a counseling approach the nurse can help to locate the cause of the difficulty; help to arrange with related workers such as psychologist, social worker or physician for additional investigation or care; or help with simple adjustments that may make the difference between serenity and conflict.

Since absence from work is to be avoided if possible, counseling may have to be scheduled during lunch or rest periods. This may necessitate adjustment of the nurse's schedule of her own daily activities so she can be available when workers are free.

Problems of general concern may be handled in group sessions—getting breakfasts that are adequate, or clothing that meets safety requirements and yet leaves the woman worker feeling attractive, or care of the common cold are examples of such problems. Sometimes counseling may be associated with screening activities; for example, a cancer-detection clinic session may be accompanied by showing films on self-examination of the breast, with interviews with the nurse for those who wish it, as well as for those who need further follow-up to establish a diagnosis.

Counseling of family members may also help, particularly when there is evidence that the worker is anxious or worried about family conditions. The family member may come to the plant or the nurse may visit him in the home. Such arrangements should be coordinated with the work of the community

17. Counseling methods are discussed in Chapter X.

public health agency; the industrial nurse should not plan to visit the pregnant wife of an industrial worker for prenatal supervision if this service is offered by the department of health or local visiting nurse service, though she might make a home visit to ascertain the need for referral.

In some instances, discussion groups may be organized for families of workers. For example, in one firm, wives of employees were invited to showings of the film on self-examination of the breast, and to discussion groups on weight control. At these sessions the nurse was available to answer questions, provide incidental information and to refer those who needed it to other agencies for further help.

Selecting and Scheduling Activities.   The work of the nurse will vary not only in accordance with the size of the industry and of her patient load, but also with the demands of the industry itself for service. The nurse in a bank, for example, will be much less concerned with accidents and first aid than with emotional problems and minor illness; the nurse in a tobacco plant employing a large Negro labor force may give first priority to tuberculosis-control activities; the nurse in a canning plant employing migratory labor may spend much time with family problems and general home hygiene and sanitation. There is no recommended specific staff-worker ratio that can be applied because of differences in hours of coverage needed per twenty-four hours and differences in exposure to hazardous processes. Brown suggests eight hours of nursing coverage per week per 100 to 2000 workers, and, in larger industries, one nurse to each additional thousand for all but very hazardous continuous-process industries.[18] However, the number of nurses actually employed is considerably below this recommended level. A study of 614 establishments in 1944 indicated a range in the average number of workers per nurse from 603 to 862.[19]

The nurse in a large plant will need to schedule the time that she is available for consultation in her office. When night workers are employed, it is important to schedule the time so it is possible to see the workers on each shift. Scheduling of physical examinations or inspections should be such that nursing

18. Brown, M. L., *Occupational Health Nursing*. New York, Springer, 1956, p. 132.

19. Whitlock, O. M., V. M. Trasko, and F. R. Kahl, *Nursing Practices in Industry*. Public Health Bulletin #283. Washington, D.C., Government Printing Office, 1944, p. 37.

time is available immediately afterward for conferences with workers and for the necessary follow-up, to see that recommendations made are actually carried out.

When the nurse covers several plants, or several installations within a single agency, she will need to schedule well in advance the times she will be at a specific place. As far as possible this should be at a regular time during the day or week, so it is easy to remember. It is generally not advisable to schedule a period shorter than two hours for an industrial visit. Time should be scheduled also for attendance at safety or health committees, and for preparing materials that may be needed for their deliberations.

An occupational health nursing approach need not be limited to industrial plants. Many of the services would apply equally well in working with the farmer who is self-employed, or with the housewife working in an occupational environment which may prove the most hazardous of all—the home. An occupational health approach in a home visit would make the nurse aware that protecting the housewife or farmer from back strain due to improper bodily posture while lifting is not different from the problem of preventing similar injury in the industrial plant.

Working in agencies organized for other purposes than health care provides a real challenge to the nurse. It demands unusual skill in organizing and coordinating nurse activities, and imagination in seeing the ways in which nursing can contribute to the major objectives of the school or industry in which the nursing is done.

SUGGESTED READINGS

PART IV

NURSING IN CLINICS

American Public Health Association, *Health Supervision of Young Children*. New York, American Public Health Association, 1955.

Bigley, Loretta I., *Community Clinics*. Philadelphia, J. B. Lippincott Co., 1947.

Carroll, Benjamin E., A Kurlander and H. Nester, Multiple Screening Pilot Study. *Public Health Reports*, 69: 1180–1184, December, 1954.

Holmes, E. M. and P. M. Bowden, Screening for Asymptomatic Disease by Health Departments. *Journal of Chronic Diseases*. 2: 384, October, 1955.

Goik, M., The Nurse in the Child Health Conference. *Children*, 1: 222–226, November-December, 1954.

Lennon, Sister Marie Isidore, *Teaching in the Out-Patient Department*. New York, G. P. Putnam's Sons, 1953.

Skinner, Mary Lou and Mayhew Derryberry, Health Education for Out-Patients. *Public Health Reports*, 69: 1107–1114, November, 1954.

School Nursing

American Association of School Administrators, *Health in Schools, Twentieth Yearbook, Revised 1951*. Washington, D.C., The Association, 1951.

American Public Health Association, *Health Supervision of Young Children*. New York, The Association, 1955.

Beckmann, G., and E. Zimmerman, A School Health Council That Works. *Nursing Outlook*, 4: 290–292, May, 1956.

Better Health for School Age Children. Washington, D.C., Children's Bureau, Department of Health, Education, and Welfare, 1952.

Bibliography, School Nursing. *Nursing Outlook*, 2: 428–429, August, 1954.

Crane, Marion and others, *Screening School Children for Visual Defects, Children's Bureau Publication No. 345*. Washington, D.C., U. S. Government Printing Office, 1954.

Cree, Margaret, Present Day Views on School Nursing. *American Journal of Public Health*, 42: 818–824, July, 1952.

Cromwell, Gertrude, *The Health of the School Child*. Philadelphia, W. B. Saunders Co., 1946.

Department of Public Health Nursing, National League for Nursing, *School Nursing Services*. New York, The League, 1956.

Expert Committee on School Health Services, World Health Organization, *Report of the First Session*. New York, Columbia University Press, 1951.

Grout, Ruth, *Health Teaching in Schools*. 2nd edition. Philadelphia, W. B. Saunders Co., 1953.

Health and Welfare Division, Metropolitan Life Insurance Company, *The School Health Program. School Health Monograph No. 12*. New York, Metropolitan Life Insurance Company, 1951.

Joint Committee on Health Problems in Education of the National Education Association and the American Medical Association, *School Health Services*. Washington, D.C., National Education Association, 1956.

Joint Committee on Health Problems in Education of the National Education Association and the American Medical Association, *The Nurse in the School*. Washington, D.C., National Education Association, or Chicago, The American Medical Association, 1956.

Kilander, H. F., *Health Services in City Schools*. Washington, D.C., U.S. Government Printing Office, 1952.

Lehne, Arthur, A School-Community Health Council. *Journal of School Health*, 26: 144–145, May, 1955.

National Conference for Cooperation in Health Education, National Committee on School Health Policies, *Suggested School Health Policies*, 3rd Edition. Chicago, The American Medical Association, 1956.

Peterson, Paul, Cooperation of Departments of Education and Health in the Administration of School Health Programs. *Public Health Nursing*, 44: 173–177, April, 1952.

Rappaport, Mary B., Cooperation of the Nurse and Teacher in the Health Program in Small Communities, *Journal of School Health*, 27: 48–52, February, 1957.

School Health Research Trends and Service Studies. *Public Health Reports*, 69: 178–182, February, 1954.

Swanson, Marie, *School Nursing in the Community Program*. New York, Macmillan Co., 1953.

Underwood, Felix, Departments of Education and Public Health Working Together. *American Journal of Public Health*, 44: 625–630, May, 1954.

The Use of School Health Records, American Journal of Public Health. *Yearbook, 1951–52*, pp. 130–32. (Part 2 of the May 1952 issue of the American Journal of Public Health.)

Wheatley, George and Grace T. Hallock, *Health Observation of School Children*. New York, McGraw-Hill Book Co., 1951.

Wishik, Samuel, Administrative Jurisdiction of the School Health Service. *American Journal of Public Health*, 41: 819–823, July, 1953.

Yankauer, Alfred, A Study of Periodic School Medical Examinations. *American Journal of Public Health*, 46: 1553–1562, December, 1956.

Yankauer, Alfred, Public Health Nursing in the Schools. *Nursing Outlook*, 2: 197–199, April, 1954.

Occupational Health Nursing

Althouse, H. L., The Dollars and Sense of Industrial Nursing. *American Journal of Nursing*, 49: 721–723, June, 1949.

American Association of Industrial Nurses, Duties and Responsibilities of the Professional Nurse in an Industrial Medical Service. *American Association of Industrial Nurses Journal*, 2: 13–14, June, 1955.

American Association of Industrial Nurses, Recommended Qualifications for a Professional Nurse Working without Nursing Supervision in an Industrial Medical Service. *American Association of Industrial Nurses Journal*, 2: 29, June, 1955.

American Nurses' Association, Functions for an Industrial Nurses in a One Nurse Service in Industry or Commerce. *American Journal of Nursing*, 54: 1130, September, 1954.

Anderson, Agnes, Changing Emphasis in Industrial Nursing. *American Journal of Nursing*, 55: 39–44, January, 1955.

Brown, Mary Louise, *Occupational Health Nursing*. New York, Springer Publishing Co., 1956.

Cameron, Dale, Human Relations in Occupational Health. *International Nursing Review*, 2: 25–28, April, 1955.

Committee on Occupational Health, *Second Report. World Health Organization Technical Report Series No. 66*. New York, Columbia University Press, July, 1953.

Doyle, Henry N., Occupational Health on Farms. *Public Health Reports*, 72: 145–148, February, 1957.

Felton, J. S. and M. D. Owens, Forecasting the Number of Employee Visits to Our Industrial Health Service. *Industrial Medicine*, 22:1–7, January, 1953.

Guiding Principles and Procedures for Industrial Nurses, *American Journal of Nursing,* 56: 192–197, 1956.

Health Maintenance for Greater Efficiency, *Small Business Management Series No. 16.* Washington, D.C., U.S. Government Printing Office, 1954.

Henricksen, Heidi, The "New Look" in Occupational Health Nursing. *Nursing Outlook,* 1: 328–331, June, 1953.

Hornung, Gertrude, The Nursing Diagnosis—an Exercise in Judgment. *Nursing Outlook,* 4: 29–30, January, 1956.

A Job Description of the Occupational Health Nurse. *Nursing Outlook,* 2: 154–156, March, 1954.

Klem, Margaret, M. F. McKiever and Walter Lear, *Industrial Health and Medical Programs.* Washington, D.C., U.S. Government Printing Office, 1954.

McGrath, Bethel, *Nursing in Commerce and Industry.* New York, Commonwealth Fund, 1946.

Small Plant Health and Medical Programs. Public Health Service Publication No. 215. Washington, D.C. U.S. Government Printing Office, 1952.

Striegel, Bernadine, Nursing in Occupational Health. *American Journal of Nursing,* 54: 445–447, April, 1954.

Williams, John K., Birmingham's Industrial Health Council. *Nursing Outlook,* 2: 244–246, May, 1954.

PART V

Professional
Responsibilities

CHAPTER XXII

Career Planning

Nurses in public health work have many reasons for selecting that particular field. Sometimes the choice is based upon a deep desire to make a social contribution and a feeling that public health offers a channel for such service; sometimes it is based on an interest in and a desire to work with people that can be satisfied best in the informal milieu of the community agency; sometimes it is just easier to combine the hours of work in public health with a second career of marriage than is true in other fields of nursing. Career planning must take account of these purposes, as well as of desirable progression within the professional field.

Career planning involves:

1. Periodic evaluation of potentials.[1]
2. Pre-service training.
3. Graded experience.
4. Training for greater responsibility.

An understanding of the competences and qualifications necessary for public health nursing is an essential base for such planning.

COMPETENCES AND QUALIFICATIONS

Professional competences necessary for public health nursing cannot be reduced to a list of qualities or academic qualifications that, once met, assure the individual of job mastery. However, certain areas of professional competence may be accepted as significant, and may be described.[2] Areas of competence in public health nursing include:

1. Evaluation is discussed in Chapter XXIII, and will not be elaborated here.

2. *Functions, Standards and Qualifications for Public Health Nurses.* New York, American Nurses' Association, 1955.

1. Competence in technical nursing and in public health.
2. Competence in interpersonal relationships.
3. Competence in leadership.
4. Competence in planning and problem solving.

These competences are inter-dependent—the absence of any one may cancel out the effectiveness of the others. For example, good competence in inter-personal relationships may cause families to like the nurse, but her capacity to help them demands that she know the content of health care, that she be able to take the lead in stimulating them to recognize and to do something about their problems, and that she be able to analyze and appraise situations and the feasibility of various possible solutions to them.

Technical Competence.   Technical competence must be current and comprehensive, dynamic rather than static. Care of arthritis, of burns, or of menopausal symptoms may be revolutionized in a matter of months. The technical skills and knowledges of nursing need constant renewal.

Thorough familiarity with and skill in performance of basic nursing procedures is a prime essential for professional competence. Since procedures carried out in the home or taught to families or patients must be adapted to the available equipment and to the widely varying competence of different families, the nurse in public health must have a firm knowledge of the principles of nursing care. With this as a base, she can suggest easy and safe modifications of procedure to meet individual situations.

Knowledge of current trends and of developments in medical practice is also fundamental, since this will affect nursing care and health instruction. It is important to recognize and be familiar with controversial or experimental as well as accepted and proved methods and treatments, since both will have to be interpreted to patients and to others in the family or community. Developments in preventive medical care as well as in the treatment of disease must be part of the nurse's knowledge. Patients will ask about fluoridation of water supplies, the Salk vaccine, the new drugs used for cancer, what kind of anesthesia they are apt to get in the hospital and a host of other questions.

The public health nurse must also be familiar with public health and epidemiologic procedures. She must know the methods of detecting and controlling diseases of public health import. She must be able to understand and interpret statistics relating to health conditions, and to make simple calculations of her own observations. She must know the community measures being applied for diagnosis, for locating cases not yet under treatment, and for securing treatment necessary to control the spread of disease, or to ameliorate its effects. These measures include the use of public information as well as laboratory or clinical measures for control.

Competence in Inter-personal Relationships. A major task in public health nursing is to help others to analyze and act upon their problems. This capacity to help is dependent upon relationships that are free from undesirable tensions or negative reactions, and upon the ability to use personal skills to guide and influence others. The nurse must also be able to work constructively with members of other agencies in the promotion of family health, and to participate effectively in group thinking and action that uses the forces generated within a group to constructive and helpful ends in family and community service.

Competence in inter-personal relationships requires *sensitivity to the needs and reactions* of others. This awareness or "feeling with" is a rather intangible quality, and difficult to define, yet for those who work intimately with people it is a skill that must be constantly developed.

Knowledge of the determinants of human behavior and ability to accept the behavior of others as an expression of their reaction to a need is also basic to competence in inter-personal relationships. Even though behavior appears unpleasant or undesirable, the public health nurse must be able to appreciate the probable roots of the action, and to accept the behavior of individuals or groups without personal resentment.

There is also need to *separate self from professional relationships*. The public health nurse must be able to compensate for strong or negative emotional response or bias that may arise from her own experience. Problems and needs must be seen and described objectively. The nurse's perfectionism or desire to dominate must not interfere with the family's right to choose the way that is right for it, nor should one's own experience distort the estimate of the effect of chronic illness or marital unhappiness upon a family's serenity.

Ability to work with others, to think and act as one of a team or group, is also essential. The public health nurse must be willing to build on the plans of others or to accept a direction not entirely her own, and still to participate fully and constructively in accomplishing the task in hand. It is necessary to act without either passive acceptance or domination, but with a free exchange of ideas and sharing of responsibility than can produce an integrated plan or activity. This sensitive, objective, cooperative approach to working with others is fundamental to the implementation of any program.

Leadership Competence. In addition to working effectively with others, public health nursing also demands the ability to exert leadership—to influence behavior. Both in family health guidance and in community planning and action, the public health nurse's expert status places her in a position where her counsel is sought, or where she may stimulate and direct appropriate action in others.

Ability to gain the confidence of others is fundamental to leadership competence. Families, employers, professional co-workers such as physicians, social workers or teachers must have confidence in the public health nurse and in her ability to give help.

Equally important is the *ability to give others confidence in themselves*. Families and individuals whom the public health nurse serves should become increasingly independent as a result of that service, and this is possible only if they have confidence in their ability to help themselves and to contribute to the welfare of their families or communities.

Ability to stir others to action is also implicit in leadership. Encouraging the young woman with syphilis to face her problem and decide what she will do; helping a group of young parents to analyze what they can do to contribute to the security and happiness of their children; stimulating the interest of high school students in studying and reducing accident hazards in school and at home—all are simple examples of application of this aspect of leadership.

Willingness to work through others is essential to leadership. To help someone else find the answer rather than tell it; to prepare the teacher or parents to handle requests for sex information rather than give a sex hygiene talk; to wait for a child study group to analyze its own problems rather than outline what the problems should be—these are ways to substitute leadership for advising.

Planning and Problem Solving. In addition to technical, inter-personal and leadership skills, the public health nurse must be able to think independently and clearly, to make sound plans on the basis of available facts and to evaluate work critically and objectively. This requires skill in handling ideas and in making judgments as well as sufficient imagination to see potential as well as obvious possibilities or difficulties.

Thinking in terms of available facts comes partly with training and partly from habit. All too often nurses have become accustomed to following the book (the agency manual, textbook or other authoritative source) or accepting procedures "as we did them in the VNA" or "in Memorial Hospital."

The professionally competent person knows and uses available facts in making decisions. If a bacteriologic study is possible, she does not depend upon previous practice to decide upon acceptable communicable disease nursing techniques. If the value of prenatal nursing visits is questioned, she does not rely upon feelings or upon preconceived ideas of the value of such supervision, but rather secures the available facts by analyzing records, by observing or questioning patients and families, or by watching other nurses at work. She determines what teaching was done, in how many instances there was evidence that nursing calls influenced the pattern of prenatal care, or what proportion of nursing reports to physicians revealed facts of significance to him in planning for care.

Ability to work in accordance with a plan is also essential to professional competence. It is important to know what should be accomplished, and the means by which defined objectives are to be achieved. This ability to plan and to follow through is basic to effective action in any phase of work—in family guidance, conferences with health officers or other workers, organizing or managing clinics, or supervising the work of students. Planning is a *way of working* rather than a step in a process.

The *ability to recognize and consider significant relationships* is also an important factor in judgmental competence. A situation must be seen in terms of its total configuration rather than as a "psychiatric case," an "uncooperative county board of commissioners" or a "low-attendance clinic." The relationship of the diagnosis of psychiatric illness to the management of the patient's household, to the child's school work, to the possible sources of the disease will create a different problem in each instance. The uncooperative county commissioners may have come into office on a promise to reduce taxes; they may have been misinformed or uninformed of health needs; they may have been subjected to a great deal of pressure for the support of other county projects. The relationship between the public health nurse's concept of what would constitute appropriate action on the part of the commissioners and their experience or the other demands made upon them is significant in securing understanding support for nursing or other health programs.

Professional competence in public health nursing is a combination of technical expertness, ability to work with and through others, to assume leadership as necessary and to plan and work with sound judgment.

It is obvious that such competences develop as the nurse herself develops on the job. However, an adequate, organized program of study is necessary as well.

QUALIFICATIONS

The American Nurses' Association has established the following as recommended qualifications for public health nurses in staff positions:

"A. Preparation in Basic Nursing
 "1. Graduation from a school of professional nursing with state accreditation at time of graduation.
 "2. Holds a current license to practice as a registered professional nurse.
"B. Preparation in Public Health Nursing as Evidenced by:
 "A degree from a university program in nursing approved by the National League for Nursing for public health nursing preparation

or

Completion of the public health content in an educational program approved by the National League for Nursing. In this case the university may certify that the credits earned by the applicant meet the requirements (viz. completion of the public health nursing content of the program).

"Such approved public health programs provide understanding, attitudes, and skills basic to competence in the following areas:
 "1. Preventive health care including such aspects as nutrition, safety, rehabilitation, mental health, environmental sanitation, and communicable disease control.
 "2. Application of basic epidemiologic and statistic principles.
 "3. Counseling, interviewing, and group work.
 "4. Individual and group teaching.

"5. Recognition and interpretation of:
  "a. Physical, mental, and social health.
  "b. Biological, occupational, and other environmental causative factors in disease.
  "c. Personality structure and development.
  "d. Patterns of human growth and development.
  "e. Family relationships.
  "f. Effects of cultural patterns on health.
"6. Program planning in relation to:
  "a. Development of nursing services in health departments, schools, and voluntary agencies.
  "b. Patterns of administration and content of public health programs including school health programs.
  "c. Patterns of community organization for planning and action in health, education, and welfare.
  "d. Trends and patterns in educational philosophy and methods including curriculum construction.
"C. Personal Competence as Shown by the Capacity to:
  "1. Express ideas clearly and in an acceptable manner.
  "2. Accept people in a nonjudgmental way.
  "3. Gain satisfaction through the development and growth of others.
  "4. Stimulate others to constructive action.
  "5. Value and use contributions of other professional groups, volunteers, and the general public, and relate these to nursing practice.
  "6. Adjust pace to realities of the situation.
  "7. Evaluate self in relation to work, and accept help from others.
  "8. Accept responsibility in professional and civic organizations.

"Personal abilities that contribute to the practice of public health nursing are apt to develop fully only with experience and maturity. However, even at the beginner's level, practice requires each of the above qualities in some degree."[3]

It is evident in sections "B" and "C" of this statement that there is a wide spread in preparation and in the possible levels of personal competences in the areas suggested. Such a spread is inevitable because of the great differences that exist in the

3. *Functions, Standards and Qualifications for Public Health Nurses.* New York, American Nurses' Association, 1955, pp. 13–14.

type, content and depth of basic nursing preparation, and because of the relatively small number of nurses in public health who have completed even one year of special preparation in public health nursing. While this proportion with such preparation has risen since 1950, when 34.1 percent were so prepared, it must be noted that in January 1955 only 37.1 percent of the 26,110 nurses reporting had completed one year or more of preparation in public health, and of the 23,044 in staff positions only 31.3 percent were so prepared.[4]

There seems little doubt that public health nursing requires at least the general and special preparation included in a university degree program. However, for the next decade it is unlikely that the majority of public health nurses could be so prepared.

Personal competence depends upon personal development as well as upon training, although it is assumed that the general preparation afforded by a degree program can do much to speed the deepening and broadening of personal skills.

PRE-SERVICE PREPARATION

The amount and type of pre-service preparation needed will, of course, depend upon the degree of independent judgment and responsibility involved in a particular position. The nurse responsible for public health nursing in a county and receiving supervisory assistance from some distance away, needs stronger pre-service preparation than does the nurse employed in a large visiting nurse association where she has immediate access to supervisory assistance and to extensive community resources for patient care.

Whenever possible the minimum of a year's academic work, planned with a university counselor to cover the basic essential content in public health, should be completed before employment. Completion of a complete university program approved by the National League for Nursing for preparation of beginning public health nurses is, of course, more desirable.

Many universities are able to help evaluate the adequacy of basic nursing preparation in terms of the demands of public health nursing, and to identify needs for clinical training in particular areas. For example, the basic nursing course may have

4. *Census of Nurses Employed for Public Health Work in the U.S., in the Territories of Alaska and Hawaii and in Puerto Rico and The Virgin Islands on January 1, 1955*. Washington, D.C., Public Health Service. 1955.

included no clinical experience in psychiatric nursing, or may have been inadequate in coverage of care of the well child, or of some phases of the maternity cycle. Deficiencies in basic nursing preparation may in some instances have been compensated for by work experience. Tests, such as those developed by the National League for Nursing, might give some indication of such competence. In many instances the combined judgment of the nurse herself and a nurse counselor from a university or employing agency may be adequate.

Such deficiencies may be repaired by planned work experience in a favorable situation, or by taking clinical courses. This, too, might better be done before entering the field of public health, since competence in nursing itself is basic. If there is no college or university prepared to help in these matters, the educational director or supervisor of a public health service, nursing bureau of the state health department, or the counseling and placement service of the state or local nurses' association might advise in a plan for strengthening preparation in basic nursing.[5]

WORK EXPERIENCE

Work assignment should afford opportunities for constantly expanding and deepening professional experience. This does not necessarily mean progression from direct service nursing to a supervisory or administrative type of position—there is a broad spread of opportunity within the staff position itself. A plan for progression toward greater independence, variety and depth of service is essential. The development of such a plan is the joint responsibility of the nurse herself and of the nursing supervisor.

Either within a particular community or by change of assignment to another area, there should be a continuous stretching of the job potential. For example, the nurse who has had a year of experience in a generalized county nursing service might plan to develop a program of group teaching or group discussion in the county, or to develop a more intensive service to school children by realignment of the duties and increased activities among the students themselves, or to develop a volunteer "patient sitting" service for chronically ill patients. These are activities which might have been difficult to undertake in the first year, but add depth and challenge to the second year's work and develop professional skill to a higher level.

5. *Facts About Nursing, 1955 Edition.* New York, American Nurses' Association, 1955, pp. 108–110.

If there is potential for and interest in advancement to supervisory or administrative work, experiences may be gradually enlarged to include more and more complex elements of a managerial or supervisory nature. For example, providing field observations for professional nursing or medical students; recruiting, training and supervisory volunteer workers; planning and evaluating nursing activities with increasing independence, all increase supervisory skills.

Sometimes ensuring proper sequence of experience demands job transfer. The nurse whose experience has been in a large urban agency may need rural experience to develop skills of community organization, planning and program evaluation; the nurse in a health department may feel the need for experience in a visiting nurse association or in a teaching hospital to deepen her patient-care skills.

There is a tendency to think of experience in terms of movement "upward" to supervisory and administrative placement. Lateral movement—change from one to another staff position— may, in fact, be more productive. The nurse who wants to be a consultant in a special field, for example, may need extended time in direct patient care in order to achieve broad competence in her field of specialization as well as in generalized public health.

TRAINING FOR NEW RESPONSIBILITIES

As new responsibilities are envisioned, plans must be made for requisite training. Such training may extend from a relatively simple self-guided program such as a few days' visit to a psychiatric hospital buttressed by a reading program or attendance at an institute, to a full graduate university course.

Training may be incorporated into the agency's in-service education program; there may be, for example, a planned program for staff nurses who will be accepting responsibility for student training, or who are beginning supervisors.

However, in most cases, there will be need for occasional off-the-job preparation. Advance planning will help place such preparation in advance but not too far ahead of the anticipated change. For example, a staff nurse with two years of experience may want to complete a graduate course in public health as a prerequisite for later supervisory placement.

The American Nurses' Association has recommended qualifications for public health nurses in administrative, supervisory and consultative positions, in addition to basic nursing preparation and preparation in public health nursing as recommended for staff nurses. These include:

"A master's degree with a major in administration, supervision, or consultation or in a special field; or a master's degree in public health from a university program approved by the American Public Health Association

or

A bachelor's degree from a university program approved by the National League for Nursing for beginning public health nurse positions which included or was supplemented by academic preparation in administration, supervision, consultation, or advanced preparation in a special field.

"Content in the fields of administration, supervision, and consultation should be sufficiently comprehensive to provide a basis for competence in the areas of:

"1. Administration of public health nursing services.

"2. Supervisory, consultative, and educational processes.

"3. Personnel administration.

"4. Research, including use of epidemiologic and administrative study procedures and statistical evaluation.

"5. Interpersonal and intergroup relations, communications, and action.

"6. Relating nursing services and programs to:

"a. Trends and developments in public health services and administration.

"b. Structure and services of local, state and federal government.

"c. Educational philosophy and methods.

"Public Health Nursing Competence as Evidenced by Satisfactory Experience

"1. For the supervisor:

"a. A minimum of two years' experience in public health nursing, at least one of which was in generalized service under public health nursing supervision.

"b. For the supervisor of school nursing, at least one of the two years of experience in public health nursing should include school nursing in either a specialized or generalized program.

"2. For the consultant:

"a. The general consultant will have need for more

experience than that demanded for the supervisor —a total of four years of experience in public health nursing of which a minimum of one year should be in a supervisory capacity.

"b. The public health nursing consultant in a special field should have a minimum of four years' experience. This experience may be in public health nursing, or in a combination of public health nursing and another type of nursing in a specialty. At least one year of the experience should be in the specialty, or in a generalized experience including the specialty, and one year in supervision in public health nursing.

"3. For the director:

"a. The director of nursing service should have a minimum of five years' experience in public health nursing, including at least three years of experience in a supervisory or consultative capacity.

"b. Experience in more than one type of agency is desirable.

"Personal Competence as Evidenced by the Capacity to

"1. Apply the personal competencies required of public health staff nurses in relatively complex and involved situations.

"2. See and work for long-range goals.

"3. Work more effectively with professional and civic leaders.

"4. Think creatively and independently about existing and anticipated needs and means of meeting them.

"**5. Accept** responsibility for decisions without undue strain."[6]

In general, the advanced work should come as close as possible to the time when supervisory appointment or supervisory activities within staff appointment are anticipated. Placed too early it may divert the nursing experiences which will deepen concepts of patient and community nursing; placed too late it forces fumbling through the first part of supervisory or administrative experience **and may** perhaps diminish interest in and capacity for the new work.

6. *Functions, Standards and Qualifications for Public Health Nurses.* New York, American Nurses' Association. 1955.

JOB AND MARRIAGE PLANNING

About half of the public health nurses working in 1951 were married.[7] Career planning must take into account this dual responsibility, recognizing the unique values and stability the married worker can bring to the service, and at the same time facing realistically the adjustments that it may demand in job sequence, training off the job, and in timing of upward movement in the organization.

There are great individual differences in the non-work demands placed upon the married nurse, and obviously no pattern can be set that meets all needs. However, in long-term career planning, the nurse who is married may decide on a short period of work followed by professional retirement; or upon an interrupted career pattern, with some years out for family care; or upon a pattern of continued employment during the childbearing period. Whatever the pattern, career plans should be realistically constructed to conserve professional skills while safeguarding the integrity of the family. Part-time employment or academic work may prove helpful in maintaining skills when the married nurse plans to return to her career after the early childbearing period.

Career planning is a joint responsibility of the nurse and the supervisory and administrative personnel. Realistic appraisal, well-placed training and comprehensive, well-savored experiences enable progression to greater nursing responsibility and to greater satisfaction in the work undertaken.

7. *Facts About Nursing.* 1955–56 Edition. New York, American Nurses' Association, 1955, p. 12.

CHAPTER XXIII

On-the-Job
Performance Improvement

Every public health nurse must be concerned with improvement of day-by-day performance. Because changing health needs and health care as well as social and economic developments are constantly remolding public health nursing, and because many facets of nursing practice can be developed fully only through personal growth and development, professional improvement must be a never-ending task. Even superior pre-service preparation may prove inadequate after a few years unless constantly re-enforced and brought up to date. While agency programs for staff development will help to improve performance, in the final analysis it is the nurse herself who must take the initiative and the responsibility for self-improvement. This responsibility may be discussed in relation to evaluation of performance, and use of supervisory and consultant services and other available resources for increasing expertness and personal-development activities.

EVALUATION OF PERFORMANCE

Evaluation of performance is a joint responsibility of the nurse and of the supervisor. It provides an opportunity for measuring performance against the professional competences expected and against service outcomes. Periodic evaluation by the responsible supervisor or administrator is frequently required as a basis for merit rating, salary adjustment and promotion, or as an accepted procedure as part of the staff-development program. If it is not required, the nurse may need to work out a plan with the appropriate supervisor or administrator for securing an evaluation at sufficiently frequent intervals to provide a base for self-improvement. Evaluation by an administrative officer who is not a nurse, while helpful, is not adequate in relation to judging and planning for improvement of professional practice—this requires nursing supervision. Good supervisory practice assumes that evaluation reports written by the supervisor are based on self-evaluation by the nurse as well as upon the supervisor's own judgment. Three types of evaluation may be identified: (1) self-evaluation, (2) self and supervisory evaluation, (3) self and group evaluation.

Self-Evaluation.   Self-evaluation should be a continuous process; as each family is discussed, each clinic session ended the nurse asks the question "How well did I do?" There is also need for a more comprehensive self-scrutiny—a look at one's whole performance, to answer the question "How well do I stack up in relation to the competences demanded for the work?" This may be undertaken in conjunction with a supervisory evaluation, or independently. It may be triggered by findings of evaluation of the nursing service. Whatever the motivating force, self-evaluation should be done unhurriedly, objectively and realistically.

If the agency has an evaluation form that suggests an approach to evaluation or indices of good performance, the nurse may use this as a guide. If not, she may write down under each major competence heading the questions she would like to consider. Such questions as these might be raised:

Have I been called upon to perform treatments or procedures in which I feel insecure?

Have I been able to answer patients' questions regarding their disease and its treatment?

Am I sufficiently familiar with the hospital treatment so as to relate home care to this effectively?

Do patients and families appear relaxed and welcoming?

Do they request service in subsequent situations where nursing care is needed?

Do families, teachers and other community workers ask my advice or call me in to participate in planning?

Have I reduced noneffective time (travel, not-at-home or unnecessary calls) as far as possible?

Can I justify the inclusion of each case in my load—should nursing be expected to make a difference?

These are, of course, suggestive and do not in any sense represent an inclusive list of the questions that might be posed.

It is usually easier to judge one's performance against the background of a specific situation, rather than in terms of generalities. For example, questions such as the above might be raised relative to a sampling of cases, perhaps taking every fifth or tenth case in the file and saying *in this case* how would these questions be answered, or, if the questions relate to administration, how did I do *this week*. In this way it is possible to find more specific indications of quality than would be possible if there were no limited point of reference.

The indices of good or poor performance need to be linked to the reason. What particular approach or action made the Jones' family shift from a negative to a positive attitude regarding the use of health services? Did it help that enough time was allowed for Mr. Jones to "blow off steam" on the first visit? Or that the nurse was able to avoid letting him refuse a second visit, and kept the door open for future contacts?

Why is there a feeling of insecurity about home care for tuberculosis—is it because of inexpertness in the procedure itself, or lack of sufficient information about the disease and its treatment, or perhaps even a lurking fear of contracting the disease one's self?

From this kind of association will come ideas for action. If "difficult" families respond when the nurse is calm and accepting, would it help to schedule visits so that such families are not seen late in the day when the nurse's fatigue may be a factor? Would further reading in the dynamics of human behavior increase awareness of signals of need for aggressive or disagreeable behavior and allow the nurse to obtain satisfaction from her capacity to understand rather than letting her own need for status in the situation provoke conflict? If insecurity arises from not being sure of the technique of administering a drug, would observation or practice in the hospital clinic help?

Thus, by looking at performance in terms of the nursing competences required, by identifying the factors that make for better or poorer performance, and by outlining the specific action which needs to be taken, the nurse's self-evaluation contributes to improved care for patients and for the community.

Self and Supervisor Evaluation.   The supervisor brings to evaluation of performance the special expertness and objectivity which grows out of her broader preparation and experience, and her competence to relate this performance to that of other nurses with comparable backgrounds and to the nurse's own previous performance.

As a basis for evaluation, the supervisor will gather information from many sources—from observation of the nurse at work in the field and in staff activities, from record review, from conferences with the nurse and others, from reports. This information will be assembled over a period of time, and as far as possible will be expressed in terms of what was done, and how this compares with best practice and with the expected level of performance for a staff nurse at this point in preparation and experience.

The staff nurse's part in this process is equally important. She will:

1. Collect such information as may be pertinent or helpful to the supervisor prior to a field visit or conference. The supervisor may be asked whether there is information she would like assembled, or the nurse herself may decide, on the basis of her own problems, what would be useful. For example, the nurse may collect information on the average number of prenatal visits per case, or the proportion of tuberculosis patients under care who are receiving medication, or the number of one- or two-visit cases.

2. Arrange field observations in such a way as to show a good cross section of the work—different types of activity, with some successes as well as some problem cases.

3. Relate the work the supervisor sees to the total program and to total care of the family or individual. The supervisor needs to know what went before and what is expected to follow if she is to evaluate what is seen at a particular point in time and to understand the program as a whole.

4. If working under the direction of a non-nurse administrative officer (health officer, school superintendent) and supervision comes from another agency's office, the nurse may arrange for a conference of the supervisor and administrator.

5. Clarify meanings and consider causes of success or failure and possible action for improvement of performance in a post-evaluation conference.

If possible, the nurse should request a copy of evaluation reports and recommendations. This will be helpful in evaluating her own subsequent progress, and provide a record of change in professional competence.

Self and Group Evaluation.   Sometimes a group of nurses or health workers can evaluate themselves through *group analysis of problems* or cases. For example, a health department might have a discussion by all field staff on reducing noneffective time. The

nurse, through discussing this problem with others, will evaluate
her own planning and may recognize parts of her work that need
further study or change.

A *case discussion*, in which a group appraises the service provided to a particular family may also prove to be a point of departure for individual evaluation. The group's suggestion that the
"uncooperative" patient may in fact be a fearful patient, or that
"middle" children often have similar problems, might lead to recognition that an approach should be changed, or that further study is
needed on the effects of family configuration.

Process recording, discussed in Chapter XI in relation to
service evaluation, may also be useful in evaluation of one's self.
Recordings or verbatim reports of interviews or visits may also be
used similarly for self-evaluation through group discussion. The
nurse may write the record herself, or an observer may do so,
setting forth what happened, including evidences or indications of
feelings as well as of overt behavior. This kind of running report
permits careful study and consideration of the possible meanings
of what happened during the visit by a group. In the course of
discussion, the nurse can evaluate her performance in the light of
the thinking and questions of others.

USE OF SUPERVISOR AND CONSULTANT

Almost every nurse will have access to continuing nursing
supervision either from her own agency or through advisory or
general consultant services offered by the division of public health
nursing of the state health department. In addition, there may be
varying numbers and types of special field consultants. Supervision may be viewed by the nurse as a necessary evil; properly
used it may become one of the most potent of tools for performance improvement. The nurse's share in the supervisory process
will make a great deal of difference in its effectiveness.

The supervisor will help with improving performance through
field observations, conferences and evaluation activities; through
channeling information and materials to the nurse; and sometimes
by correspondence.

The nurse has a real part to play in making the field supervisory visit, or supervisory conference, a success. She can:

1. Prepare in advance for the supervisor's visit, selecting activi-
    ties or patients for the supervisor to see or to discuss, includ-
    ing some successes and some problems. She can ask the
    supervisor whether there are special aspects of work she
    would like to see or discuss.

2. In an agency under other than nursing direction, talk with the administrator (health officer, medical director or school officer) about the supervisor's impending visit and ask him whether he has problems to suggest for discussion and whether he would like a conference with the supervisor.

3. Review the program as a whole, and jot down special problems with which she'd like help; assemble service reports or other data she may want to see.

4. Review previous evaluation or supervisory field visit reports to see whether follow-up of suggestions made in them should be reported or progress evaluated with the supervisor.

Much of the supervisor's capacity to help depends upon the freedom the nurse feels in presenting and discussing problems. The nurse should recognize that she and the supervisor have a common objective—to improve the care families receive. Centering attention on this, rather than on fear that the supervisor is "checking up," will make for a more productive activity.

The specialized supervisor or consultant may be used in much the same way to observe performance, suggest improved methods or areas for further study and to provide materials.

USE OF OTHER RESOURCES FOR INCREASING PROFESSIONAL EXPERTNESS

In urban centers, *university extension* classes or *continuation courses* may be available in nursing subjects or in related fields such as education, human relations, or anthropology. These regularly organized courses may or may not carry university credit, and are often scheduled to permit attendance on a part-time basis. "Week-end workshops" or late afternoon and evening classes are frequently offered. In many instances, universities are equipped to set up special courses upon request, and if a group of nurses or other professional workers wants a course in group dynamics or in health appraisal of school children, such courses may be made available.

Nurses' associations may also offer continuing educational activities. Opportunities for this self-initiated type of educational effort may be increased if nurses participate fully in the work of their professional organizations and see in that organization a powerful potential for improving nursing service. Regular attendance at meetings of professional associations may be an excellent source of new ideas on nursing or medical care. Even though the meetings are centered on something else, the informal interchange of ideas with other nurses is in itself productive.

Regular professional reading is a necessity for any professional worker. The public health nurse should familiarize herself with the publications that are of most use to her.

American Journal of Nursing, Nursing Outlook, The American Journal of Public Health, and *Public Health Reports* are basic sources of information. In addition to these the nurse in industry may want to read some publication in the general field of industrial health, such as *Industrial Medicine;* the school will want to include something in the field of education such as the *Journal of School Health, Physical Education and Recreation,* or the *Journal of Educational Research. Social Casework, The Journal of the American Medical Association,* and *Hospitals* are related publications that frequently carry material of special interest to public health nurses. Journals in special fields, such as *Children* and *Mental Hygiene,* may also prove helpful. Local public or medical libraries or state health department libraries may have or borrow periodicals or books in the general field of medicine, nursing or public health, and librarians may also suggest new sources of information. It is important to have a plan for reading. One evening a week is not too much to devote to reading in nursing or related fields. If this reading is done thoughtfully and widely, it will provide stimulation and professional refreshment that will open new vistas in daily work.

A nursing office *reference library* may be built around a few basic textbooks and inexpensive pamphlets or reprints. An informational file may be used to provide ready reference to current materials on the various aspects of nursing and medical care. Reprints, pamphlets or abstracts, or significant current literature may be filed under subject headings in a regular letter-size file.

Local hospitals or schools of nursing are invaluable resources in maintaining nursing skills. Sometimes it is possible to attend in-service training sessions for hospital personnel that have a bearing on the public health program—for example, a seminar on drug therapy in schizophrenia, or on interviewing for personnel at a tuberculosis hospital. Some nurses have been able to spend a few days at work in the hospital as a means of refreshing basic nursing skills or securing practice in new kinds of treatments which are used in the home as well as in the hospital.

USING IN-SERVICE EDUCATION OPPORTUNITIES FULLY

Most agencies will have a definite program for *in-service education.* This may be an agency-wide program for all workers such as physicians, engineers, health educators and social case workers, or a program for the nursing staff only. In some states the division of public health nursing of the state health department may organize in-service educational projects on a state-wide basis, available to all public health nurses in the state. Staff nurses will be expected to make suggestions for the content of such programs, and it is often possible to arrange for seminars, institutes, lectures or demonstrations that center about changing medical or nursing procedures.

Full participation in such activities will result in much greater benefit than just saying "present" when the attendance roll is called. Advance preparation makes it possible to take full advantage of the program. For example, if the subject for discussion is rheumatic fever, the nurse may review her case load and analyze the problems encountered to find needs or possibilities for better diagnostic care through the school health program, or to find lack of suitable educational materials. With such background information it is possible to participate actively, to appreciate the significance of the materials presented and to see applications to current work situations.

A PROGRAM FOR PERSONAL DEVELOPMENT

In the definition of professional competence it is apparent that success in public health nursing must depend in large measure upon personal qualities and abilities. Such personal effectiveness is difficult to define and to learn, yet without it technical competence is of relatively little value. Planning for personal development must include: (1) a program for health maintenance, (2) a program for broadening cultural appreciation, (3) a program for building communication skills and (4) a program for increasing planning and analytical ability.

Health Maintenance. Most types of public health nursing require more than usual physical stamina and emotional maturity, yet the health habits of nurses are all too often typical not of the best but of the least desirable practice.

Good habits of daily living—proper nutrition, rest and sleep—are, of course, basic. Even these simple requirements may require some planning if food must be procured in small-town restaurants, where selection is limited, or when long distances between homes to be visited or activities necessitate night travel by car or hard driving to meet schedules.

In addition to this, nursing has its own particular hazards. Immunization procedures should be completed as recommended by the physician in accordance with the degree of exposure and particular geographic factors. Good posture habits are essential to prevent strain or other injury in lifting or moving patients or equipment. Good work methods and sometimes establishment of short periods for rest or relaxation are necessary to avoid unnecessary fatigue. Proper instruction in driving is essential for the nurse who uses a car, especially in areas where the climate is severe or special driving hazards are present.

Emotional health is essential for one who aspires to help others. The cultivation of a variety of interests and recreational pursuits helps to maintain a healthy balance between work and play. Most public health nurses, too, must learn how to face the compromises that must be made when it is not possible to meet all of the nursing needs that are recognized. Satisfaction in work must be achieved within the limits imposed by lack of time, of training, or of supporting services.

Broadening Cultural Appreciations.   Present-day nursing exists in the midst of a culture that is peculiarly our own and of our time. The fully competent nurse must relate herself to this culture. Through the arts—music, literature and painting—or through other media such as handicrafts, nature study, or group activities such as singing, discussion, or team sports, the public health nurse may broaden the base of her understanding and appreciation.

Active participation or creative activity is generally more satisfying than observation or listening; one learns to enjoy and appreciate painting more if there are opportunities to paint or sketch.

Time to live—to do things for fun—is not a luxury for the professional worker; it is part of the maintenance cost of professional competence.

Building Communication Skills.   To be able to communicate one's ideas effectively to others through speech, written words or use of figures is an indication of personal and professional competence. Public health nursing makes frequent demands for use of communication skills, and the public health nurse should cultivate the ability to speak and write effectively, and to use numbers to interpret quantitative ideas with accuracy and clarity. Courses in public speaking, writing, elementary statistics, and in group work may help. Speeches and written materials can also be analyzed for readability.[1] Another good plan is to try out a speech or talk on non-nurse friends.

1. Flesch, R., *The Art of Plain Writing.* New York, Harper & Bros., 1949.

Process recording or actual recording of visits may also be analyzed for evidence of failures in communication.

Building, Planning and Analytical Ability. The ability to analyze situations and to plan with good judgment may be learned by practice. Most people who "don't think straight" or who "have poor judgment" are those who do not take the time or trouble to tackle problems correctly. Planning and analytical ability may be cultivated by conscious attention, and by using every opportunity for critical study of nursing cases or situations. It will help to:

1. Plan time for planning. Set aside a definite time for planning work, analyzing service or reviewing needs of particular families or services, such as school or industrial programs. Planning should be considered an integral part of all work to be done.
2. Obtain all available pertinent facts.
3. Use opportunities to present analyses of cases or services to supervisor or advisory nurses, to administrators, to boards or committees, or at nursing meetings. Such activities require critical study and will develop skill in analysis and broaden the base for planning nursing care.
4. Make decisions deliberately when necessary. Gather all the essential facts, mull them over, then decide. Good judgment depends on having all the facts, seeing their relationships and acting in accordance with them. The person who can make immediate decisions is not always soundest in thinking and action.
5. Take a chance on being wrong, provided being wrong cannot harm anyone. If wrong judgments are recognized and studied, they may improve later decisions.

Maintaining professional competence is a continuing task. While supervisors, administrators and consultants may help, the final responsibility for achieving full professional skill must rest with each individual nurse herself.

CHAPTER XXIV

Contributing to the

Development of Nursing

Today as never before the development of nursing must rest on the excellence of performance of each individual nurse and the degree to which she exercises judgment and skill. Conversely, the capacity of any nurse to achieve excellence of performance is dependent upon the status of nursing as a profession. Each nurse must be cognizant of her responsibility for contributing to the development of nursing as a whole.

PROFESSIONAL ACTION CHANNELS

The public health nurse must see the essential relationships between public health nursing and preparation for basic nursing and to nursing in other fields. Public health nursing suffers when recruitment for basic nursing is inadequate, or when opportunities for advanced preparation of teachers and supervisors in schools of nursing lag. Public health nursing as well as patient care suffers if salaries of hospital nurses are so low that there are too few hospital nurses to provide necessary patient care and instruction in the hospital.

Through her professional associations and through participation in community and agency planning and action groups, and through research and service studies, the public health nurse should play her part in improving nursing in all fields. She may interpret nursing and its needs to related professional workers in her agency or community, participate in recruitment activities for schools of nursing through her contacts with school counselors and students, serve on study groups or committees to survey nursing needs or resources, or know and interpret the needs for nursing service in hospitals.

Through the public health nursing section of the American Nurses' Association the nurse can play a part in shaping nursing practice. Through the National League for Nursing she can work with lay members and nurses from other fields on problems of service and nursing education.

Membership in related organizations may also be an important part of contributing to nursing. The American Public Health Association provides a channel for interpreting nursing to other members of the public health team; the National Education Association or other organized teacher groups offer an opportunity for relating nursing to educational efforts.

Attendance and active participation at meetings of professional organizations are essential. Paying dues is not enough; it is the thinking and sustained activity of the membership itself which makes professional associations a real force for human betterment. Action left in the hands of a few may well become disassociated from the realities of the situation. For example, a small number of highly qualified administrators and teachers may have a completely different concept of the functions of a staff nurse than do the nurses themselves. Only as a large number of staff nurses themselves think, talk, and decide can a true and realistic picture emerge.

The nurse must also contribute to professional development by analyzing and sharing her own experience. For example, if she finds very different patterns of child rearing in two neighborhoods, she might present this experience at a hospital case conference or to a planning committee when maternal and child health services are being discussed. The nurse director of the hospital might welcome discussion of a study of the types of cases referred by the hospital to the public health agency at a staff meeting, or at a meeting of the medical board of the hospital. Success or failure in special kinds of group approaches might be written up for discussion at an agency staff meeting.

Reporting through articles in professional journals is another way of sharing experiences and influencing professional development. A report of results from spacing visits to tuberculosis patients differently, or of using a group approach in teaching may encourage others to try a similar program.

Many public health nurses will marry and have several years in which they are not actively engaged in nursing. During this interval, the nurse is a particularly valuable member of her profession, for she sees nursing from both the professional and consumer viewpoint.

By maintaining her interest in organization activities, and perhaps by serving on committees or advisory groups, the nurse may make the kind of contribution not possible under other circumstances. For example, working with a Future Nurses' Club or with a Parent-Teacher Association health committee, the homemaker-nurse can bring to the members the value of her own experience. At the same time she may herself gain new skills in working with groups, in speaking or counseling.

RESEARCH AND SERVICE STUDIES

Research has been defined as "seeking the answer to a question pressing for solution."[1] In public health nursing there are a multitude of such questions—some simple, some complex; some small, some big; some of general import and some of purely local significance.

Some of these questions relate to nursing practice. What should be the function of the public health nurse in relation to home care of the psychiatric patients; how far should her efforts be involved in therapy or restricted to supportive services? Is a nondirective approach in prenatal conferences more productive than a directive one? Does allowing a period of dependence on the nurse speed up or delay self-help in the long-term disabled patient? Is using the family's thermometer better than carrying one for home care? What is a safe thermometer technique?

Other questions relate to public health practice. Do behavior problems vary in type and incidence in relation to the child's place in the family? Is absenteeism in industry connected with particular cultural or educational factors? Will group work with venereal disease patients result in locating a larger proportion of contact cases?

Still other questions relate to administration. Are one- or two-visit family contacts effective in providing comprehensive nursing care? Will telephone follow-up of school absences be effective in selecting children who need home care? Could record work be reduced? Is group teaching of diabetic patients more or less costly

1. Arnstein, Margaret, Improving Nursing Service. *Canadian Nurse,* 52: 869–874, November, 1956.

than individual teaching? Is volunteer direction of volunteer activities a factor in regularity and continuity of service?

Some of these questions can be answered only by intensive and highly skilled research done by a group of researchers from different professions. Others can be studied by the nurse on the job, with help from those with greater study skills than her own. While special study and training in analysis and tests of logical thinking, or in the intricacies of social or biological science, are required to *direct* research, most nurses can participate in planning and conducting research studies, and can initiate and complete simple research or service studies.

Research is not only for the experts. Kittinger calls it "essentially a state of mind—a friendly welcoming attitude toward change—going to look for it instead of waiting for it to come."[2]

Research may be distinguished from simple thinking about a problem by:

1. Its dependence upon facts or observable occurrences as opposed to personal bias or opinion.
2. Its systemic organization for assembling and analyzing the facts.
3. Its limitation of conclusions to those which are inherent in the facts, and which are tested for significance.

Research should be repeatable, that is, another research worker or team should be able to follow the steps outlined and, given the some conditions, would be expected to obtain the same answer.

Service studies or action research are sometimes distinguished from more formal research by the limitations of their method or of the universality of their application. For example, a county health nurse may study several mothers' classes using a lecture-demonstration method and a demonstration-discussion method in alternate classes. Based upon patients' judgments, an analysis of their responses and questions, her own judgment and simple oral tests, she may find that the group using the demonstration-discussion method consistently did better. Such a study would not show that demonstration-discussion was *generally* better than lecture-demonstration. Properly planned, however, it might indicate that with *this* subject matter, *this* type of instructor and in *this* type of class and community, demonstration-discussion was the more effective method. Such a finding has significance for application in the situation, and may have a very real effect on service outcomes despite its limitations.

2. *Nursing Research*, 2: 40, June, 1953.

SELF-CONDUCTED STUDIES

The nurse who uses research as a means of improving service must be willing to plan carefully and realistically for systematic study. The following guides may help:

1. Select a problem which it is assumed can be answered by a research or study approach. Theoretically, a research approach can be applied to any problem. However, in public health nursing there will be many questions that are best answered in other ways, either because the units of measurement cannot be defined without long and involved study, or because satisfactory methods of objective study have not been developed. For example, it may not be possible to gauge the temper of a community regarding use of preventive services by way of an expensive full-scale opinion study based on a reliable statistical sample of the population. The answer will not be sought in a study, but rather a more feasible approach may be made by combining the opinions of field and administrative staff, talking with a relatively small number of individuals and agencies and thinking about the situation in relation to similar factors. However, it is certainly safe to say that a study approach is used much less frequently than it might be.

The following questions may help to decide whether a study is indicated:

a. Are the facts on which to base the study available?

b. Are the facts sufficiently accessible so they can be collected with the staff and in the time available?

c. Are the facts sufficiently easy to identify and classify so that they do not require unusual preparation or research skill?

d. Are the facts sufficiently pertinent so that, when collected, they will give a true answer to the problem?

e. Will the facts available cause a limitation of coverage in the problem that might lead to a fragmentary and possibly misleading answer?

2. Define the problem clearly. The question to be answered should be specifically and clearly stated, with the limits set. For example, the question "How can maternal and child health nursing service be improved?" is less subject to exact study than is the question "Is a patient-directed interview more effective than a nurse-directed interview in changing health behavior in relation to prenatal care?"

3. Decide what information should be gathered. What must be known to answer the question? For example, in the question posed above, what information, facts and observations will show *change*

in behavior? How pertinent to this is change in knowledge? What facts are needed regarding previous behavior before the service is started? Are judgmental as well as objective data necessary?

4. Decide how data will be analyzed before collecting them. For example, it may be important to see whether the differences in learning about prenatal care vary in accordance with the age or educational background of the patient. If analysis is to be made in relation to these factors, the information needed can be easily collected if planned in advance. If such data are not collected in the course of the study, it may be difficult or impossible to secure them at a later date, and the value of the entire study may be lessened because the import of this factor cannot be evaluated.

5. Select a study group. Decide how large a group is to be studied, and over how long a period of time. For example it may be decided to study 100 tuberculosis home visits or six mothers' classes.

The group studied should be representative of the whole. For example, quite different reactions to group work might occur in a neighborly suburban community than in a crowded city; the findings in one situation might not hold true in the other. If the purpose is to find out how suburban dwellers react, the study group can be limited to this set. If a more generalized answer is needed a more representative cultural and socio-economic group would be required.

A statistician can help to decide how large and diverse a group must be to represent a typical sample of the population and whether it would provide a fairly reliable base for drawing conclusions.

6. Use a control group, if possible, when the effect of a particular action is to be measured. In this way it is possible to compare what happens when a particular action is taken with what happens without it. For example, if the effects of intensive home visiting undertaken early after diagnosis of long-term illness is to be measured, a study group might receive the intensive early placed service, while a control group might receive "usual" or limited care.

The control group should be like the study group in all respects save the one factor being studied. For example, if those receiving intensive care included a larger proportion of young persons than did the control group, a difference of outcome might be due to greater motivation in the young group, and not to the method by which nursing service was provided.

There are many ways of assuring the comparability of groups used for study and for control, through matching procedures or random selection. The statistician's help may be needed for this. Often, however, simple methods such as using alternate patients for the study and the control group, or selecting every third (or fifth or tenth) patient for study will produce reasonably comparable groups for study. Whatever method of selection is used, the study and control groups should be analyzed to be sure that they are comparable.

7. Be sure the data collected include a baseline—information regarding the status at the beginning of the study. What did the expectant mothers know before the class started? How did the disabled patient feel about his condition before visits were made? How much had the family availed itself of preventive services before nursing service was instituted?

8. Decide how many observations should be made and for how long a period to give a reliable answer for *the purposes of the study*. For example, a study of the home nursing needs of twenty-five diabetic patients might not be adequate for generalization on the needs of diabetic patients in a large teaching hospital or for a city nursing service. It might, however, provide an adequate index for program planning in a one-nurse county service.

9. Put the facts or observations in some systematic order that will show the essential relationships. For example, in studying needs of diabetic patients, did age or sex make a difference? Did duration of illness have any effect on nursing needs? Did different nurses appraise needs differently?

10. Study the findings for their implication for action. Are they sufficiently clear to cause a change in procedure, or are they supportive rather than conclusive? If the answer is in the affirmative, should the new procedure be tested out as new facts are collected?

Do the findings show that the method of the study was not satisfactory? For example, it might be found that the estimate of nursing needs of diabetic patients showed no consistency in relation to the judgment of patients, of different nurses, or of nurse and physician. This may mean that the method of study was inadequate. Perhaps a prior agreement, regarding classification and identification of needs, by the nurses and physicians involved would produce more reliable data.

It is obvious from a review of the above that the nurse who is going to engage in self-directed studies will need to seek the help of those more experienced than herself in study procedures. Advice may be secured from many sources, depending on the type of problem. The supervising nurse or special consultant, the biostatistician or statistician in the health department or in a college or university, the university staff in educational or social research, all have had training and competences that might be useful. Sometimes a nursing organization or community council member may be interested in the study, and may have competences or facilities within the staff or membership to help. The nurse should think through the question she needs to have answered, and the possible approach. Then, *before* starting the study, she should confer with available advisors.

PARTICIPATING IN TEAM RESEARCH

Often the nurse will participate in studies done by someone else, or may serve as one member of a research team. As a research team member or participant the nurse may:

1. Suggest areas that need research.
2. Participate in planning for the study and in formulating procedures.
3. Assist in the collection of data.
4. Teach and supervise others who are collecting data.
5. Help to interpret findings.

Suggesting New Areas for Research.   The public health nurse, because of her closeness to the community and to the patient, has a unique opportunity to see research needs. For example, she may notice that attendance at a cancer diagnosis clinic is skewed in the direction of the upper economic group, and raise the question as to what motivates attendance and what promotional measures might be devised to reach a wider group; or she may observe that receptivity to home care of the patient with long-term illness varies greatly even when facilities for such care are judged to be adequate, and raise the question as to the effect of the family's feelings and of hospital and medical support on this attitude.

Participation in Planning.   The nurse can bring to the research planning group an intimate knowledge of people and their needs. For example, she would probably know how and where people shop, which would make a difference in the way food-purchasing data might be collected; or how people feel about their responsibility as community members, which might affect their willingness to undergo physical or laboratory tests while well; or what response might be anticipated to group attendance at film showings.

The nurse will also be useful in working out procedures for collecting data or arranging for examinations or treatment. She will know how communities are organized, where leadership resides, where and how people tend to assemble in groups. All of these may make a difference in designing a research project.

Assisting in the Collection of Data.   Nurses are frequently asked to collect data for studies. In doing this they need to understand the purpose and general plan of the study, and the way in which the information is expected to be used. In this way they can observe more intelligently.

The nurse may also observe in the course of collecting data certain factors not included in the study which seem to have pertinence. For example, if afternoon temperatures are being studied, she may note that the time set for recording temperature coincided with return of children from school, predinner activity and maximum stress of the homemaker. This may result in delay in recording or inadequate attention to timing and hence to inaccurate recording.

Teaching and Supervising Others Collecting Data or Carrying Out Procedures.   The public health nurse is accustomed to teaching and supervising families and hence may be called upon to do so when families are asked to keep a record of illnesses, or of food actually eaten by each member of the family or of patients' reactions to a particular drug or therapy. Such teaching may be on a group or community, as well as on a family, basis.

Interpretation of Findings.   The nurse may also be important in interpreting the findings of a study. For example, she may recognize the influence of cultural patterns in causing geographic differences within a city in relation to the numbers of patients who remain under home care for long-term illness; or in opposing community forces, such as a small group of untrained midwives, who may have been counteracting teaching done by health department personnel.

Working with a research team has all of the problems and requires all of the skills of team work in general. There is need to try to understand the other person's point of view and to interpret his professional vocabulary; to establish relationships of mutual confidence and trust; and to accept responsibility for full participation rather than simply collecting information for some one else to use.

It takes every nurse, working with related professional workers and with the public, to push nursing to new achievements. Through individual deliberative thinking and reporting, through joint action, research and study, and constant interpretation of nursing as a whole, the public health nurse takes her part in the development of her profession.

SUGGESTED READINGS

Part V

Alcott, Louise, M. R. Moore and Honora Camden, Combining Marriage and Nursing. *American Journal of Nursing*, 55: 1344–1349, November, 1955.

American Nurses' Association, Functions, Standards and Qualifications, Educational Administrators, Consultants and Teacher's Section. *American Journal of Nursing*, 56: 1586–1588, December, 1956.

American Nurses' Association, *Functions, Standards and Qualifications for Public Health Nurses*. New York, The Association, 1955.

American Nurses' Association, *Wherever You Are, Nurse*. New York, The Association, 1955.

Arnstein, Margaret, Improving Nursing Service, *Canadian Nurse*, 52: 869–874, November, 1956.

Bixler, Geneveive, What Is Research? *Nursing Research*, 1: 7–8, June, 1952.

Brandt, E. J., Building Expertness in a Clinical Field. *Public Health Nursing*, 41: 143–147, March, 1949.

Ferguson, Marion, Research in Nursing. *American Journal of Public Health*, 41: 716–719, June, 1951.

Flesch, Rudolph, *The Art of Plain Writing*. New York, Harper & Bros., 1949.

Florentine, H. G., Are Supervisors Necessary? *American Journal of Nursing*, 54: 845–847, 1954.

Frasher, Charles, ABC's of the Merit System. *Public Health Nursing*, 42: 473–479, May, 1950.

Greenblatt, Milton, The Nurse in Research. *Nursing Research*, 1: 36–40, February, 1953.

Lentz, E. M., What Is a Supervisor. *Nursing Outlook*, 4: 336–337, June, 1956.

Leone, Lucille, The Ingredients of Research, *Nursing Research*, 4: 51, October, 1955.

McKiever, Nell, How to Use a Consultant. *Adult Leadership*, 3: 14–16, April, 1955.

McManus, R. Louise, What Colleges and Universities Offer the Practicing Nurse. *American Journal of Nursing*, 54: 1478–1480, December, 1954.

Roberts, D. I., A Psychiatrist Helps Them Understand Their Patients. *American Journal of Nursing*, 56: 1586–1588, December, 1956.

Robinson, Virginia, *Supervision in Social Case Work*. Chapel Hill, University of North Carolina Press, 1946, Chapter 3, "The Development of a Professional Self in Social Case Work."

Safford, Beverly, My experience with Self-Evaluation. *Nursing Outlook,* 3:30–31, January, 1955.
This is Your N.L.N. New York, National League for Nursing, 1956.
Toward New Frontiers in Public Health. The American Public Health Association Story. New York, The Association, 1956.

Index

Note: In this index "nurse" shall mean "public health nurse" unless otherwise specified, and "nursing" shall mean "public health nursing."

427